Rainer Scheer, Susanne Alban, André-Michael Beer,
Wolfgang Blaschek, Reinhild Klein, Wolfgang Kreis, Gero Leneweit,
Harald Matthes, Günther Spahn, Rainer Stange (Hrsg.)

Die Mistel in der Tumortherapie 6

Herausgeberinnen und Herausgeber:
Dr. Rainer Scheer, Carl Gustav Carus-Institut, Allmendstr. 55, 75223 Niefern-Öschelbronn

Prof. Dr. Susanne Alban, Pharmazeutisches Institut, Abtlg. Pharmazeutische Biologie, Christian-Albrechts-Universität zu Kiel, Gutenbergstr. 76, 24118 Kiel

Prof. Dr. med. André-Michael Beer, Klinik für Naturheilkunde, Klinik Blankenstein, Universität Bochum Lehrbereich Naturheilkunde, Abtlg. Allgemeinmedizin, Im Vogelsang 5–11, 45527 Hattingen

Prof. Dr. Wolfgang Blaschek, Vogteiweg 13 B, 24119 Kronshagen

Prof. Dr. med. Reinhild Klein, Universitätsklinikum Tübingen, Medizinische Klinik, Abteilung für Hämatologie, Onkologie, Rheumatologie, Klinische Immunologie, Pulmologie, Otfried-Müller-Str. 10, 72076 Tübingen

Prof. Dr. Wolfgang Kreis, An den Weiherwiesen 12, 91334 Hemhofen

PD Dr. Gero Leneweit, Carl Gustav Carus-Institut, Allmendstr. 55, 75223 Niefern-Öschelbronn

Prof. Dr. med. Harald Matthes, Gemeinschaftskrankenhaus Havelhöhe, Kladower Damm 221, 14089 Berlin

Dr. med. Günther Spahn, Internist, Onkologe, Hämatologe, Trimed Mainz, Helix Medical Excellence Center, Haifa-Allee 24, 55128 Mainz

Dr. med. Rainer Stange, Charité-Universitätsmedizin Berlin und Immanuel-Krankenhaus, Naturheilkunde, Königstr. 63, 14109 Berlin-Wannsee

Die Mistel in der Tumortherapie 6

Aktueller Stand der Forschung und klinische Anwendung

Rainer Scheer, Susanne Alban, André-Michael Beer,
Wolfgang Blaschek, Reinhild Klein, Wolfgang Kreis, Gero Leneweit,
Harald Matthes, Günther Spahn, Rainer Stange (Hrsg.)

KVC | VERLAG

KVC Verlag | Natur und Medizin e. V.
Am Deimelsberg 36, 45276 Essen
Tel.: (0201) 56305 70, Fax: (0201) 56305 60
www.kvc-verlag.de

Scheer, R.; Alban, S.; Beer, A.-M.; Blaschek, W.; Klein, R.; Kreis, W.; Leneweit, G.; Matthes, H.; Spahn, G.; Stange, R. (Hrsg.)
Die Mistel in der Tumortherapie 6 –
Aktueller Stand der Forschung und klinische Anwendung

Wichtiger Hinweis: Für Angaben über Dosierungsanweisungen und Applikationsformen kann vom Verlag keine Gewähr übernommen werden. Jede Dosierung oder Applikation erfolgt auf eigene Gefahr des Benutzers. Geschützte Warennamen (Warenzeichen) werden nicht besonders kenntlich gemacht.

ISBN 978-3-96562-089-6

Umschlaggestaltung: eye-d Designbüro, Essen
Druck: Rudolf Glaudo GmbH & Co. KG, Wuppertal

Inhalt

Vorwort/ Foreword XVII

I. Biologie, Pharmazie, Phytochemie, Galenik
I. Biology, Pharmacy, Phytochemistry, Galenic ___________ 1

Hartmut Ramm, Konrad Urech:

"Few Can Imagine That Mistletoe is One of the Most Interesting Plants." – 100 Years of Karl von Tubeuf's *Monograph on Mistletoe*

„Wenige wissen, dass die Mistel eine der allerinteressantesten Pflanzen ist." – 100 Jahre *Monographie der Mistel* des Karl von Tubeuf 3

Konrad Urech, Alejandro Casteller, Stephan Baumgartner:

Distribution and Abundance of *Viscum album* ssp. *album* in France

Verbreitung und Häufigkeit von *Viscum album* ssp. *album* in Frankreich 13

Matthias F. Melzig, Catharina Delebinski, Georg Seifert, Wenyan Xie:

Selected Aspects on Biological Properties of miRNA From *Viscum album* L.

Ausgewählte Aspekte zu biologischen Eigenschaften von miRNA aus *Viscum album* L. 19

Lucie Schröder, Jennifer Senkler, Hans-Peter Braun:

The Energy Metabolism of European Mistletoe (*Viscum album* L.)

Der Energiestoffwechsel der europäischen Mistel (*Viscum album* L.) 35

Valter Paes de Almeida, Irailson Thierry Monchak, João Vitor da Costa Batista, Mirio Grazi, Hartmut Ramm, Vijayasankar Raman, Stephan Baumgartner, Carla Holandino, Jane Manfron:

Microscopic Characterization of European Mistletoe (*Viscum album* L. subspecies *album*) 45

Angelika Heinze, Anton Berg, Gero Leneweit:

In welchen Phasen ihrer Entwicklung bildet *Viscum album* L. Statolithenstärke?

In Which Phases of its Development Does *Viscum album* L. Form Statolithic Starch? 57

Josanna Kaufmann, Harden Rieger, Gero Leneweit:

Liposomale Verkapselung von Mistelextrakten für die Therapie des Glioblastoms

Liposomal Encapsulation of Mistletoe Extracts for the Therapy of Glioblastoma 67

Gero Leneweit, Josanna Kaufmann, Larissa Lubitz, Harden Rieger:

Novel Formulations of Mistletoe Extracts for Targeted Cancer Therapies

Neuartige Formulierungen von Mistelextrakten für zielgerichtete Krebstherapien 79

II. Präklinik: Immunologie, Zytologie, *in vitro*- und *in vivo*-Untersuchungen

II. Preclinic: Immunology, Cytology, *In Vitro* and *In Vivo* Studies ______ 89

Sebastian Wolfshöfer, Martina Gast, Friedemann Schad, Hedwig Lammert, Michael Hummel, Sebastian Stintzing, Patricia Grabowski:

Inhibition of Colorectal Cancer Cell Line Growth by Mistletoe Extracts

Hemmung des Wachstums von Kolorektalkarzinomzelllinien durch Mistelextrakte 91

Michelle Nonato de Oliveira Melo, Alan Clavelland Ochioni, Patricia Zancan, Adriana Passos Oliveira, Mirio Grazi, Rafael Garrett, Carla Holandino, Stephan Baumgartner:

Viscum album Mother Tinctures Interrupted the Warburg Effect in Breast Cancer Cells: Metabolite Profile and Antitumoral *In Vitro* Mechanisms 103

Ilona Zilkowski, Claudia Turek, Nora Mörbt, Peter Vögele, Florian C. Stintzing:

In Vitro Mutagenicity Assessment of Aqueous *Viscum album* L. Preparations

Bewertung der *in vitro*-Mutagenität von wässrigen *Viscum album* L.-Zubereitungen 117

Ulrike Weissenstein, Bettina Leonhard, Stephan Baumgartner:

A Fermented Mistletoe Extract Elicits Endoplasmic Reticulum Stress Driven Immunogenic Cell Death in Breast Cancer and Melanoma Cells

Ein fermentierter Mistelextrakt induziert einen durch Stress im Endoplasmatischen Retikulum hervorgerufenen immunogenen Zelltod in Brustkrebs- und Melanomzellen 125

Michael Schink, Eugenia Violeta Díez García de Olalla, Alexander Sebastian Franzén, Martin J. Raftery, Sabine Rieger, Gabriele Pecher:

Einfluss eines Mistelextrakts in Kombination mit einer Checkpoint-Inhibitor-Therapie auf die Aktivität der natürlichen Killerzellen gegen Brustkrebsspheroide

Effect of Mistletoe Extract on the Activity of Natural Killer Cells in Combination With Checkpoint Inhibitor Therapy Against Breast Cancer Spheroids 129

III. Klinische Anwendung
a) Studien, Fallberichte, klinische Erfahrung

III. Clinical Application
a) Studies, Case Reports, Clinical Experience __________ 133

Shiao Li Oei, Anja Thronicke, Hannah Wüstefeld, Christian Grah, Friedemann Schad:

Improvement of Quality of Life in Lung Cancer Patients Receiving Targeted Oncological Treatment in Combination With *Viscum album* L.

Verbesserung der Lebensqualität von Lungenkrebspatienten unter zielgerichteter onkologischer Therapie in Kombination mit *Viscum album* L. 135

Friedemann Schad, Diana Steinmann, Anja Thronicke, Christian Grah, Shiao Li Oei:

Verbesserung der Lebensqualität von Lungenkrebspatienten nach Bestrahlung und additiver *Viscum album* L.-Therapie: Eine Real-World Data-Studie

Improvement of Quality of Life in Lung Cancer Patients Receiving Radiotherapy in Combination With *Viscum album* L.: A Real-World Data Study 149

Anja Thronicke, Shiao Li Oei, Patricia Grabowski, Friedemann Schad:

Kombination von zielgerichteter Therapie und Helixor *Viscum album* L. bei Patientinnen mit Brust- oder anderen gynäkologischen Tumoren

Combination of Targeted Therapy and Helixor *Viscum album* L. in Breast and Gynecological Cancer Patients 163

Shiao Li Oei, Klaudia Kunc, Marcus Reif, Ulrike Weissenstein, Timo Weiß, Hannah Wüstefeld, Harald Matthes, Christian Grah:

Prospektive Beobachtungsstudie zur Kombinationstherapie von Immun-Checkpoint-Inhibitoren und *Viscum album* L. beim fortgeschrittenen Lungenkarzinom (PHOENIX-III)

Prospective Observational Study of Advanced Lung Cancer Patients Treated With a Combination of Immune Checkpoint Inhibitors and *Viscum album* L. Extract (PHOENIX-III) 173

Jennifer E. Felenda, Claudia Turek, Florian C. Stintzing:

Sicherheit, Verträglichkeit, therapeutische Wirksamkeit und Lebensqualität (LQ) von Patienten mit malignen urogenitalen Tumorerkrankungen unter der Behandlung mit Iscucin® Populi – Ergebnisse einer nicht interventionellen Studie (NIS)

Safety, Tolerability, Therapeutic Efficacy and Quality of Life (QoL) Assessment of Patients With Malignant Urogenital Tumors Upon Treatment With Iscucin® Populi – Results of a Non-interventional Study (NIS) 185

Chang Moo Kang:

Viscum album as Potential Adjuvant Role in Standard Care of Resected Pancreatic Cancer 203

Ann-Kathrin Lederer, Michael Schink, Sabine Rieger, Roman Huber:

Pharmakokinetik von Mistellektinen nach intravenöser Applikation von Helixor® P bei gesunden Probanden

Pharmacokinetics of Mistletoe Lectins After Intravenous Administration of Helixor® P in Healthy Volunteers 205

Timotheus Haeck, Ana-Paula Simões-Wüst, Sibylle Creutz v. Essen, Florian Strasser, Matthias Kröz:

Mistletoe Therapy in Context of a Multimodal Treatment in a Patient With Severe Cancer-Survivorship-Fatigue-Syndrome With Comorbid Sleep Disorder: A Case Report

Misteltherapie im Rahmen einer multimodalen Behandlung bei einer Patientin mit schwergradigem Cancer-Survivorship-Fatigue-Syndrom und komorbider Schlafstörung: Ein Fallbericht 215

Joon Beom (John) Park, Inmyung Oh, Sunjoo Chung, Taek Joon Yoon, JongBae Kim:

Clinical Regression of Chondrosarcoma Applying High Doses of *Viscum album* Extracts (VAE) by Intratumoral Injection: A Case Report 227

Devra Davis, Dugald Seely, Christopher Morash, Mikail Kogan, Nasha Winters, Jeffrey A. Jones:

Mistletoe and Pharmacological Ascorbate: An Innovative Integrative Oncology Protocol for BCG-Refractory High-grade Bladder Cancer 241

Karolina Königsberger, Wilfried Tröger, Marcus Reif, Dorothea Schläpfer, Konrad Urech, Marion Debus, Thomas Meisermann, Andrea Diehl, David D. Martin, Stephan Baumgartner:

Anwendung eines lipophilen Extraktes aus *Viscum album* bei aktinischer Keratose, kutanem Plattenepithelkarzinom und Basalzellkarzinom

Viscum album Lipophilic Extract in Actinic Keratosis, Cutaneous Squamous Cell Carcinoma and Basal Cell Carcinoma 251

Markus Reif, Roland Zerm, Christoph Gutenbrunner, Matthias Kröz:

Classification and Minimum Clinically Important Difference of the German Version of the Cancer Fatigue Scale (CFS-D)

Klassifikation und minimale klinisch relevante Differenz der deutschen Version der Cancer Fatigue Scale (CFS-D) 261

Ana Paula Simões-Wüst, Daniel Krüerke:

Mistletoe Therapy During Pregnancy: A Historical Review

Misteltherapie während der Schwangerschaft: Ein historischer Rückblick 281

Frank Meyer:

Misteltherapie als hausärztliche Basismaßnahme bei Krebserkrankungen: Eine integrative Perspektive

Mistletoe Therapy as a Primary Care Intervention in Cancer Treatment: An Integrative Perspective 293

Annika Mascher, Florian Pelzer, Lorna J. Duncan, David D. Martin, Stephan Baumgartner, Bettina Berger:

Das Erleben der Misteltherapie aus Patientensicht – Eine qualitative Interviewstudie

The Introspective Patient Experience of Mistletoe Therapy in Cancer – A Qualitative Study 301

Friedemann Schad, Anja Thronicke, Marion Debus, Maike Kergel, Yván Villegas, Georg Soldner:

Die Webseite für die Misteltherapie in der Onkologie – www.mistel-therapie.de

The Website for Mistletoe Therapy in Oncology – www.mistel-therapie.de 315

Andreas Arendt, Marion Debus, Johannes Gutsch, Lydia Garnitschnig, Markus Karutz, Angela Kuck, Mathias Sauer, Reinhard Schwarz, Georg Soldner, Markus Sommer:

Individualisierte Behandlung mit Mistelpräparaten bei onkologischen Erkrankungen: Weiterentwicklung des Vademecums

Individualized Treatment With Mistletoe Preparations in Oncology – Further Development of the Vademecum 325

Katharine Offer, Marcus Reif, Karen Moody:

European-US Collaboration to Put Iscador in the Pediatric Oncology Pipeline: Lessons Learned

Europäisch-amerikanische Zusammenarbeit zur Einführung von Iscador in die pädiatrische Onkologie: Ein Erfahrungsbericht 333

III. Klinische Anwendung
b) Übersichtsreferate und Reviews klinischer Studien

III. Clinical Application
b) Survey Articles and Reviews of Clinical Studies ______ 339

Annette Bopp:

Krankheit als Impuls des Lebens

Illness as an Impetus of Life 341

Ralf Hofheinz:

Integrative Oncology: How Can we Implement it Into Daily Practice?

Integrative Onkologie: Wie können wir sie in die tägliche Praxis umsetzen? 357

Harald Matthes:

Die Zukunft der Misteltherapie – Eine Übersicht

The Future of Mistletoe Therapy – An Overview 361

Johannes Wilkens:

Das Meridiansystem als neue Basis für die Misteltherapie

The Meridian System as the New Basis of Mistletoe Therapy 377

Matthias Rostock, Mirjam Wüsthof, Alena Krause, Alina Busch:

Die klinische Studienlage zur Misteltherapie in der Onkologie – in systematischen Reviews, Metaanalysen und Leitlinien

Current State of Clinical Studies on Mistletoe Therapy in Oncology – Including Systematic Reviews, Meta-Analyses and Guidelines 391

Friedemann Schad:

Die Mistel in der klinischen Anwendung – Real-World Data und Leitlinien

Mistletoe in Clinical Practice – Real-World Data and Guidelines 407

Harald Walach, Daniela Paepke, Martin Loef:

Lebensqualität von Brustkrebspatientinnen unter Mistelextrakt-Behandlung: Eine systematische Übersichtsarbeit und Metaanalyse

Quality of Life in Breast-Cancer Patients Treated With Mistletoe Extracts: A Systematic Review and Meta-Analysis 423

IV. Anwendung bei nichtonkologischen Erkrankungen
IV. Use in Non-oncological Diseases ____ 433

Christian Grah, Irina Gatov, Shiao Li Oei, Marcus Reif, Hannah Wüstefeld, Annika Marzok:

Neue Therapie der Sarkoidose mit verdünnten Vielstoffgemischen, insbesondere Iscucin Salicis und *Ferrum chloratum* comp.

New Therapy of Sarcoidosis With Diluted Multi-Substance Mixtures, Especially Iscucin Salicis and *Ferrum chloratum* comp. 435

V. Anwendung bei Tieren
V. Use of Mistletoe in Animals ____ 449

Anke Beermann, Ulrike Biegel, Marcus Reif, Lucia Unger, Ophélie Clottu, Christoph Koch:

Therapy Response of Equine Sarcoid-bearing Horses When Treated With Orally Administered Mistletoe Extract Compared to Administration by Subcutaneous Injection or Placebo, Respectively

Ansprechen von Pferden mit equinen Sarkoiden auf die Behandlung mit oral eingenommenem Mistelextrakt im Vergleich zur subkutanen Injektion oder einem Placebo 451

Ophélie Clottu, Ulrike Biegel, Marcus Reif:

Fallserie einer oralen Anwendung der Misteltherapie (Iscador® P) zur Behandlung von Equinen Sarkoiden

Case Series on the Oral Use of a Mistletoe Extract (Iscador® P) in Equine Sarcoid 455

Ulrike Biegel, Meike Mevissen, Simone Schuller, Katja Ruess, Ophélie Clottu, Hannah Ayrle, Christoph Koch, Michael Walkenhorst:

Could *Viscum album* L. Be a Therapeutic Option for Companion Animals Suffering From Neoplastic Diseases? A Systematic Review

Könnte *Viscum album* L. eine therapeutische Option für Haustiere mit neoplastischen Erkrankungen sein? Eine systematische Literaturübersicht 467

Autorenverzeichnis/ Contributing Authors 471

Stichwortverzeichnis 475

Keyword Index 482

Vorwort

Glück gehabt: Auf Grund des vierjährigen Turnus fand im November 2023 auch das 8. Mistelsymposium ohne pandemiebedingte Beschränkungen statt, erneut in der Europäischen Akademie Otzenhausen (Nonnweiler/Saarland) und mit über 100 Teilnehmenden. In zahlreichen Übersichts- und Kurzreferaten sowie auf Postern wurden aktuelle Daten aus relevanten Gebieten der Biologie, Pharmazie und Pharmakologie, der Präklinik und Klinik, Erkenntnisse aus therapeutischer Erfahrung sowie klinische Studien präsentiert. Auch nicht onkologische Anwendungen der Mistel und ihre Anwendung bei Tieren kamen zur Sprache. Schwerpunkt des klinischen Teils waren diesmal onkologische Immuntherapien in Kombination mit einer Misteltherapie. Erstmals bei diesem Symposium wurde eine Online-Fortbildung zur „Praxis der Misteltherapie" als Hybrid-Veranstaltung angeboten.

Die Veröffentlichung der Beiträge des 8. Mistelsymposiums erfolgt in drei Teilen:

1. Zuerst die Abstracts der Vorträge und Poster vorab in einem Sonderheft des Journal of Integrative and Complementary Medicine (JICM). Sie sind bis Oktober 2026 online frei zugänglich (siehe unter doi.org/10.1089/jicm.2023.29117.abstracts).
2. Die Videomitschnitte der Online-Vorträge stehen auf der Symposiums-Homepage www.mistelsymposium.de für Fachpublikum frei zur Verfügung.
3. Im vorliegenden Buch werden die Beiträge des 8. Mistelsymposiums in ausführlicher Form publik gemacht. Die Herausgeber dieses Buches danken allen Autorinnen und Autoren von Vorträgen und Postern beim 8. Mistelsymposium, die mit ihren Manuskripten zu diesem Buch beigetragen haben.

Unsere Mistelsymposien geben nicht nur einen breit gefächerten Überblick, sondern auch neue Impulse und einen Motivationsschub für weitere Forschung. Sie sind ein Forum für den gemeinsamen Diskurs, der biologisches, pharmazeutisches und klinisches Fachwissen vereint, um Synergien zu nutzen und um eine treibende Kraft für weitere Studien und Ansätze in der Forschung zu sein. Entsprechend sollten der Dialog und die Zusammenarbeit zwischen konventioneller und komplementärer Onkologie weiter ausgebaut und Vertrauen gegenseitig gestärkt werden. Dazu möchten die Mistelsymposien, zusammen mit den Symposiums-Büchern und den anderen genannten Veröffentlichungen, Grundlage und Beitrag sein für eine Integrative Onkologie, eine Medizin der Zukunft.

So ist beabsichtigt, die Reihe dieser Veranstaltungen 2027 mit dem 9. Mistelsymposium fortzusetzen.

Für die Herausgeber:
Dr. rer. nat. Rainer Scheer, Niefern-Öschelbronn
Prof. Dr. med. Harald Matthes, Berlin
im Sommer 2024

Foreword

We were lucky: due to the four-year cycle, the 8th Mistletoe Symposium took place in November 2023 without pandemic-related restrictions, once again at the European Academy Otzenhausen (Nonnweiler/Saarland) and with more than 100 participants. Current data from relevant areas of biology, pharmacy and pharmacology, preclinical and clinical research, findings from therapeutic experience and clinical studies were presented in numerous overview and short presentations and on posters. Non-oncological applications of mistletoe and its use in animals were also discussed. This time, the clinical part focused on oncological immunotherapies in a combination with mistletoe therapy. For the first time at this symposium, an online training course on the "Practice of mistletoe therapy" was offered in hybrid.

The contributions to the 8th Mistletoe Symposium will be published in three parts:

1. First, the abstracts of the lectures and posters in advance in a special issue of the Journal of Integrative and Complementary Medicine (JICM). They will be freely accessible online until October 2026 (see doi.org/10.1089/jicm.2023.29117.abstracts).
2. The video recordings of the online presentations are freely available to the professional audience on the symposium website www.mistelsymposium.de/english/organizers,-objectives.aspx.
3. In this book the contributions to the 8th Mistletoe Symposium are published in a comprehensive form. The editors of this book would like to thank all the authors of lectures and posters at the 8th Mistletoe Symposium who contributed to this book with their manuscripts.

Our Mistletoe Symposia not only provide a wide-ranging overview, but also new impulses and motivation for further research. They are a forum for joint discourse, bringing together biological, pharmaceutical, and clinical expertise to exploit synergies and to be a driving force for further studies and approaches in research. Accordingly, the dialog and cooperation between conventional and complementary oncology should be further expanded and the mutual trust should be strengthened. The Mistletoe Symposia, together with the symposium books and the other publications mentioned, would like to be the basis and contribution to an integrative oncology, a medicine of the future.

The intention is to continue the series of these events in 2027 with the 9th Mistletoe Symposium.

On behalf of the editors:
Dr. rer. nat. Rainer Scheer, Niefern-Öschelbronn
Prof. Dr. med. Harald Matthes, Berlin
Summer 2024

I. Biologie, Pharmazie, Phytochemie, Galenik

I. Biology, Pharmacy, Phytochemistry, Galenic

“Few Can Imagine That Mistletoe is One of the Most Interesting Plants.” – 100 Years of Karl von Tubeuf’s *Monograph on Mistletoe*

„Wenige wissen, dass die Mistel eine der allerinteressantesten Pflanzen ist.“ – 100 Jahre *Monographie der Mistel* des Karl von Tubeuf

Hartmut Ramm, Konrad Urech

Summary

In 1923, the *Monograph on Mistletoe*, comprising well over 800 pages, was published. The botanist Karl von Tubeuf had thus created a standard work through the breadth of topics and his precise descriptions, which has remained the basis for research on white-berried mistletoe (*Viscum album* L.) to this day. Interestingly, *V. album* was introduced into medicine as an injectable around the same time and became the most widely used remedy in complementary cancer treatment in the 20th century. Tubeuf’s accurate documentation of French locations of the exceptionally rare oak mistletoe made even possible in 1927 to produce an oak mistletoe preparation (Iscador® Qu). His investigations into the occurrence of *V. album* on various tree species in Europe were also intended as a means of regulating the rampant spread of mistletoe, which is currently once again in the critical focus of public attention due to climate change. Tubeuf’s detailed studies of chorology, morphology and physiology led him to the conclusion that mistletoe differs from botanical normality in almost all respects. Current research has deepened this exceptional position, for example by revealing a lack of complex I in the respiratory chain of the mitochondria and correspondingly in photosystem I of the chloroplasts.

In the meantime, several monographs have been published describing the entirety of parasitic flowering plants, including well over thousand species of mistletoe distributed all over the globe. However, the diversity of the literature on mistletoe research, which has increased exponentially in recent decades, is hardly reflected in these monographs. True to Tubeuf’s statement

that "such a work is actually never finished", it seems timely to respond to the currently growing worldwide interest in research on *V. album* with a new monograph that is as comprehensive as it is in-depth.
Keywords: Tubeuf, monograph, mistletoe, *Viscum album*, cancer remedy, oak, botany, distribution

Zusammenfassung
Im Jahr 1923 erschien die weit über 800 Seiten umfassende *Monographie der Mistel*. Der Botaniker Karl von Tubeuf hatte damit durch die Breite der Themen und seine präzisen Beschreibungen ein Standardwerk geschaffen, das bis heute die Grundlage für die Erforschung der Weißbeerigen Mistel (*Viscum album* L.) ist. Interessanterweise wurde *V. album* etwa zur gleichen Zeit als Injektionspräparat in die Medizin eingeführt und entwickelte sich zum meistverwendeten Mittel in der komplementären Krebstherapie. Tubeufs genaue Dokumentation französischer Standorte der äußerst seltenen Eichenmistel ermöglichte 1927 dann auch die Herstellung eines Eichenmistelpräparats (Iscador® Qu).
Seine Untersuchungen zum Vorkommen von *V. album* auf verschiedenen Baumarten in Europa sollten damals auch dazu dienen, die starke Ausbreitung der Mistel einzudämmen, die u.a. aufgrund des Klimawandels aktuell erneut in den Fokus der Öffentlichkeit rückt. Tubeufs detaillierte Studien zur Chorologie, Morphologie und Physiologie führten ihn zu dem Schluss, dass sich die Mistel in fast allen Aspekten von der botanischen Normalität unterscheidet. Aktuelle Forschungen haben diese Ausnahmestellung noch vertieft, indem sie beispielsweise das Fehlen von Komplex I in der Atmungskette der Mitochondrien und im Photosystem I der Chloroplasten aufzeigen konnten.
Inzwischen sind mehrere Monographien erschienen, welche die Gesamtheit der parasitären Blütenpflanzen beschreiben, darunter weit über tausend weltweit verbreitete Mistelarten. Die Vielfalt der Literatur zur Mistelforschung, die in den letzten Jahrzehnten exponentiell zugenommen hat, spiegelt sich in diesen Monographien jedoch kaum wider. Getreu der Aussage von Tubeuf, dass „ein solches Werk eigentlich nie fertig ist", scheint es an der Zeit, auf das derzeit weltweit wachsende Interesse an der Erforschung von *V. album* mit einer neuen, ebenso umfassenden wie tiefgehenden Mistel-Monographie zu reagieren.
Stichworte: Tubeuf, Monographie, Mistel, *Viscum album*, Krebsmedikament, Eiche, Botanik, Verbreitung

Background

In 1923, the botanist Karl von Tubeuf (1862–1941) published a *Monograph on Mistletoe* (Fig. 1), comprising well over 800 pages (Tubeuf 1923). In this book he compiled all the knowledge on mistletoe (*Viscum album* L.) at that time. Through the breadth of topics and his precise descriptions he created a standard work that work has remained the basis for research on white-berried mistletoe to this day.

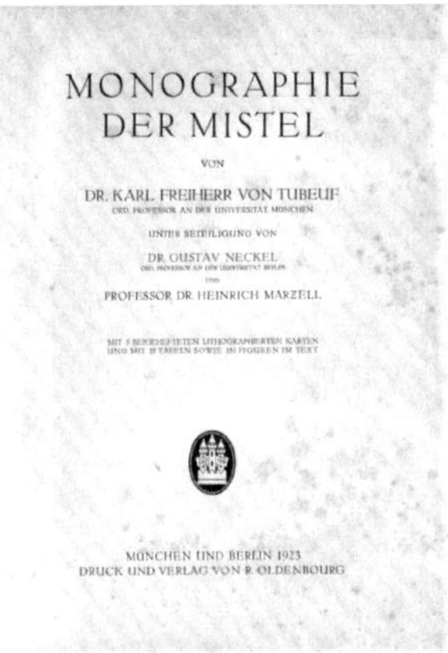

MONOGRAPHIE
DER MISTEL
VON
DR. KARL FREIHERR VON TUBEUF
UNTER BETEILIGUNG VON
DR. GUSTAV NECKEL
UND
PROFESSOR DR. HEINRICH MARZELL
MÜNCHEN UND BERLIN 1923
DRUCK UND VERLAG VON R. OLDENBOURG

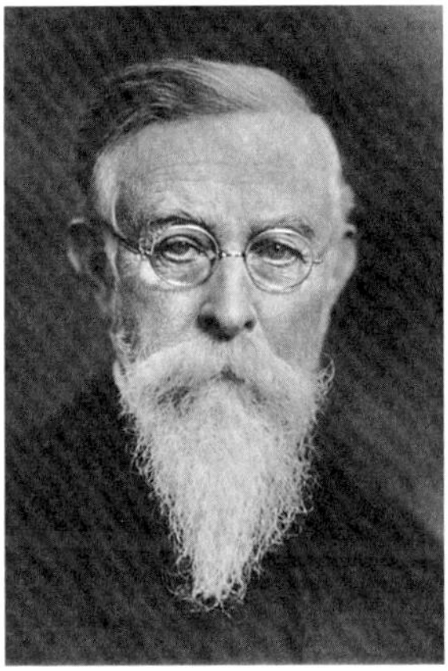

Fig. 1: Cover page of the *Monography of Mistletoe* (left), published by Karl von Tubeuf (right) in 1923

Historical coincidence

Mistletoe became a popular motif in Art Nouveau, which emerged at the end of the 19th century (Becker, Schmoll 1986) and as a new artistic movement was regarded as countermovement to backward-looking historicism as well as to the soulless industrialization. It was during this period that Tubeuf began his scientific work with mistletoe in Berlin. In 1907 he called from his chair in Munich for collaboration on a survey of mistletoe distribution, initially regional but eventually extended to the whole of Germany and Europe. Coinciding in time, Rudolf Steiner (1861–1925) started a new approach to mistletoe from 1904 onwards, based on his goetheanistic research methods. In 1916 he recommended to the physician Ita Wegman that mistletoe, known since ancient times as "all-healing", would be specifically suitable for cancer therapy (Ramm 2015). When after delays because of World War I, Tubeuf's *Monograph* was finally published in 1923 key elements of mistletoe pharmacy as inaugurated by Steiner were realized for the first time (Selg 2016; Ramm *et al.* 2019).

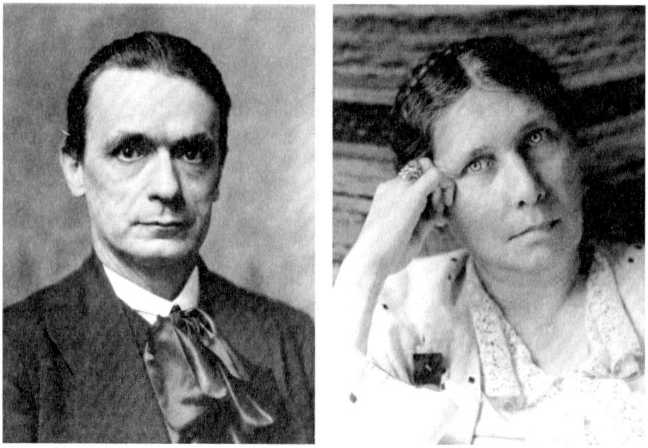

Fig. 2: Rudolf Steiner (left), Ita Wegman (right).

Implication on mistletoe therapy

Tubeuf had thoroughly studied and described mistletoe's germination, growth, flowering, and fruiting and its interaction with the host tree. He was the first to provide evidence of the three "races" (today: subspecies) of *V. album* and thus recognized an important aspect for the significance of host trees in mistletoe therapy for cancer. Based on his detailed documentation of mistletoe-bearing oaks (*V. album* growing on *Quercus robur* and *Q. petraea*) in France (Fig. 3), Ita Wegman could then provide the oak mistletoe preparation Iscador® Qu as early as 1927 (Urech 2002).

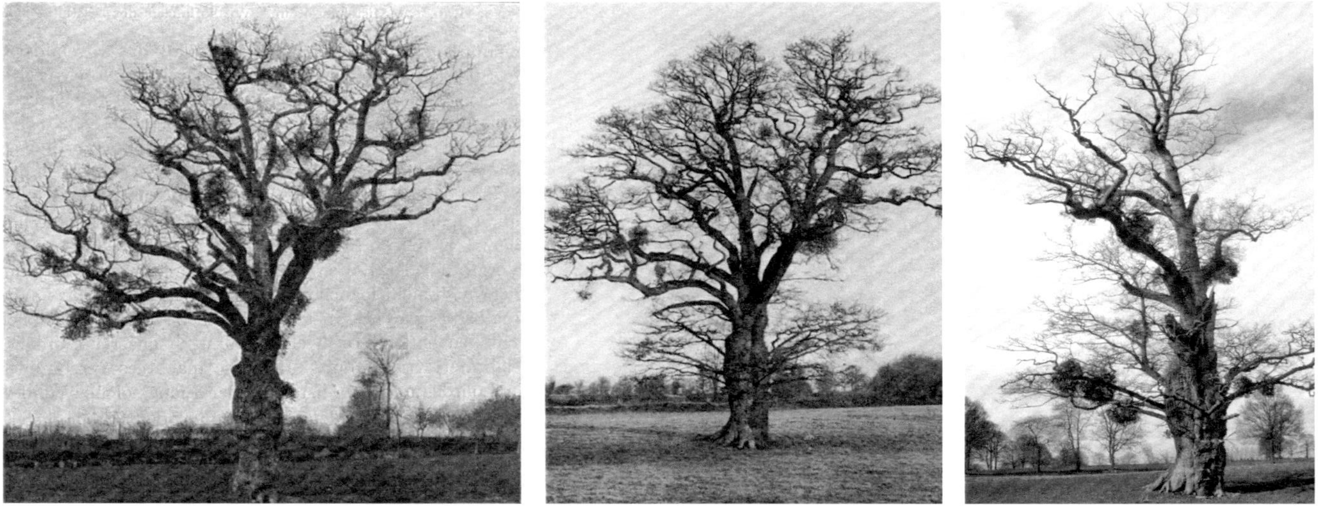

Fig. 3: The white-berried Mistletoe (*Viscum album*) on the oak (*Quercus robur*) from Isigny-le-Buat in 1898 (left; from Tubeuf (1923)), in 1959 (middle; photo: Hiscia Institute) and in 1999 (right, photo: K. Urech)

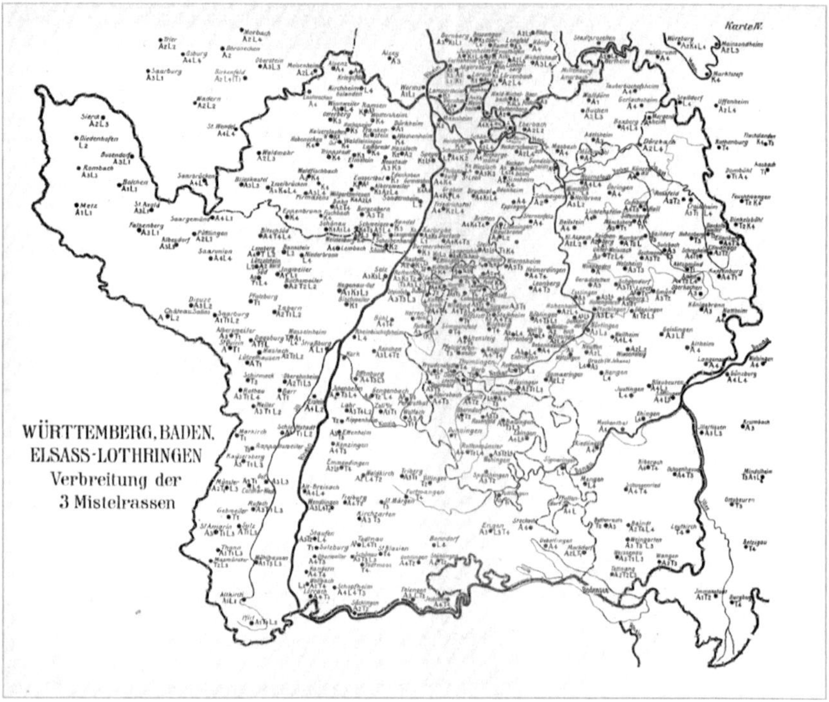

Fig. 4: A map from Tubeuf (1923), presenting the occurrence of the three subspecies of *V. album* in the Southwest of Germany at the beginning of the 20th century: A = apple tree, L = deciduous trees, T = fir, K = pine; the occurrence is ranging from 1 = very frequent, 2 = rather frequent, 3 = occasionally, 4 = rare.

Practical relevance

In his days, Tubeuf was at the forefront of practical mistletoe research. His success in cultivating mistletoe inspired subsequent professional cultivation of *V. album* for pharmaceutical purposes (Ramm *et al.* 2000). Being the first to document the occurrence of *V. album* on various tree species in Europe (Fig. 4), Tubeuf had intended his investigations also as a means for regulating the rampant spread of mistletoe, which probably due to climate change is currently again in the critical focus of public attention all over Europe, (Lech *et al.* 2020).

Missing link

Birds being most relevant for the spreading of mistletoe, Tubeuf discussed various species and their relationship to *V. album* and identified especially mistle trush (*Turdus viscivorus*), fieldfare (*T. pilaris*) and waxwing (*Bombycilla garrulus*) as main distributors of mistletoe (Fig. 5). Interestingly, Tubeuf missed the blackcap (*Silvia atricapilla;* Fig. 5), which nowadays, due to its flexible reaction on climate change, is assumed as highly effective in the spreading of *V. album* (Ramm 2017; Briggs 2021).

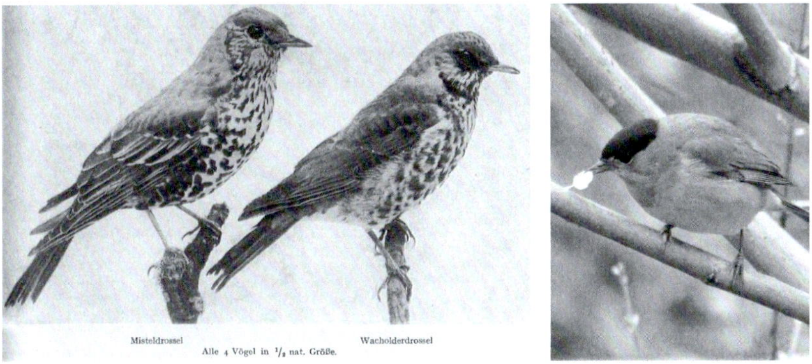

Fig. 5: Mistle trush and fieldfare (left, from Tubeuf 1923) and blackcap (right; photo: H. Ramm)

Among mistletoe-related insects, Tubeuf identified the honeybee as a pollen predator and "useless visitor to the mistletoe flower" that does not contribute to pollination. But he did not discuss the importance of pollen-bearing mistletoe bushes for the hive, which nowadays often awakens already in late winter. Therefore, the importance of mistletoe for ecology and biodiversity also deserves an updated assessment (Nickrent 2011).

Exceptional botany

Tubeuf's detailed studies of chorology, morphology and physiology led him to the conclusion that mistletoe differs from botanical normality in almost all aspects. Well known since long as poisonous plant, only research in the 1980ies revealed that *V. album* exhibits two poisonous substances and that viscotoxins and mistletoe lectins present strict polarities in spatial and seasonal concentrations (Urech *et al.* 2004). Current research has even deepened the exceptional position of *V. album*, for example by revealing extraordinary characteristics of its genome (Zonneveld 2010). Most stunningly, with respect to mistletoe being a "through and through green plant" (Tubeuf 1923), is a reduced photosynthesis capacity due to the lack of complex I in photosystem I of the chloroplasts (Schroeder *et al.* 2022). These authors do even conclude that «[t]he importance of the host trees supplying *V. album* with carbohydrates may have been underestimated so far». With this statement they emphasize the call for more comprehensive research especially on physiology and pharmacology of *V. album* that was only at its rise a century ago when Tubeuf published his *Monograph on Mistletoe.*

Conclusion and outlook

In the meantime, several monographs have been published describing the entirety of parasitic flowering plants (Kuijt 1969; Heide-Jørgensen 2008), including well over thousand species of mistletoe distributed all over the globe, or specific genera of the Santalaceae (Büssing 2000). However, the diversity of the literature on research about the white-berried *mistletoe*, which has increased exponentially in recent decades, is hardly reflected in these monographs. True to Tubeuf's statement that "such a work is actually never finished", it seems timely to respond to the currently growing worldwide interest in research on *V. album* with a new monograph that is as comprehensive as it is in-depth.

Conflict of interest

The authors declare no conflicts of interest.

Literature

Becker H, Schmoll H: Mistel. Arzneipflanze, Brauchtum, Kunstmotiv im Jugendstil. Stuttgart: Wiss. Verlagsgesellschaft; 1986.

Briggs J: Mistletoe, Viscum album (Santalaceae), in Britain and Ireland: a discussion and review of current status and trends. British & Irish Botany. 2021; 3 (4): 419–454.

Büssing A: Mistletoe, The Genus Viscum. Amsterdam: Harwood Press; 2000.

Heide-Jørgensen HS: Parasitic Flowering Plants. Leiden: Brill; 2008.

Kuijt J: The biology of parasitic flowering plants. Los Angeles: University of California Press; 1969.

Lech P, Zółciak A, Hildebrand R: Occurrence of European Mistletoe (Viscum album L.) on Forest Trees in Poland and Its Dynamics of Spread in the Period 2008–2018. Forests. 2020; 11 (1): 83.

Nickrent DL: Santalales (Including Mistletoes). In: Encyclopedia of Life Sciences (ELS). Chichester: John Wiley & Sons, Ltd; 2011: DOI:10.1002/9780470015902.a0003714.pub2.

Ramm H, Grazi G, Scheibler M, Urech K: Cultivation and development of Viscum album L. In: Büssing A: Mistletoe, The Genus Viscum. Amsterdam: Harwood Press; 2000: 75–94.

Ramm H: Mistletoe through Cultural and Medical History: The All-Healing Plant Proves to Be a Cancer-Specific Remedy. In: Zänker KS, Kaveri SV (eds.): Mistletoe – From Mythology to Evidence-Based Medicine. Basel: Karger; 2015: 1–10.

Ramm H: Zum Verhalten mistelverbreitender Vögel. In: Ramm H, Urech K: Aus der Arbeit mit der Mistel – Erfahrungen, Ergebnisse, Perspektiven. Arlesheim: Verlag des Ita Wegman Instituts; 2017: 145–161.

Ramm H, Schaller G, Urech K, Baumgartner S: Iscador – Pharmazeutische Grundlagen und spirituelles Verständnis für die Verarbeitung der Mistel zum Krebspräparat. Merkurstab. 2021; 74 (3): 219–226.

Schröder L, Hegermann J, Pille P, Braun HP: The photosynthesis apparatus of European mistletoe (Viscum album). Plant Physiology. 2022; 00: 1–19.

Selg P: Mensch und Mistel. Berlin: Salumed; 2016.

Tubeuf KFv: Monographie der Mistel. München, Berlin: Oldenbourg; 1923.

Urech K: Die Eiche von Isigny-Le-Buat – Wahrzeichen der Eichenmistel in Frankreich. Mistilteinn. 2002; 3: 4–13.

Urech K, Jäggy C, Schaller G, Baumgartner S: Giftsubstanzbildung und Wachstumsdynamik der Mistel (Viscum album L.). Mistilteinn. 2004; 5: 20–35.

Zonneveld BJM: New record holders for maximum genome size in eudicots and monocots. J Bot. 2010; 527357.

Dr. Hartmut Ramm, Dr. Konrad Urech
Society for Cancer Research, Hiscia Institute, Kirschweg 9,
4144 Arlesheim, Switzerland

Corresponding author:
h.ramm@vfk.ch

Distribution and Abundance of *Viscum album* ssp. *album* in France

Verbreitung und Häufigkeit von *Viscum album* ssp. *album* in Frankreich

Konrad Urech, Alejandro Casteller, Stephan Baumgartner

Summary

The geographic distribution and abundance of *Viscum album* ssp. *album* in the highly heterogenous environment of France have been visually assessed. The recording of the distribution and abundance was made from a moving car along the roads passed through in the period of February and March (1980–2001). The presence of the well visible mistletoe plants on the defoliated host trees was assessed within intervals of 7–9 km according to a semi-quantitative abundance scale by defining six abundance classes: (0) absent, (1) rare, (2) occasional, (3) frequent, (4) common and (5) abundant. The survey points were plotted on IGN (Institut Géographique National, 1:200'000) maps and analysed using GIS (Geographic Information System). Nearly 11900 survey points were assessed covering most parts of France except namely some peripheral northern regions. Roughly north of 46th parallel area-wide presence of *V. album* ssp. *album* was registered with the exception of a few outstanding areas devoid of mistletoe (e.g. the Beauce). High mistletoe densities were recorded in the central regions of Franche-Comté, Bourgogne, Centre and Pays de la Loire and along rivers often lined with poplars. South of the 46th parallel there was a more or less coherent mistletoe-free area with interspersed conspicuous mistletoe centers (*e.g.*, in the Périgord, the area around Saintes, near Bordeaux and near Toulouse). Mistletoe abundance increased towards the northern slope of the Pyrenees. The highly differentiated spatial patterns of mistletoe distribution detected in the present study in addition to previous cartographic work can be the basis for the identification of physical and biotic factors crucial for the presence and thriving of *V. album* ssp. *album*.

Keywords: *Viscum album* ssp. *album*, France, geographic distribution, abundance

Zusammenfassung
Die geografische Verbreitung und Häufigkeit von *V. album* ssp. *album* in den unterschiedlichen Landschaften Frankreichs wurden visuell bonitiert. Die Erfassung der Verbreitung und der Häufigkeit erfolgte aus einem fahrenden Auto heraus entlang der im Zeitraum Februar und März (1980–2001) befahrenen Straßen. Innerhalb einer Fahrstrecke von jeweils etwa 7–9 km wurde das Vorhandensein der gut sichtbaren Mistelpflanzen auf den entlaubten Wirtsbäumen nach einer semiquantitativen Häufigkeitsskala bonitiert, wobei sechs Häufigkeitsklassen definiert wurden: (0) fehlend, (1) selten, (2) gelegentlich, (3) verbreitet, (4) häufig und (5) Massenvorkommen. Die Index-Werte wurden in Karten des IGN (Institut Géographique Nationale 1:200.000) eingetragen und mit Hilfe von GIS (Geografisches Informationssystem) ausgewertet. Mit nahezu 11900 Erhebungspunkten wurden die meisten Teile Frankreichs mit Ausnahme namentlich einiger nördlicher Randregionen erfasst. Ungefähr nördlich des 46. Breitengrades wurde ein flächendeckendes Vorkommen von *V. album* ssp. *album* festgestellt, mit Ausnahme einiger weniger Gebiete, in denen keine Misteln vorkommen (z. B. in der Beauce). Hohe Misteldichten wurden in den zentralen Regionen Franche-Comté, Bourgogne, Centre und Pays de la Loire sowie entlang der oft von Pappeln gesäumten Flüsse festgestellt. Südlich des 46. Breitengrades gab es ein mehr oder weniger zusammenhängendes mistelfreies Gebiet mit vereinzelten auffälligen Mistelzentren (z. B. im Périgord, in den Gebieten um Saintes, bei Bordeaux und bei Toulouse). Gegen den Nordhang der Pyrenäen zu stieg die Häufigkeit der Mistel. Die sehr differenzierten räumlichen Muster der Mistelverbreitung, die in der vorliegenden Studie festgestellt wurden, können in Ergänzung zu früheren kartografischen Arbeiten als Grundlage für die Ermittlung physikalischer und biotischer Faktoren dienen, die für das Vorhandensein und Gedeihen von *V. album* ssp. *album* entscheidend sind.
Schlüsselwörter: *Viscum album* ssp. *album*, Frankreich, geographische Verbreitung, Häufigkeit

Introduction

At the beginning of the last century Tubeuf (1923) collected all available data on the geographical distribution of *V. album* in France. He stated that most coastal areas and the northern departments were void of mistletoe. It was in 1990 that Dupont published his "Atlas partiel de la flore de

France" were the notifications of the presence of *V. album* in a coarse grid are presented although according to his own criticism with insufficient recordings in certain regions and without differentiating between the three subspecies of *V. album, V. album* ssp. *album, V. album* ssp. *abietis* and *V. album* ssp. *austriacum*.

The work presented here concentrated on the subspecies of *V. album* ssp. *album* growing exclusively on deciduous trees in France. The objective was not only the geographic range but also the abundance. Distribution and abundance of *V. album* ssp. *album* have been visually assessed. This project has been carried out within the framework of a systematic search for pharmaceutically interesting mistletoe on rare hosts in France. Patterns of the distribution and abundance in the highly heterogenous environment of France might be the basis of subsequent work for the identification of physical and biotic factors crucial for the presence and thriving of *V. album* ssp. *album*.

Methods

Distribution and abundance of *V. album* ssp. *album* was assessed from a moving car along the roads passed through in the period of February and March (1980 – 2001). The presence of the well visible mistletoe plants on the defoliated host trees and shrubs was classified within a driving distance of about 7–9 km each according to the semi-quantitative abundance scale A.C.F.O.R. of Morris and Therivel (1995) by defining six abundance classes: absent (0), rare (1), occasional (2), frequent (3), common (4) and abundant (5). The survey points were plotted on IGN (Institut Géographique National, 1:200,000) maps and analysed using ArcGIS (Geographic Information System).

Results and discussion

Nearly 11900 survey points were assessed covering most parts of France except namely some peripheral northern regions (see Fig. 1). France appeared to be divided approximately along the 46th parallel into a northern part with an almost coherent area-wide occurrence of *V. album* ssp. *album* and a southern part of vast almost mistletoe-free landscapes with interspersed centers of high concentrations of mistletoe. The most remarkable southern centers with high mistletoe densities could be found, *e.g.*, in the Périgord, in the area around Saintes, near Bordeaux and near Toulouse. Mistletoe abundance increased towards the northern slope of the Pyrenees. In the northern part of France above the 46th parallel the following striking patterns of mistletoe abundances have been observed. A few areas absolutely free of mistletoe are interspersed in mistletoe-permeated landscapes. The most conspicuous area devoid of mistletoe is the Beauce south of Paris. Remarkably high densities of mistletoe were recorded in the central regions of Franche-Comté, Bourgogne, Centre and Pays de la Loire. Rivers often lined with poplars are favoured habitats that permeate the landscape like mistletoe veins: *e.g.*, the large rivers Loire, Allier, Cher, Vienne, Seine, Marne but also smaller watercourses.

The method of visual assessment of the abundance used in the present work proved to be well suited for the detection of epiphytic mistletoe. The moving view from a moving car is appropriate to capture also poorly visible specimens of green mistletoe providing that the trees and shrubs are in a defoliated state. All survey points have been assessed by one and the same person thus avoiding inter-individual differences.

Still, the method of visual assessment of the abundance used in the present work has some limitations. It has to be taken into account that the recorded abundance indices correspond to the presence of mistletoe in the vicinity of 7 to 9 km roads passed through so that the abundance class may also depend on the direction in which a particular region is traversed. If one crosses, *e.g.*, a river associated with masses of mistletoe the index will be lower than if a road parallel to the river is followed. Utmost attention was required when setting the abundance class zero, as the occurrence of concealed individual mistletoe can never be completely ruled out. However, the absence of visible mistletoe over a distance of 7–9 km gives a high but not an absolute certainty that there is no mistletoe. The method is particularly suitable for recording gradients in mistletoe abundance.

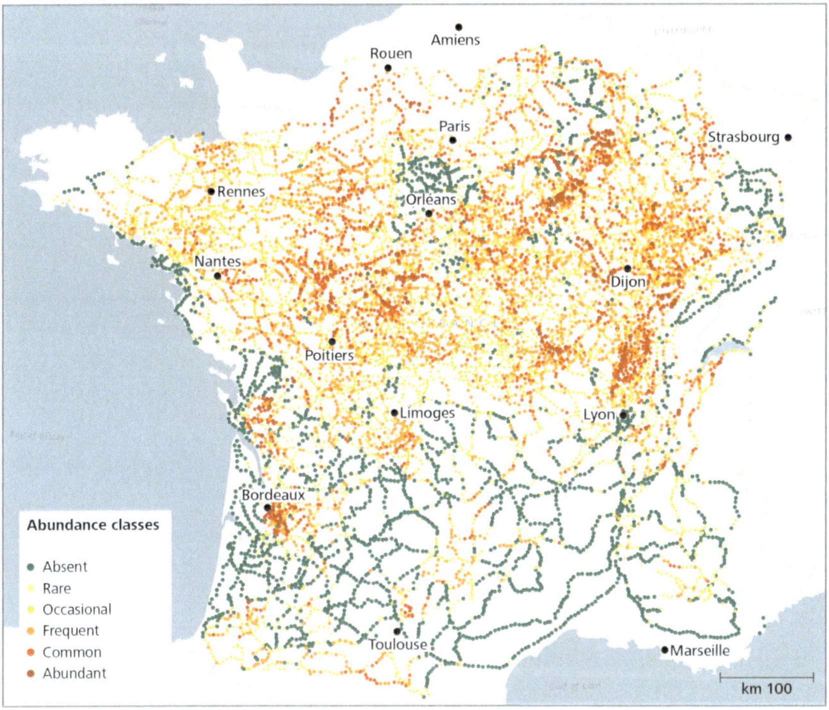

Fig. 1: Geographical distribution and abundance of *Viscum album* ssp. *album* in France. Abundance has been visually assessed along the roads passed through by means of six abundance classes as specified in Methods and in the figure above.

The highly differentiated spatial patterns of mistletoe distribution detected in the present study in addition to previous cartographic work (Dupond 1990) can be the basis for the identification of physical and biotic factors crucial for the presence and thriving of *V. album* ssp. *album*. In particular, the impact of geological, edaphic, hydrological and climatic factors and of biotic interactions (host trees, birds, pests, etc.) on the chorology of mistletoe awaits to be investigated.

Conflict of interest

We confirm that there is no conflict of interest and no financial support that could have influenced the outcome of this work.

Literature

Dupond P: Atlas Partiel de la Flore de France. Collections Patrimoines Naturels, Vol. 3. Paris: Musée National d'Histoire Naturelle de Paris; 1990.

Morris P, Therivel R: Methods of environmental assessment. London: University College London Press; 1995.

Tubeuf K v: Monographie der Mistel. München, Berlin: Verlag R. Oldenbourg; 1923.

Dr. Konrad Urech, Dr. Alejandro Casteller,
Prof. Dr. Stephan Baumgartner
Society for Cancer Research, Hiscia Institute, Kirschweg 9,
4144 Arlesheim, Switzerland

Corresponding author:
k.urech@vfk.ch

Selected Aspects on Biological Properties of miRNA From *Viscum album* L.

Ausgewählte Aspekte zu biologischen Eigenschaften von miRNA aus *Viscum album* L.

Matthias F. Melzig, Catharina Delebinski, Georg Seifert, Wenyan Xie

Summary
Pioneering studies indicate the possibility of cross-kingdom regulation of plant miRNAs on human health and diseases. In *Viscum album* L. from apple tree we identified 29 most genuine novel miRNAs. To evaluate their bioactivity, we selected six of these miRNAs with the most abundant expression. These miRNAs were synthesized and transfected into different tumor cell lines to check their biological effects in different tumor cell lines in comparison with three conserved miRNAs which were expressed not only in mistletoe, but also rich in many other plants to check the selectivity of mistletoe miRNAs effects. As a result, val-miR218 significantly reduced cell viability among various tumor cell lines, especially in osteosarcoma U2OS, SAOS-2 and 143B cells, indicating its promising therapeutic potential. Val-miR218 strongly inhibited osteosarcoma cell proliferation, induced cell apoptosis and arrested cells at G0/G1 phase. Extracellular vesicles (EVs) play an essential role in mediating the function of miRNAs. Mistletoe EVs has been successfully isolated and examined for their effects in protecting and transportation of val-miR218. As expected, val-miR218 was packaged in mistletoe EVs. After the uptake of mistletoe EVs by cells, val-miR218 was delivered into the cytoplasm and interacted with its target genes.
Keywords: Mistletoe; miRNA; osteosarcoma cells; cell proliferation; extracellular vesicles

Zusammenfassung
Neuartige Studien verweisen auf die Möglichkeit des Einflusses von pflanzlichen miRNAs auf Prozesse, die Gesundheit und Krankheit des Menschen regulieren. In *Viscum album* L. (Wirtsbaum Apfel) identifizierten wir 29 neue miRNAs, die für diese Misteln spezifisch sind.

Um ihre Bioaktivität zu bewerten, wählten wir sechs dieser miRNAs aus, die am stärksten exprimiert wurden. Für die weiteren biologischen Studien wurden diese miRNAs synthetisiert und in verschiedene Tumorzelllinien übertragen. Um die Selektivität der Wirkungen von mistelspezifischen miRNAs zu überprüfen, wurden als Vergleich dazu drei konservierte miRNAs eingesetzt, die auch in anderen Pflanzen gebildet werden. Die Ergebnisse zeigten, dass vor allem val-miR218 die Vitalität verschiedener Tumorzelllinien signifikant hemmte, insbesondere bei den Osteosarkomzelllinien U2OS, SAOS-2 und 143B, was auf ein therapeutisches Potenzial hinweist. Val-miR218 hemmte signifikant auch die Proliferation von Osteosarkomzellen und arretierte sie in der G0/G1-Phase. Zudem induzierte diese miRNA Apoptose in diesen Zellen. Extrazelluläre Vesikel (EVs) spielen eine wesentliche Rolle bei der Vermittlung der Wirkung von miRNAs. Mistel-EVs mit enthaltener val-miR218 wurden erfolgreich aus Frischpflanzen isoliert und hinsichtlich ihre Schutzfunktion beim Transport von miRNA untersucht. Nach der Aufnahme von Mistel-EVs durch kultivierte Zellen wurde val-miR218 ins Zytoplasma transportiert und trat in Wechselwirkung mit seinen Zielgenen.
Schlüsselwörter: Mistel, miRNA, Osteosarkomzellen, Zellproliferation, Extrazellulärvesikel

Introduction

MicroRNAs (miRNAs) are naturally occurring, small single-stranded non-coding RNA molecules that regulate gene expression by binding to various parts of mRNA (5′UTR, CDS, and 3′UTR), inducing their cleavage or translational repression. In both plants and animals, miRNA-mediated gene silencing is biochemically based on the principle of recognition and loading of miRNAs onto argonaute (AGO) proteins to form an RNA-protein complex that targets complementary mRNAs and regulates protein synthesis (Zhu *et al.* 2022; Nielsen *et al.* 2022). They are essential in various biological events, including cell proliferation, metabolism, development, and survival (Voinnet 2009; Friedman *et al.* 2009).

Our previous studies revealed a large number of miRNAs presented in *Viscum album* L., including conserved and mistletoe-specific miRNAs. The bioinformatics analysis indicated that these miRNAs are able to influence the expression of genes involving a range of biological processes, contributing to human diseases such as cancer, cardiovascular diseases, and neurological disorders (Xie *et al.* 2017). Some mistletoe miRNAs were found stable during the herbal preparation process (Xie, Melzig 2018), indicating their integrity prior to gastrointestinal digestion or subcutaneous injection, are the common application routes for mistletoe preparations (Steele *et al.* 2015; Marvibaigi 2014). In this study, we screened eight miRNAs (three conserved miRNAs and five mistletoe-specific miRNAs) with relatively high expression in mistletoe for their anti-tumor effects *in vitro*, identified the most effective one, and performed a first animal experiment as proof of concept.

Materials and methods

Cell culture and miRNA mimics

The U2OS, SAOS-2, HepG2, and HT29 cell lines were obtained from the German Collection of Microorganisms and Cell Cultures GmbH (Leibniz Institute DMSZ, Braunschweig, Germany). The cell lines 143B, Colo320R, U-87, SK-N-SH were purchased from American Type Culture Collection (ATCC, Manassas, VA, USA). Mesenchymal stem cells (MSCs) were obtained from Merck Millipore (Burlington, MA, USA). Cells were cultured with recommended media supplied with 10 % fetal bovine serum (FBS) in a humidified 5 % CO2 incubator at 37 °C. Human embryonic lung fibroblasts Fi301, kindly offered by Prof. Dr. Christian Hagemeier, Labor für Pädiatrische Molekularbiologie, Charité – Universitätsmedizin Berlin, Germany, were maintained in Eagle's minimum essential medium (EMEM) supplemented with Earle's balanced salt solution, 25 mM HEPES, 1 mM sodium pyruvate, 2 mM L-alanyl-L-glutamine, non-essential amino acids, 0.75 ‰ (w/v) sodium bicarbonate, 50 µg/ml gentamicin and 10 % fetal bovine serum (FBS). The Allstar negative control miRNA (NC miRNA), biotinylated val-miR218, val-miR218 inhibitor and negative control inhibitor were designed and purchased from Qiagen (Hilden, Germany). The miRNA mimics (Xie *et al.* 2023) were synthesized by Metabion International AG (Planegg/Steinkirchen, Germany).

Transfection and viability assays

Invitrogen™ Lipofectamin RNAiMAX (ThermoFisher Scientific, Waltham, MA, USA) was used to achieve miRNA transfection. For cell viability assays, cells were seeded in 48-well plates at a concentration of 2×10^4/well. After 24 h incubation, cells were transfected with miRNA mimics (20 nM). Cell viability was measured by using MTT assay at 72 h post-transfection. For real-time cell proliferation analysis, cells were seeded at a density of 2×10^4 cells per well in 8-well E-Plate (ACEA Biosciences; San Diego, CA, USA), and cell proliferation was monitored by xCELLigence™ real-time analysis (ACEA Biosciences) for five days. For cell apoptosis assays, cells were seeded in 12-well plates at a concentration of 1×10^5/well. Apoptosis was evaluated 72 h and 120 h post-transfection by detection of annexin V (APC) and propidium iodide (PI) by Cytoflex flow cytometer (Beckman Coulter Inc., Fullerton, California, USA).

Mistletoe EV isolation and characterization

Mistletoe leaves growing on *Malus sylvestris* (L.) Mill. were collected from Botanic Garden (Berlin, Germany) in February 2020. The leaves (5 g) were washed and grounded in 50 mL PBS buffer (pH 7.4), supplied with 1 mM DTT and cOmplete, EDTA-free protease inhibitor cocktail (Roche, Germany). The raw extract was centrifuged at 1000 g for 10 min, 4000 g for 20 min, 15000 g for 90 min to remove large fiber and cell debris. The supernatant was filtered through a 0.8 µm filter. The EVs were concentrated and purified from the filtrate using the OptiPrep cushion procedure and gradient density ultracentrifugation (Zhuang *et al.* 2015). Briefly, the filtrate was added to the centrifuge tube with 2 mL of 60 % iodixanol (Sigma-Aldrich, St. Louis, MO, USA) at the bottom to form a cushion layer. After spinning at 40000 rpm (118000 g) for 70 min using a Beckman Ti70 rotor, a volume of 3 mL from the bottom of the ultracentrifuge tubes was collected, resulting in a mixture of 40 % iodixanol. A discontinuous gradient was created by placing 3 mL of 5 % iodixanol solution at the bottom. Subsequently, underlay 3 mL of 10 % iodixanol, 3 mL of 20 % iodixanol, 3 mL of 40 % iodixanol solution containing mistletoe EVs, followed by 1 mL of 60 % iodixanol. After centrifuging the tubes in an SW41 Ti rotor at 36000 rpm (164000 g) for 18 h in Beckman Optima LE-80K ultracentrifuge (Beckman Coulter), gently collect 13 individual 1 mL fractions from the top of the tubes. The fractions 9–11 that were located within the density range of 1.13–1.20 g/mL were combined and washed by cushion ultracentrifugation in PBS and resuspended in PBS for further application. Mistletoe EVs were placed on Formvar-Carbon coated grids (Electron Microscopy Sciences, Hatfield, PA, USA), stained with Uranyless (Electron Microscopy Sciences), and observed under scanning electron microscopy (Hitech, Tokyo, Japan) in TEM mode. TEM imaging was performed using 30 kV acceleration voltage. The size of EVs was measured by Nanoparticle Tracking Analysis NTA (Malvern Panalytical, Malvern, UK), and the protein concentration of EVs was determined by BCA assay (Thermo Scientific). To investigate if mistletoe EVs could rescue the cytotoxicity of val-miR218, U2OS cells were seeded in 96-well plate at 1×10^4 cells per well and treated with mistletoe EVs (10 μg/mL) or negative control miRNA inhibitor (NC inhibitor, 50 nM) or val-miR218 inhibitor (50 nM) or the combinations, MTT assay was performed 72 h after the treatment. The inhibitors were miRCURY LNA miRNA inhibitors (Qiagen, Hilden, Germany).

Confocal microscopy

The mistletoe EVs were stained with red fluorescent lipid dye PKH26 (Merck Millipore, Burlington, MA, USA), and the free dye was removed by ultracentrifugation (at 40000 rpm for 70 min). Furthermore, FAM-labeled val-miR218 was transfected into mistletoe EVs using Exo-Fect siRNA/miRNA Transfection Kit (SBI System Biosciences, Palo Alto, CA, USA). After 24 h incubation with either stained EVs or the EVs transfected with FAM labeled val-miR218, U2OS cells were stained with Hoechst 33342 (Merck Millipore) and Alexa Fluor 594-phalloidin (Abcam, Cambridge, United Kingdom) and imaged under a confocal microscope (SP8, Leica Microsystems, Wetzlar, Germany).

Animal xenograft experiment

Eight-week-old female NOG mice (NOD.Cg-Prkdcscid Il2rgtm1Sug/JicTac; Taconic Biosciences GmbH, Germany) were housed in a pathogen-free facility in IVC (Tecniplast, Italy) cages and fed an autoclaved standard diet (Ssniff, Soest, Germany) with acidified drinking water ad libitum. SAOS-2 cells (1×10^6) were subcutaneously injected in PBS:Matrigel (1:1) into the left flank of six mice per treatment or control group. Intra-tumoral injections with single-stranded val-miR218 (0.75 mg/kg) or vehicle were started with palpable tumors (day15 post cell transplantation). Injections were applied at 2–3 different areas directly into the tumor (5 mm under the skin). Compound or vehicle was administered twice per week. Body weight was measured before each treatment, and mice were carefully monitored for health and symptoms of toxicity. Animals were sacrificed by cervical dislocation at the end of the experiment. Animal experiments were performed in accordance with the German Animal Welfare Act and all procedures were approved by local authorities (Landesamt für Gesundheit und Soziales, LAGeSo Berlin, Germany) under approval number A-0010/19 for preclinical tumor experiments.

Statistics

All *in vitro* experiments were performed in three independent experiments. MiRNA treated groups were compared to NC miRNA-treated group using t-tests, while statistical comparisons among multiple groups were performed using one-way analysis of variance (ANOVA) followed by multiple post-hoc comparisons (t-test). All results with $p \leq 0.05$ were considered significant.

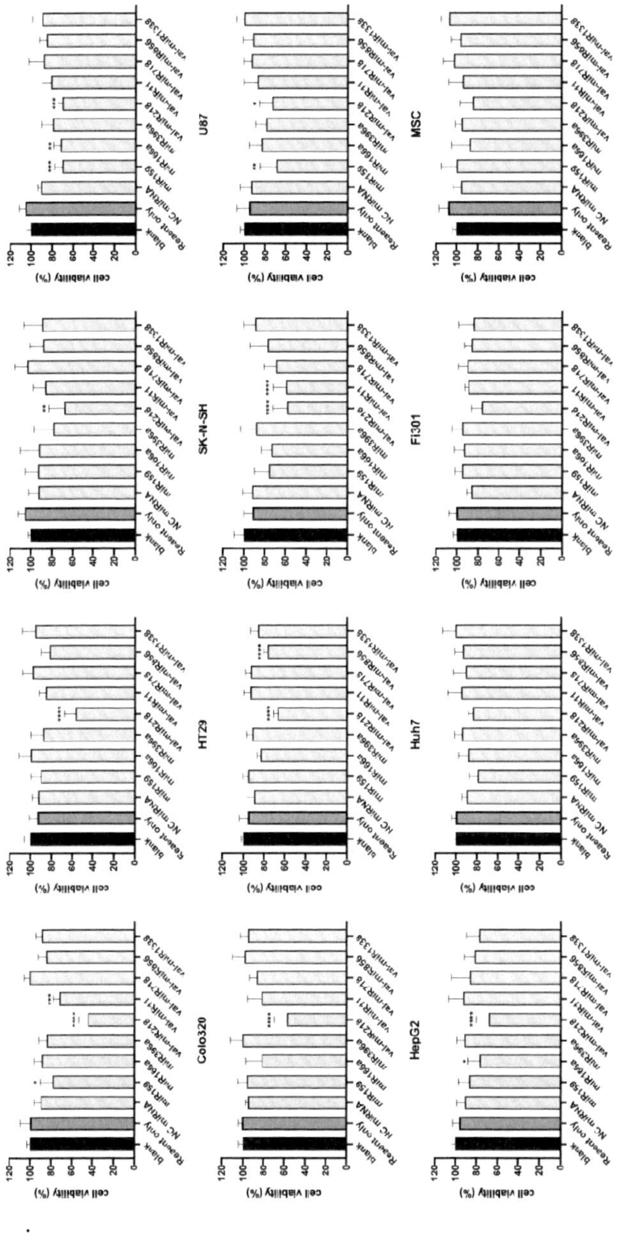

Fig. 1: Bioactive mistletoe miRNAs screen for cytotoxic effects. Cells were seeded in 48-well plates at a density of 2×10^4 cells per well and transfected with various miRNA mimics at a concentration of 20 nM.Cell viability was determined by MTT assay 72 h after transfection. N = 3. Compared with cells treated with NC miRNA, *$p<0.05$; **$p<0.01$; ***$p<0.001$; ****$p<0.0001$.

Results

Screening bioactive mistletoe miRNAs

To analyze the bioactivity of mistletoe-specific miRNAs, three conserved miRNA and five mistletoe-specific miRNAs with the most abundant expression were selected. These includes miR159, miR166a, miR396a, val-miR218, val-miR11, val-miR718, val-miR856 and val-miR1338. The miRNAs were transfected into the different tumor or non-tumor cells to check their cytotoxic effects. As shown in Figure 1, val-miR218 significantly reduced cell viability in most tested tumor cell lines, mainly in the osteosarcoma cell lines U2OS, SAOS-2 and 143B. Especially val-miR218 induced almost 50 % viability in osteosarcoma cells U2OS and SAOS-2, respectively.

There was no obvious toxicity of val-miR218 in human fibroblast cell line Fi301 and human mesenchymal stem cells (MSCs), indicating the specificity of val-miR218. Besides, some other miRNAs possessed cytotoxicity in specific cell lines too. Consistent with a previous report (Chin *et al.* 2016), conserved miRNA miR159 inhibited the growth of JIMT-1, U2OS, and U-87 cells. Val-miR11 decreased cell viability in U2OS and SK-N-SH cells. Here in this study, we mainly focus on investigating the bioactive effects of val-miR218

Val-miR218 mimics strongly inhibited osteosarcoma cell growth and induced their apoptosis

To evaluate the effect of val-miR218 on the proliferation of osteosarcoma cells U2OS, SAOS-2, and 143B, cells were transfected with val-miR218 and constantly monitored for 7 days. As shown in Figure 2A, the NC miRNA had no pronounced effect on cell proliferation, while val-miR218 mimics significantly inhibited proliferation in a time and concentration-dependent manner. For U2OS and SAOS-2, the cell index reduced up to 80 % after val-miR218 transfection time-dependently (Fig. 2A). For 143B, a decrease in cell proliferation was observed, especially after 20 nM val-miR218 treatment compared to NC. To determine the induction of apoptosis, val-miR218 treated cells were analysed by annexin V/PI staining and FACS analysis. Apoptosis was enhanced with the increase of incubation time (Fig. 2B). SAOS-2 cells were more sensitive to val-miR218, which showed 10 % more apoptotic cells in response to val-miR218, compared to U2OS cells. For 143B, no prominent apoptosis was induced three days after transfection.

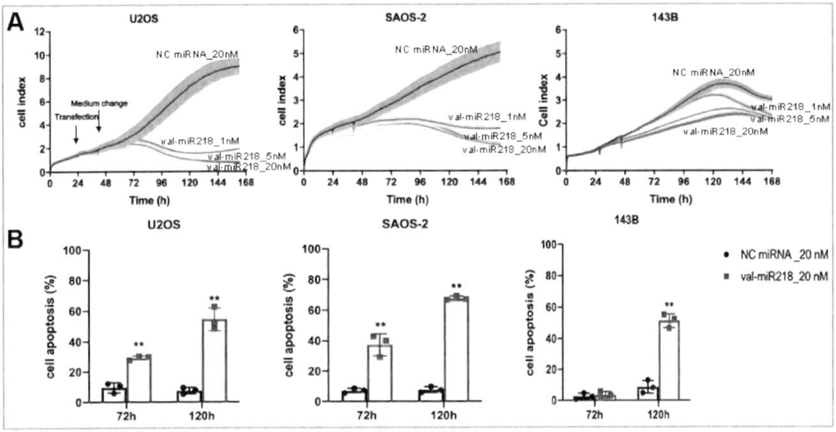

Fig. 2: Val-miR218 inhibits cell proliferation and induces cell apoptosis in osteosarcoma cells in a time and concentration-dependent manner. (A) Osteosarcoma cells were seeded at a density of 2×10^4 cells/ well in 8-well E-Plate (ACEA Biosciences, USA) and transfected with either val-miR218 or NC miRNA.
The medium was changed 24 h after transfection. Cell proliferation was monitored by xCELLigence real-time analysis (ACEA Biosciences, USA) for a total of 7 days. (B) Cells were seeded at a density of 1×10^5 cells/ well in 12-well plates and transfected with either val-miR218 or NC miRNA. Cell apoptosis was determined after depicted incubation periods by Annexin V/PI and FACS Flow cytometry. N = 3. Compared cells treated with NC miRNA, **$p<0.01$.

Mistletoe EVs carry and transport val-miR218 to recipient cells

In order to evaluate whether mistletoe EVs mediate the function of val-miR218, mistletoe EVs were isolated from mistletoe extracellular fluid using gradient density ultracentrifugation. They showed typical round and cup-shaped structures under SEM, with an average diameter of 119 nm

(Fig. 3A, B). To evaluate if mistletoe EVs mediate the function of val-miR218, U2OS cells were either incubated with mistletoe EVs alone or in combination with val-miR218 inhibitor, negative control miRNA inhibitor, respectively. The incubation with mistletoe EVs caused a 40 % reduction of cell viability.

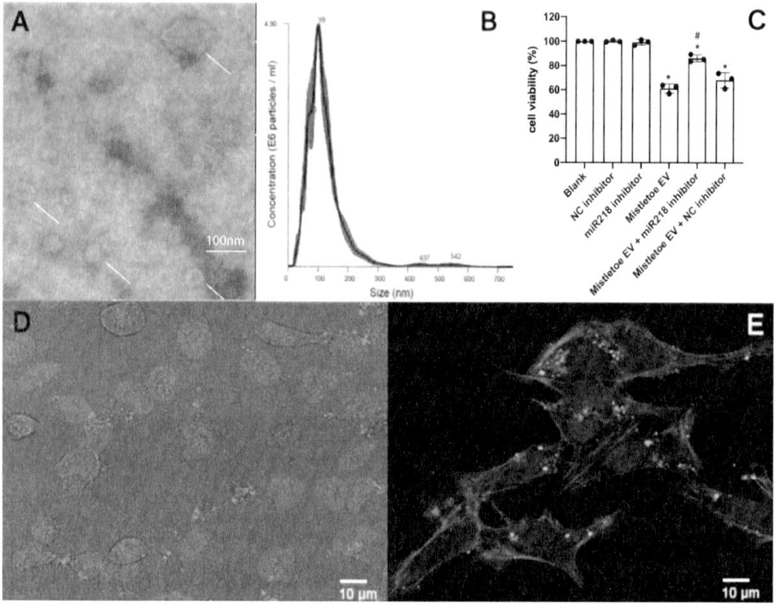

Fig. 3: Mistletoe EVs might mediate cell uptake of val-miR218. (A) Visualization of mistletoe EVs under TEM. (B) Size distribution of mistletoe EVs. (C) U2OS cells were seeded in 96-well plate at 1×10^4 cells per well and treated with mistletoe EVs (10 µg/mL) or negative control miRNA inhibitor (NC inhibitor, 50 nM) or val-miR218 inhibitor (50 nM) or the combinations, MTT assay was performed 72 h after the treatment. Compared with blank cells, $^*p<0.05$; compared with cells treated with EVs, #$p<0.05$. (D) U2OS cells were incubated with PKH26 stained mistletoe EVs for 24 h, and cell uptake of EVs was checked under a confocal microscope. (E) FAM-labeled val-miR218 was transfected into EVs and then incubated with U2OS cells for 24 h. The cell nucleus was stained by Hoechst 33342, and cell skeleton was stained by Phalloidin. N = 3.

As shown in Figure 3C, the NC inhibitor did not influence the effect of mistletoe EVs whereas the val-218 inhibitor significantly rescued the EVs caused cytotoxicity. However, val-miR218 inhibitor did not completely inhibit the impact of EVs; around 15 % of cells were still found dead in the cells co-treated with EVs and val-miR218.

To check if mistletoe EVs transport val-miR218 into mammalian cells, we first labeled EVs with red fluorescent lipid dye PKH26 and incubated them with U2OS cells. As shown in Figure 3D, EVs were successfully taken by U2OS cells after 24 h incubation. Furthermore, FAM-labeled val-miR218 was transfected into mistletoe EVs. After 24 h incubation with EVs, the uptake of val-miR218 by U2OS was directly observed under confocal microscope (SP8, Leica microsystems, Germany). The data suggest that mistletoe EVs facilitate the uptake of val-miR218 by U2OS cells.

Val-miR218 reduces tumor growth *in vivo*

To investigate the therapeutic potential of val-miR218, the efficacy was tested *in vivo*. For this purpose, Saos-2 xenografts were intratumorally treated nine times for approximately four weeks with single-stranded val-miR218. Val-miR218 treatment led to a significant reduction of tumor weight and tumor volume in comparison to the control group (Fig. 4). The mice in the experiments did not show significant changes in body weight or signs of toxicity during the study, which means the val-miR218 treatment was well tolerated.

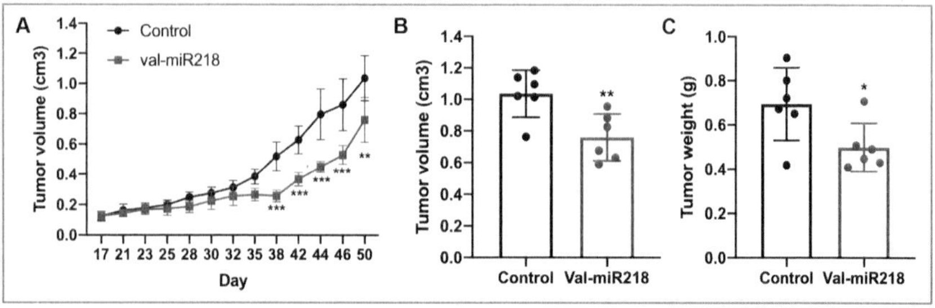

Fig. 4: Val-miR218 reduces tumor weight and tumor volume *in vivo*. Xenografts were treated intratumorally with 0.75 mg/kg of val-miR218 twice weekly. The application was given in a total of 9 times. (A) Tumor volume was measured every 3 days. (B) and (C) Tumor volume and tumor weight were determined one day after the last injection. Compared to control group, *P<0.05, **P<0.01, *** P<0.001.

Discussion

Recent research has revealed the presence of intact and functional plant-derived miRNAs in human fluids and tissues, suggesting possible cross-kingdom regulatory effects (Zhang *et al.* 2012; Chin *et al.* 2016; Chen *et al.* 2021). The idea of cross-kingdom and gene regulation in humans by plant miRNAs serves as a promising treatment strategy for treating malignant tumors and matches the use of mistletoe preparation. Here, we identified bioactive miRNAs from mistletoe and confirmed anti-cancer effects of mistletoe-specific miRNAs for the first time. As the most abundant mistletoe-specific miRNAs, val-miR218 showed significant cytotoxicity in most tested tumor cells, especially osteosarcoma U2OS, SAOS-2, and 143B cells. In addition, val-miR218 effectively inhibited osteosarcoma cell proliferation and induced cell apoptosis time-dependently, indicating its promising potential for cancer treatment therapy. It is well known that naked miRNAs are extremely sensitive in herbal preparations and the mammalian circulation system. Our previous study detected val-miR218 in various mistletoe extracts and indicated the relative stability of val-miR218 (Xie, Melzig 2018). Being packed into EVs, mistletoe miRNAs could be transferred to the circulating system or directly reach receipt cells via EVs. In the present study, val-miR218 inhibitors could significantly reverse mistletoe EV-induced cytotoxicity, indicating val-miR218 is associated with mistletoe EVs. Being loaded inside EVs, val-miR218 could be efficiently delivered into human cells. The data from the animal experiment indicated val-miR218 as a promising miRNA for tumor treatment *in vivo*. The mechanism underlying will be further investigated in future studies. However, the development of chemical modifications for miRNA used as drug (e. g., the addition of a 2'-O-methyl group or locked nucleic acids) and delivery systems (e. g., neutral lipid emulsions, plant or human cell-derived EVs) for miRNA mimics and anti-miRs remains a crucial challenge for their *in vivo* applications (Rupaimoole, Slack 2017).

In conclusion, we have demonstrated for the first time the high potential of val-miR218 in inhibiting proliferation in various tumor cell lines *in vitro*, as well as for osteosarcoma *in vivo*. Further studies are needed to identify the miRNA and protein profile in mistletoe EVs. The mistletoe EVs not only offer an efficient vehicle but also a naturally derived combination of various bioactive ingredients.

Acknowledgements

This work was supported by German Research Foundation (DFG, XI174/2-1) and Software AG-Stiftung (SAGST, Darmstadt, Germany). We would like to thank Experimental Pharmacology & Oncology Berlin-Buch GmbH for carrying out the animal experiment.

Conflict of interest

The authors declare that there is no conflict of interest.

References

Chen X, Liu L, Chu Q et al.: Large-scale identification of extracellular plant miRNAs in mammals implicates their dietary intake. PLoS One. 2021; 16: e0257878.

Chin AR, Fong MY, Somlo G et al.: Cross-kingdom inhibition of breast cancer growth by plant miR159. Cell Res. 2016; 26: 217–228.
Friedman RC, Farh KK-H, Burge CB et al.: Most mammalian mRNAs are conserved targets of microRNAs. Genome Res. 2009; 19: 92–105.
Marvibaigi M, Supriyanto E, Amini N et al.: Preclinical and clinical effects of mistletoe against breast cancer. Biomed Res Int. 2014; 2014: 785479.
Nielsen AF, Bindereif A, Bozzoni I et al.: Best practice standards for circular RNA research. Nature Methods. 2022; 2022: 1–13.
Rupaimoole R, Slack FJ: MicroRNA therapeutics: towards a new era for the management of cancer and other diseases. Nat Rev Drug Discov. 2017; 16: 203–222.
Steele ML, Axtner J, Happe A et al.: Use and safety of intratumoral application of European mistletoe (Viscum album L.) preparations in oncology. Integr Cancer Ther. 2015; 14: 140–148.
Voinnet O: Origin, biogenesis, and activity of plant microRNAs. Cell. 2009; 136: 669–687.
Xie W, Adolf J, Melzig MF: Identification of Viscum album L. miRNAs and prediction of their medicinal values. PLoS One. 2017; 12: e0187776.
Xie W, Melzig MF: The stability of medicinal plant microRNAs in the herb preparation process. Molecules. 2018; 23: 919.
Xie W, Delebinski D, Gürgen D et al.: Inhibition of osteosarcoma by European Mistletoe derived val-miR218. Extracell Vesicles Circ Nucleic Acids. 2023; 4: 306–322.
Zhang L, Hou D, Chen X et al.: Exogenous plant MIR168a specifically targets mammalian LDLRAP1: evidence of cross-kingdom regulation by microRNA. Cell Res. 2012; 22: 273–274.
Zhu Y, Zhu L, Wang X et al.: RNA-based therapeutics: an overview and prospectus. Cell Death & Disease. 2022; 13: 1–15.
Zhuang X, Deng Z-B, Mu J et al.: Ginger-derived nanoparticles protect against alcohol-induced liver damage. J Extracell Vesicles. 2015; 4: 28713.

Prof. Dr. Dr. h. c. Matthias F. Melzig[1], Dr. Catharina Delebinski[2],
Prof. Dr. Georg Seifert[3], Dr. Wenyan Xie[1]

[1] Institut für Pharmazie der Freien Universität Berlin, Pharmazeutische Biologie, Germany

[2] Department of Pediatric Oncology/Hematology, Otto-Heubner-Centre for Pediatric and Adolescent Medicine (OHC), Charité – Universitätsmedizin Berlin, corporate member of Freie Universität Berlin and Humboldt Universität zu Berlin, Berlin 13353, Germany.

[3] Charité, Universitätsmedizin Berlin, Germany

Corresponding author:
melzig@zedat.fu-berlin.de

The Energy Metabolism of European Mistletoe (*Viscum album* L.)

Der Energiestoffwechsel der europäischen Mistel (*Viscum album* L.)

Lucie Schröder, Jennifer Senkler, Hans-Peter Braun

Summary

In 1923, the Munich botanist Professor Karl von Tubeuf published his highly regarded book "Monographie der Mistel". On almost 1000 pages, he summarized the knowledge about *Viscum album* at that time and came to the much-quoted conclusion: "Nothing about this plant is normal". *V. album* is an evergreen obligate semi-parasitic flowering plant that grows on numerous trees. Its life cycle fundamentally differs from that of other flowering plants, and also from other parasitic flowering plants. *V. album* is meanwhile intensively investigated at the molecular level. It has been found to contain an extremely large genome consisting of almost 100 billion base pairs (nucleotide pairs). The genome has not yet been sequenced, but most of the protein-coding regions are meanwhile known. It turned out that the nucleotide composition of the protein-coding genes of *V. album* is unusual for dicot plants, as the proportion of the nucleotides deoxyguanosine monophosphate (G) and deoxycytidine monophosphate (C) is comparatively high. This implies increased DNA stability, but at the same time a considerable higher energy demand for the transcription of its genes. Cell division in *V. album* also requires a great amount of energy, as the genome has to be duplicated beforehand. How can *V. album* provide this energy? It was found that *V. album* mitochondria, which are responsible for the formation of the energy-rich compound adenosine triphosphate (ATP), lack a key protein complex (NADH dehydrogenase; complex I) that is considered indispensable for ATP formation. In the meantime, we have investigated the energy metabolism of *V. album* chloroplasts. We found that the chloroplasts also have a limited capacity to form ATP. This gives us a picture that *V. album* can live with a comparatively reduced energy metabolism despite an increased energy requirement for its genetic system. It is concluded that the host trees must supply *V. album* with energy-rich compounds to a greater extent than previously thought.

Keywords: Energy metabolism; cellular respiration, photosynthesis, mitochondria, chloroplasts, genome, *Viscum album*

Zusammenfassung
Im Jahr 1923 veröffentlichte der Münchner Botaniker und Professor Karl von Tubeuf sein viel beachtetes Buch „Monographie der Mistel“. Auf fast 1000 Seiten fasste er das damalige Wissen über *Viscum album* zusammen und kam zu dem vielzitierten Schluss: „Nichts an dieser Pflanze ist normal“. *V. album* ist eine immergrüne, obligat halbparasitäre Blütenpflanze, die auf zahlreichen Bäumen wächst. Ihr Lebenszyklus unterscheidet sich grundlegend von dem anderer Blütenpflanzen sowie dem anderer parasitischer Blütenpflanzen. *V. album* wird inzwischen intensiv auf molekularer Ebene untersucht. Es wurde festgestellt, dass sie ein extrem großes Genom mit fast 100 Milliarden Basenpaaren (Nukleotidpaaren) besitzt. Das Genom ist noch nicht sequenziert, aber die meisten der proteinkodierenden Regionen sind inzwischen bekannt. Es zeigte sich, dass die Nukleotidzusammensetzung der proteinkodierenden Gene von *V. album* für zweikeimblättrige Pflanzen ungewöhnlich ist, da der Anteil der Nukleotide Desoxyguanosinmonophosphat (G) und Desoxycytidinmonophosphat (C) vergleichsweise hoch ist. Dies impliziert eine erhöhte DNA-Stabilität, gleichzeitig aber auch einen erheblich höheren Energiebedarf für die Transkription ihrer Gene. Auch die Zellteilung in *V. album* erfordert einen hohen Energieaufwand, da das Genom zuvor verdoppelt werden muss. Wie kann *V. album* diese Energie bereitstellen? Es wurde festgestellt, dass den Mitochondrien von *V. album*, die für die Bildung der energiereichen Verbindung Adenosintriphosphat (ATP) verantwortlich sind, ein wichtiger Proteinkomplex (die NADH-Dehydrogenase; Komplex I) fehlt, der als unentbehrlich für die ATP-Bildung gilt. In der Zwischenzeit haben wir den Energiestoffwechsel der Chloroplasten von *V. album* untersucht. Wir fanden heraus, dass die Chloroplasten ebenfalls eine begrenzte Kapazität zur Bildung von ATP haben. Daraus ergibt sich das Bild, dass *V. album* trotz eines erhöhten Energiebedarfs für sein genetisches System mit einem vergleichsweise reduzierten Energiestoffwechsel leben kann. Daraus wird geschlossen, dass die Wirtsbäume *V. album* in größerem Umfang als bisher angenommen mit energiereichen Verbindungen versorgen müssen.
Schlüsselwörter: Energiestoffwechsel, Zellatmung, Photosynthese, Mitochondrien, Chloroplasten, Genom, *Viscum album*

Introduction

Photosynthesis is in the very center of the plant energy metabolism. In addition, however, plant cells also carry out cellular respiration. With regard to gas metabolism, photosynthesis and respiration are complementary processes: photosynthesis involves the fixation of carbon dioxide (CO_2) and the release of oxygen, whereas respiration involves the consumption of oxygen and the liberation of CO_2. Both processes, photosynthesis, which takes place in the chloroplasts, and respiration, for which the mitochondria are responsible, enable the synthesis of energy-rich compounds, in particular adenosine triphosphate (ATP). Almost all energy-requiring processes in plant cells are driven by ATP. Here, we review particularities of the energy metabolism of *V. album*.

The respiration of *V. album*

V. album has a very special mode of cellular respiration (Senkler *et al.* 2018; Maclean *et al.* 2018; Schröder *et al.* 2020). The final step of cellular respiration takes place at the inner mitochondrial membrane (IMM) and is based on the activities of five enzyme complexes, namely complexes I, II, III, IV, and V. The first four complexes establish an electron transport chain (the 'respiratory chain') which enables formation of a proton gradient across the IMM. Complex V utilizes this proton gradient to form ATP. Surprisingly, it was found that complex I of the respiratory chain is absent in *V. album*. This complex, which is an NADH dehydrogenase, not only channels a large proportion of electrons into the respiratory chain, but also strongly contributes to the proton gradient. Until now, complex I has generally been considered essential for cellular respiration in higher organisms. In fact, *V. album* is currently the only example of a multicellular eukaryote that can live without complex I. It meanwhile has been found that the respiratory chain of *V. album* is remodeled in two respects: first, enzymes that can replace the function of complex I (albeit only imperfectly, as they do not contribute to the generation of the proton gradient across the IMM) are particularly abundant. Second, the complexes III and

IV form stable supercomplexes, which enable the last segment of the respiratory chain to proceed particularly effectively. Due to the absence of complex I, *V. album* may save the energy necessary for building this complex, which is actually very large and consists of almost 50 protein subunits in plants (Klusch *et al.* 2021). At the same time, however, the reduction of the respiratory chain in *V. album* limits the mitochondrial capacity to form ATP. It has been concluded that the mitochondrial ATP provision for the cell is significantly reduced in *V. album*.

The energy metabolism in the cytosol and the nucleus

In plant cells, mitochondrially produced ATP is the main energy supply for processes in the cytosol and nucleus. In the cytosol, ATP is used for the formation of uridine triphosphate (UTP), which facilitates sucrose biosynthesis from the end products of photosynthesis (mainly activated trioses). Sucrose is the most important transport form of sugar. It is exported by leaf cells to cell types that cannot carry out photosynthesis. Sucrose also is the building block for cellulose and therefore is required for plant growth. In the nucleus, ATP is required for DNA replication, as well as transcription of genes. Transcripts are subsequently used for protein biosynthesis in the cytosol. Both DNA replication and gene transcription are very energy-intensive, as are sucrose and protein biosynthesis in the cytosol.

DNA replication in *V. album* even has to be considered particularly energy-demanding. It has been found that the *V. album* genome is exceptionally large compared to other eukaryotes (Zonneveld 2010). The haploid genome consists of around 100 billion base pairs (nucleotide pairs). In comparison, the human genome consists of only 3 billion base pairs and that of the model plant *Arabidopsis thaliana* of 0.15 billion base pairs. As a consequence, every cell division of *V. album* is associated with an extremely large investment of energy. This might be compensated to some extent by the fact that *V. album* only grows slowly and therefore has prolonged cell cycles. However, there are phases in which *V. album* grows faster, especially in spring (Urech *et al.* 2004).

The genetic system of *V. album*

Recently, projects have been carried out to sequence and characterize the *V. album* genome (Schröder *et al.* 2022a; 2023). However, as direct sequencing of its large genome is very elaborate, a strategy based on systematic sequencing of gene transcripts has been carried out. This has at least clarified the sequence information of all areas of the genome that code for proteins. The data of this project are accessible on our *V. album* genome project website (https://viscumalbum.pflanzenproteomik.de). It turned out that *V. album* transcripts (and thus also the DNA of the transcribed sections) contain increased amounts of the nucleotides deoxyguanosine monophosphate (G) and deoxycytidine monophosphate (C), compared to other dicot plants. Increased GC contents mean that the DNA is especially stable. At the same time, however, energy demands for transcribing the corresponding DNA segments are increased. It can therefore be concluded that in *V. album* not only the process of DNA replication but also that of transcription is particularly energy-intensive.

Taken together, this creates a special situation in *V. album*, as formation of the energy-rich compound ATP by mitochondria is limited, but at the same time important energy-requiring processes, such as DNA replication and transcription, are to be categorized as particularly energy-intensive. How this works is currently a mystery.

The photosynthesis of *V. album*

In addition to mitochondria, also the chloroplasts in plant cells can produce ATP, provided that light is available. Is the chloroplast capacity to produce ATP increased in *V. album*? To address this question, chloroplasts from *V. album* leaves were biochemically purified and characterized (Schröder *et al.* 2022b). Electron microscopic examinations of the isolated organelles revealed reduced amounts of endogenous membranes, the so-called thylakoid membranes, inside the chloroplasts (Fig. 1). These thylakoid membranes are necessary for the 'light reaction', which provides energy for the subsequent CO_2 fixation by the Calvin-Benson-cycle. Analogous to the mitochondrial respiratory chain, the chloroplast light reaction is also based on the presence of enzyme complexes: the photosystems I and II, and the cytochrome b_6f complex. These protein complexes constitute an electron transport chain and enable formation of a proton gradient across the thylakoid membrane, which is used for ATP synthesis by a chloroplast ATP synthase complex.

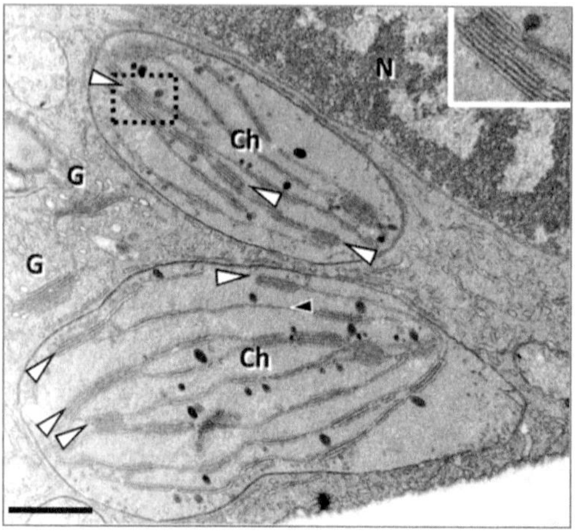

Fig. 1: Transmission electron microscopy (TEM) image of part of a *V. album* leaf cell. White arrowheads, grana; black arrowhead, single layered thylakoid; N, nucleus; G, Golgi; Ch, chloroplast. The scale bar corresponds to 1 µm in the image and to 0.5 µm in the inset (boxed area). Image taken from Schröder *et al.* 2022b, modified.

A systematic characterization of the chloroplast protein complexes of *V. album* has now shown that the ATP production capacity of the light reaction is reduced compared to other plants (Schröder *et al.* 2022b). In particular, it was found that a protein complex, which is homologous to mitochondrial complex I and referred to as the chloroplast NADH-dehydrogenase-like complex (NDH complex), also is completely absent in *V. album* (Fig. 2). Corresponding indications had already emerged during a sequencing project of the *V. album* chloroplast genome, when genes coding for subunits of this protein complex could not be identified (Petersen *et al.* 2015).

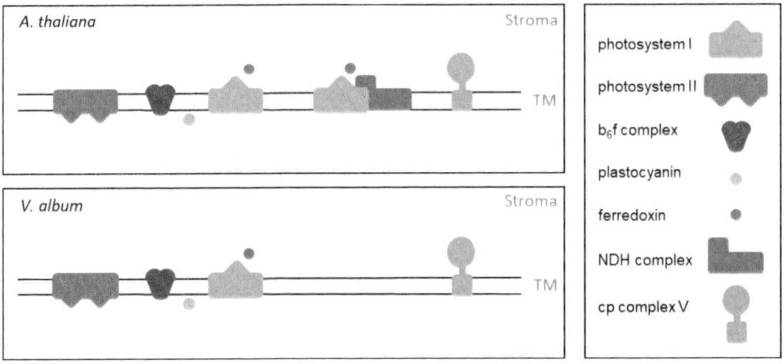

Fig. 2: The protein complexes and protein supercomplexes of the light reaction of photosynthesis in the model plant *Arabidopsis thaliana* (top) and *Viscum album* (bottom). The identities of the complexes are given to the right of the two boxes. TM, thylakoid membrane. Image taken from Schröder *et al.* 2022b, modified.

The NDH complex is required for a special mode of the light reaction in which electrons are cycled around photosystem I. This process contributes to the formation of the proton gradient across the thylakoid membrane. Due to the absence of the NDH complex and the fact that photosystem I is present in comparatively low amounts, it can be concluded that the chloroplast capacity to form ATP is also limited in *V. album*. This is consistent with physiological results obtained for isolated *V. album* chloroplasts, which also revealed a comparatively low activity of protein complexes involved in the photosynthetic light reaction (Tuquet, Sallé 1996).

Conclusion

The energy metabolism of *V. album* is very special. The capacities of its mitochondria and chloroplasts to produce ATP are limited. At the same time, some processes in *V. album* are particularly energy-intensive, such as the replication of its comparatively huge genome and the transcription of its comparatively GC-rich genes. "Nothing about this plant is normal"

– this realization by Karl Freiherr von Tubeuf (Tubeuf 1923) also applies to the molecular biology of *V. album*. It is possible that the cytosol of *V. album*, in which the metabolic pathway of glycolysis takes place, is particularly involved in ATP formation, for which there are indeed indications (Maclean *et al.* 2018). But where do the sugars come from that are needed as substrates for glycolysis? They certainly can come from the photosynthesis of *V. album*, but to meet its energy requirement, substantial import of sugars (and probably other organic compounds) from the host trees additionally must take place. This conclusion is supported by previous biochemical studies (e.g. Escher *et al.* 2004). *V. album* carries out photosynthesis by itself but is supplied by its host trees not only with water and minerals, but above all with products of their photosynthesis. This may have been underestimated in the past. The interaction between *V. album* and its host trees definitely deserves further attention.

Conflict of interest

We hereby confirm that there are no known conflicts of interest associated with this publication and there has been no significant financial support for this work that could have influenced its outcome.

References

Escher P, Eiblmeier M, Hetzger I, Rennenberg H: Seasonal and spatial variation of carbohydrates in mistletoes (Viscum album) and the xylem sap of its hosts (Populus x euamericana and Abies alba). Physiol Plant. 2004; 120 (2): 212–219. doi: 10.1111/j.0031-9317.2004.0230.x.

Maclean AE, Hertle AP, Ligas J, Bock R, Balk J, Meyer EH: Absence of Complex I Is Associated with Diminished Respiratory Chain Function in European Mistletoe. Curr Biol. 2018; 28 (10): 1614–1619.e3. doi: 10.1016/j.cub.2018.03.036.

Klusch N, Senkler J, Yildiz Ö, Kühlbrandt W, Braun HP: A ferredoxin bridge connects the two arms of plant mitochondrial complex I. Plant Cell. 2021; 33 (6): 2072–2091. doi: 10.1093/plcell/koab092.

Petersen G, Cuenca A, Seberg O: Plastome Evolution in Hemiparasitic Mistletoes. Genome Biol Evol. 2015; 7 (9): 2520–2532. doi: 10.1093/gbe/evv165.

Schröder L, Senkler J, Braun HP: Special features of cellular respiration in Viscum album. In: Scheer R, Alban S, Becker H et al. (Hrsg.): Die Mistel in der Tumortherapie 5. Essen: KVC; 2020: 3–13.

Schröder L, Hohnjec N, Senkler M, Senkler J, Küster H, Braun HP: The gene space of European mistletoe (Viscum album). Plant J. 2022a; 109 (1): 278–294. doi: 10.1111/tpj.15558

Schröder L, Hegermann J, Pille P, Braun HP: The photosynthesis apparatus of European mistletoe (Viscum album). Plant Physiol. 2022b; 190: 1896–1914. doi: 10.1093/plphys/kiac377

Schröder L, Rupp O, Senkler M, Rugen N, Hohnjec N, Goesmann A, Küster H, Braun HP: The Viscum album Gene Space database. Front Plant Sci. 2023; 14:1193122. doi: 10.3389/fpls.2023.1193122

Senkler J, Rugen N, Eubel H, Hegermann J, Braun HP: Absence of Complex I Implicates Rearrangement of the Respiratory Chain in European Mistletoe. Curr Biol. 2018; 28 (10): 1606–1613.e4. doi: 10.1016/j.cub.2018.03.050

Tubeuf K: Monographie der Mistel. R. Oldenbourg Verlag, München/Berlin; 1923.

Tuquet C, Sallé G: Characteristics of chloroplasts isolated from two mistletoes originating from temperate (Viscum album) and tropical (Tapinanthus dodoneifolius) areas. Plant Physiol Biochem. 1996; 34: 283–292.

Urech K, Jäggy C, Schaller G, Baumgartner S: Giftsubstanzbildung und Wachstumsdynamik der Mistel (Viscum album L.) im Jahreslauf. Mistilteinn 2004; 5: 20-35. https://www.vfk.ch/informationen/broschueren/mistilteinn/

Zonneveld BJM: New record holders for maximum genome size in eudicots and monocots. Journal of Botany 2010: 1-4. doi: 10.1155/2010/527357

Dr. Lucie Schröder, Dr. Jennifer Senkler, Prof. Dr. Hans-Peter Braun
Institute of Plant Genetics, Leibniz Universität Hannover
Herrenhäuser Str. 2, 30419 Hannover, Germany

Corresponding author:
braun@genetik.uni-hannover.de

Microscopic Characterization of European Mistletoe (*Viscum album* L. subspecies *album*)

Valter Paes de Almeida, Irailson Thierry Monchak, João Vitor da Costa Batista, Mirio Grazi, Hartmut Ramm, Vijayasankar Raman, Stephan Baumgartner, Carla Holandino, Jane Manfron

This contribution is a summary of Almeida VP de *et al.*: Investigations on the morpho-anatomy and histochemistry of the European mistletoe: *Viscum album* L. subsp. *album*. Scientific Reports. 2023; 13: 4604. https://www.nature.com/articles/s41598-023-29799-z

Summary
Viscum album L. (*Santalaceae*) is an important medicinal plant commonly used to treat cancer and various other ailments. As hemi-parasite it is growing on the branches of several host trees and shrubs. This work illustrates the anatomical and histochemical features of the leaves, stems, berries, and seeds of *V. album* subsp. *album* (*Santalaceae)* growing on the branches of *Malus domestica* (Suckow) Borkh. (*Rosaceae*). The leaves are isobilateral, amphistomatic with paracytic stomata, and showed straight anticlinal epidermal cell walls, and thick cuticles with epicuticular wax crystalloids. The midrib is flat on both sides and has a single vascular bundle, whereas the petiole is concave-convex in shape and contains five bundles. The stems show a ring of nine vascular bundles enclosing the pith. Four morphotypes of calcium oxalate crystals were observed in different plant parts. The results of this study provide new microscopy information that can help in the authentication of mistletoe plant materials.
Keywords: Anatomy, energy dispersive X-ray spectroscopy, light microscopy, scanning electron microscopy

Introduction

The genus *Viscum* (*Santalaceae*) comprises about 111 species (POWO 2024). *Viscum* species, popularly called "mistletoes", are shrubby hemiparasites growing on the aerial parts of host trees and shrubs (Iscador-AG 2024). *Viscum album* grows on more than 450 different species of hosts through its three subspecies, *V. album* subsp. *album*, *V. album* subsp. *austriacum* (Wiesb.) Vollm., and *V. album* subsp. *abietis* (Wiesb.) Abrom., with distinct host preferences and, to some extent, specific geographic distribution (Barney *et al.* 1998).

Viscum album is an important medicinal plant. It was utilized in complementary oncological therapy in the early 1900s (Ramm 2015). Since then, many reports have been published describing its medicinal properties (Ostermann *et al.* 2020). Besides carcinosis, mistletoe is used to treat cardiovascular diseases, epilepsy, infertility, menstruation problems, spleen diseases and ulcers (Peñaloza *et al.* 2020). The plant is reported to contain several pharmacologically active compounds, such as amino acids, flavonoids, phenolic acids, polysaccharides, terpenoids, viscotoxins and mistletoe lectins (Melo *et al.* 2022).

Viscum album subsp. *album* is commonly known as "European mistletoe"(Iscador-AG 2024). Since there is only limited information on the anatomy, micromorphology or histochemistry of *Viscum album* subsp. *album* growing on *Malus domestica* (Suckow) Borkh. available so far, the present study aimed to fill this gap and provide pharmacognostic data for authentication and quality control of mistletoe plant materials.

Material and methods

Plant specimens were collected in Switzerland (Rütti, Himmelried) and deposited (C.H. Quaresma 18.332) in the Herbarium of the Universidade Estadual do Rio de Janeiro, Brazil. The methods used in this study are extensively described in a previous publication by Almeida *et al.* (2023).

Results and discussion

The leaves, on surface view, evidenced straight and thin anticlinal cell walls on both adaxial and abaxial epidermises (Fig. 1a, d), covered externally by thick cuticle (Fig. 1e). Paracytic stomata (Fig. 1a, d) and epicuticular wax crystalloids (Fig. 1f) were observed on both sides. These features are common in *Viscum* species (Andronache *et al.* 2006; Khan *et al.* 2009; Mehrvarz *et al.* 2012), however, anomocytic stomata were found in *V. album* subsp. *austriacum* (Elkiran 2022). Thus, the stomata type can be used as an anatomical marker to distinguish between subspecies.

In cross-section (CS), the leaf epidermis was unilayered with cutinized external cell walls on both sides (Fig. 1e, i). The mesophyll was undifferentiated and comprised polygonal cells (Fig. 1g, h). However, dorsiventral mesophyll was found in *V. album* subsp. *album* collected from a host plant *Tilia cordata* Mill. (Andronache *et al.* 2006) and *V. album* subsp. *austriacum* growing on *Pinus* sp. (Elkiran 2022). The mesophyll cells contained several starch grains (Fig. 1i, k), as reported in various species and subspecies of *Viscum* (Elkiran 2022). The midrib was flat on both sides (Fig. 1g) and contained a central collateral vascular bundle (Fig. 1g). Fibers were found abutting the xylem and phloem (Fig. 1g, j). Bicollateral vascular bundles were found in *V. album* and *V. cruciatum* Sieber ex Boiss. in a study by Khan *et al.* (2009).

The petiole, in CS, had a concave-convex shape with two wings on adaxial side (Fig. 2a). The epidermal cells were covered by a thick cuticle (Fig. 2b). The vascular system was collateral and represented by five bundles organized in an open arc (Fig. 2a). A cap of perivascular fiber adjoined the xylem and phloem (Fig. 2c).

The stem was circular in CS (Fig. 2d) with an unilayered epidermis (Fig. 2g). The external wall was thick and fully cutinized (Fig. 2g), and papillate (Fig. 2e, g). The cortex was wide and collenchymatous (Fig. 2e). The vascular system showed nine bundles forming a ring delimiting the pith (Fig. 2d). One cap of perivascular fibers was attached to the xylem and another to the phloem (Fig. 2d–f, i). Cortical, vascular and medullary parenchyma are filled with starch grains (Fig. 2g–i).

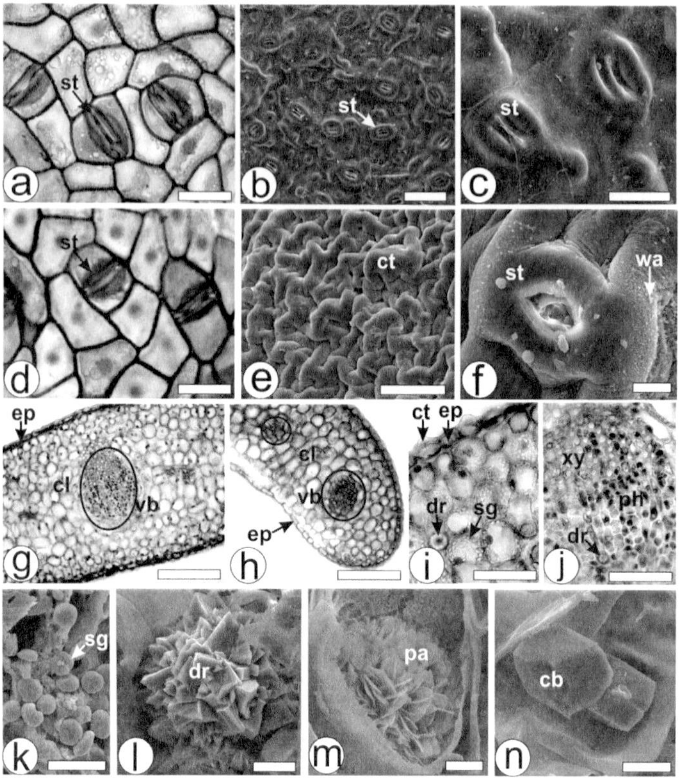

Fig. 1: Anatomy of the leaves of *Viscum album* subsp. *album*: (a, d, g–j) light microscopy and others SEM. (a–f) Leaf in surface view; (a–c) adaxial and (d–f) abaxial side; (g–n) transverse sections. Cb cubic-shaped crystal, cl chlorenchyma, ct cuticle, dr druse, ep epidermis, ph phloem, pa platy aggregation cluster crystal, sg starch grain, st stomata, vb vascular bundle, wa epicuticular wax, xy xylem.

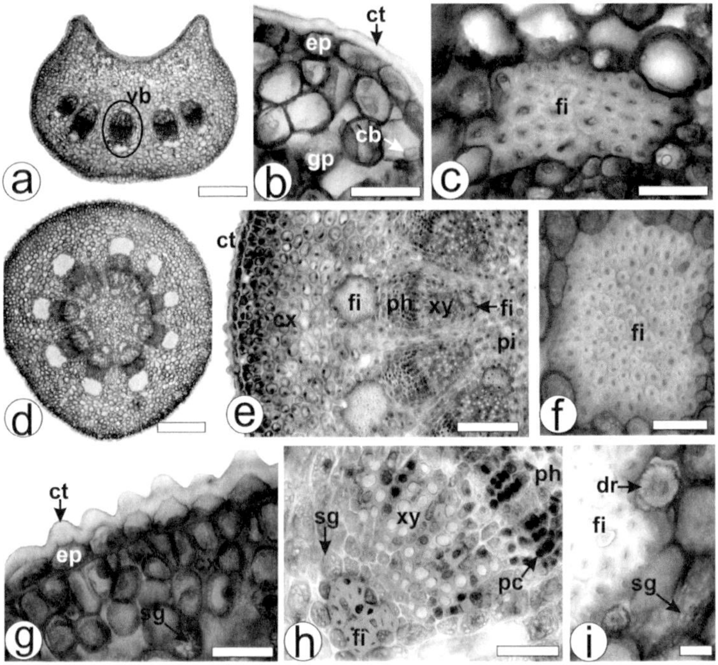

Fig. 2: Petiole (a–c) and stem (d–i) anatomy of *Viscum album* subsp. *album* in CS: (a–i) light microscopy. cb cubic-shaped crystal, ct cuticle, cx cortex, dr druse, ep epidermis, fi fiber, gp ground parenchyma, pc phenolic compounds, ph phloem, pi pith, pr quadrangular prismatic crystal, sg starch grain, vb vascular bundle, xy xylem.

The berries, in CS, presented the exocarp formed by an unilayered epidermis covered by a smooth cuticle and 3–4 layers of angular collenchyma (Fig. 3a, b). In the medial region, small collateral vascular bundles were present (Fig. 3a). The mesocarp contained an outer fleshy layer and an inner viscin tissue (Fig. 3a, c), which composed of strongly vacuolated globular cells (Fig. 3c–e) and highly viscous, sticky, and extensible, long cells with spirally thickened walls located towards the endocarp (Fig. 3f). These cells contained a few starch grains.

The seed, in CS, showed an unilayered epidermis containing starch grains and covered externally by a cuticle (Fig. 3h). The endosperm cells were large, parenchymatous and contained chlorophyll and large amounts of starch grains (Fig. 3g–i). The seed usually had two embryos, each with two cotyledons and a hypocotyl (Fig. 3i). The number of embryos per berry varies in *Viscum album* (Ramm *et al.* 2004).

Different morphotypes of crystals, such as druses, quadrangular prismatic crystals, cubic-shaped crystals and platty aggregation cluster crystals, were found in almost all organs of *V. album* subsp. *album* (Fig. 1i, j, l–n). The presence of crystals was commonly reported in *Viscum* (Andronache *et al.* 2006; Khan *et al.* 2009). In the present study, the EDS spectra of druses exhibited prominent peaks for calcium (Ca), carbon (C), and oxygen (O) showing that these were made of calcium oxalate. Magnesium (Mg), phosphorous (P), and potassium (K) were also found in minor concentrations. This is the first study of the elemental chemical composition of crystals of *Viscum* species using EDS.

The microchemical tests detected lipophilic compounds in the cuticles of all organs analyzed (Fig. 4a–e). In addition, oil bodies were found in the leaf epidermis and mesophyll (Fig. 4a), epidermis and ground parenchyma of the petiole (Fig. 4b), various tissues of the stem (Fig. 4c), and exocarp cells of the berry (Fig. 4d). Oil bodies stained in red with Nile blue, indicating that the bodies contained neutral fats (Fig. 4f). Phenolic compounds were found in the vascular bundles of the leaves (Fig. 4g, h) and stems (Fig. 4j), and cortex of the stems (Fig. 4i).

Polysaccharides were detected in the epidermis, mesophyll and midrib ground parenchyma (Fig. 4m) of the leaf, phloem and pith of the stem (Fig. 4n), exocarp and mesocarp of the berry, and all the cell walls of the seed. Starch grains were found in epidermis and mesophyll of the lamina (Fig. 4o) and ground parenchyma of the midrib, spread in the cortex, medullary rays and pith of the stem (Fig. 4p), in mesocarp of berry (Fig. 4q) and endosperm of seed (Fig. 4r). Proteins were evidenced in the proteins corpuscles presents in the leaves (Fig. 4s), stems (Fig. 4t), berries (Fig. 4u,w), and especially in the endosperm of the seeds (Fig. 4v, x). No histochemical tests were previously reported for *V. album* subsp. *album*.

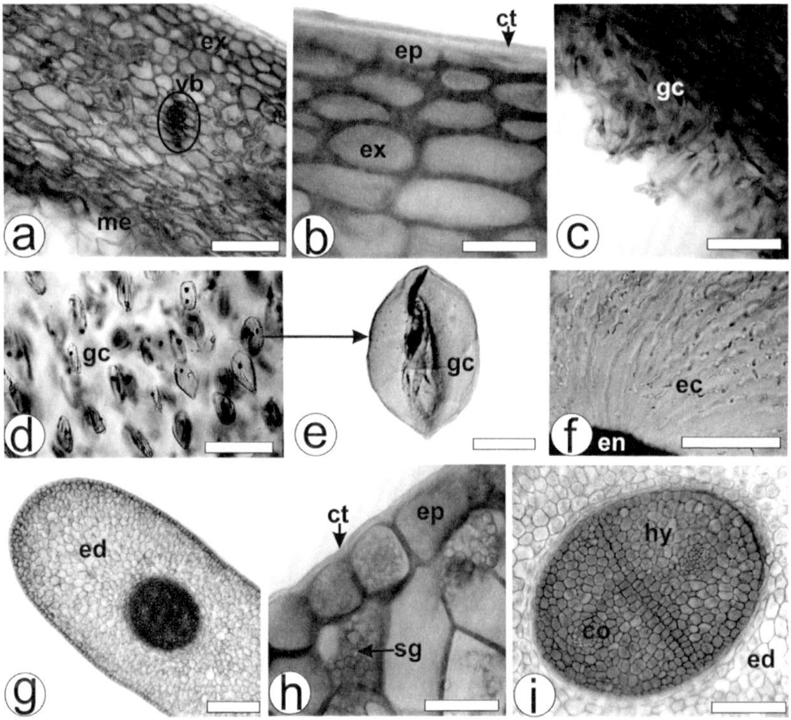

Fig. 3: Fruit (a–f) and seed (g–l) anatomy of *Viscum album* subsp. *album* in CS. ct cuticle, co cotyledon, ec elongated cells with spiral thickening, ep epidermis, ed endosperm, en endocarp, ex exocarp, gc globular cells, hy hypocotyl, me mesocarp, sg starch grain, vb vascular bundle.

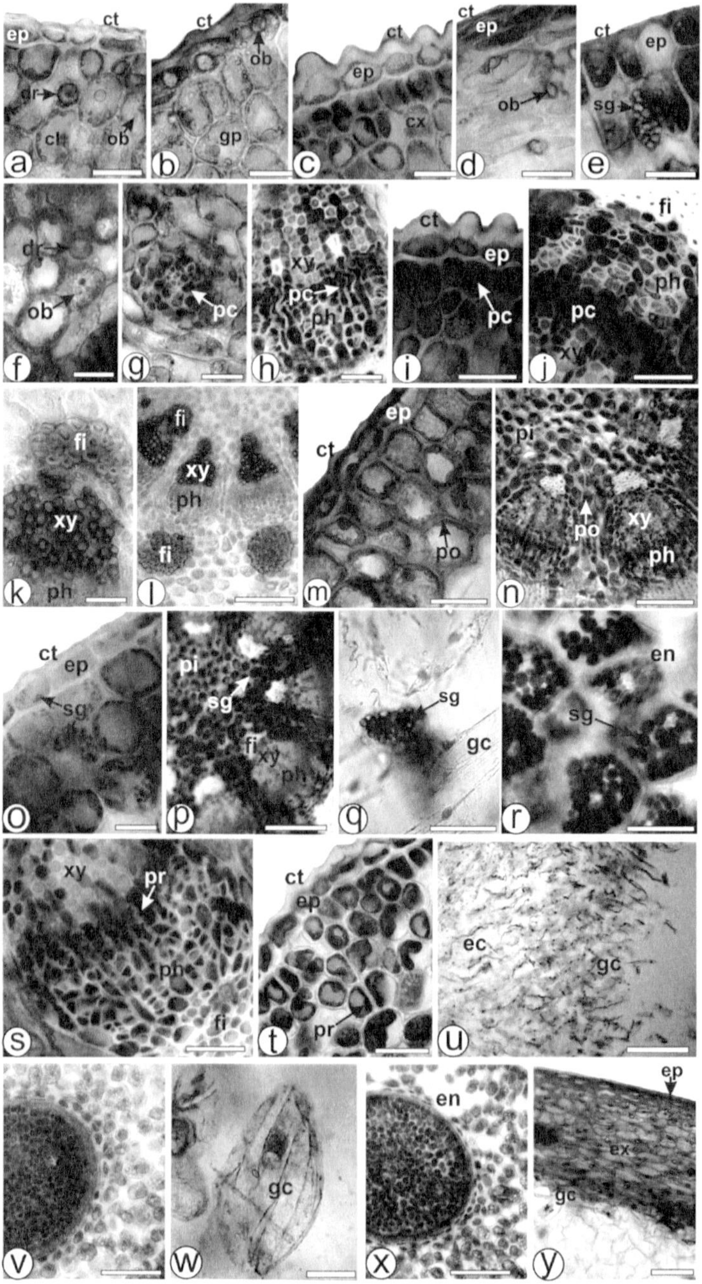
a ep ct dr cl ob
b ct ob gp
c ct ep cx
d ct ep ob
e ct ep sg
f dr ob
g pc
h xy pc ph
i ct ep pc
j fi ph pc xy
k fi xy ph
l fi xy ph fi
m ep ct po
n pi po xy ph
o ct ep sg
p pi sg fi xy ph
q sg gc
r en sg
s xy pr ph fi
t ct ep pr
u ec gc
v
w gc
x en
y ep ex gc

Fig. 4 (p. 52)**:** Microchemical tests of *Viscum album* subsp. *album*. (a, g, o) Lamina, (f, m, k, s) Midrib, (b, h) Petiole, (c, i, j, l, n, p, t) Stem, (d, q, u, w, y) Berry, (e, r, v, x) Seed. Reagents: (a–e) Sudan III. (f) Nile blue. (g, h) Potassium dichromate. (i, j) Ferric chloride. (k, l) Phloroglucinol/HCl. (m, n) PAS (periodic acid-Schiff reagent). (o–r) Iodine solution. (s–v) Xylidine Ponceau. (w, x) Coomassie Brilliant blue. (y) Ruthenium red. cl chlorenchyma, ct cuticle, cx cortex, dr druses, ec palisade-like elongated cells with spirally thickened walls, en endosperm, ep epidermis, ex exocarp, fi fibers, gc globular cells, gp ground parenchyma, hy hypocotyl, ob oil bodies, pc phenolic compounds, ph phloem, pi pith, po neutral polysaccharides, pr protein, sg starch grain, xy xylem.

Conclusion

This study provides valuable information on the anatomical and microchemical characteristics of *Viscum album* subsp. *album*. The anatomy features of the leaf, stem, berry, and seed are significant, and this study reveals several attributes of taxonomic importance at the genus and species levels. The present study will also provide a basis for future studies involving other taxa in the family for a better understanding of the morpho-anatomy, interaction with host plants, and phylogeny of this interesting group of hemi-parasitic plants.

Acknowledgements

We acknowledge the C-Labmu Center at the State University of Ponta Grossa forSEM/EDS facilities. This study was funded by Coordenação de Aperfeiçoamento de Pessoal de Nível Superior of Brasil (CAPES; Finance Code 001; 88887.569108/2020-00) and Fundação de Amparo à Pesquisa do Estado do Rio de Janeiro (FAPERJ; BPP 201.004/2022).

Conflict of interests

The authors declare no conflicts of interest.

References

Almeida VP, Monchak IT, Batista JVC et al.: Investigations on the morpho-anatomy and histochemistry of the European mistletoe: Viscum album L. subsp. album. Sci Rep. 2023; 13: 4604.

Andronache A, Toma I, Toma C: The structure of vegetative organs in Viscum album and Loranthus europaeus. Analele Stiinţ ale Univ. 2006; 2: 13-18.

Barney CW, Hawksworth FG, Geils BW: Hosts of Viscum album. Eur J For Pathol. 1998; 8: 187–208.

Elkiran O: Comparative anatomical study of Viscum album L. subsp. album and Viscum album subsp. austriacum (Wiesb.) Vollman. Ejons Int J Math Eng Nat Sci. 2022; 21: 12–17.

Iscador AG: Die Welt der Iscador AG https://iscador.com/download/die-welt-der-iscador-ag/ (accessed: 18.01.2024).

Khan MA, Sharif T, Ahmad M et al.: Anatomical characterization of parasitic plants of Pakistan. Pak J Bot. 2009; 41: 2661–2669.

Mehrvarz SS, Shavvon RS, Golmohammadi N: Notes on the genus Viscum (Viscaceae) in Iran: A new combination based on morphological evidence. Afr J Agric Res. 2012; 7: 1694–1702.

Melo MNO, Ochioni AC, Zancan P et al.: Viscum album mother tinctures: Harvest conditions and host trees influence the plant metabolome and the glycolytic pathway of breast cancer cells. Front Pharmacol. 2022; 13: 1027931.

Ostermann T, Appelbaum S, Poier D et al.: A systematic review and meta-analysis on the survival of cancer patients treated with a fermented Viscum album L. extract (Iscador): An update of findings. Complement Med Res. 2020; 27 (4): 260–271.

Peñaloza E, Holandino C, Scherr C et al.: Comprehensive metabolome analysis of fermented aqueous extracts of Viscum album L. by liquid chromatography–high resolution tandem mass spectrometry. Molecules. 2020; 25 (17): 4006–4020.

POWO: Plants of The World Online https://powo.science.kew.org/taxon/urn:lsid:ipni.org:names:30000304-2 (Accessed 18.01.2024).

Ramm H: Mistletoe through cultural and medical history: The all-healing proves to be a cancer-specific remedy. In: Zanker KS, Kaveri SV (Ed.): Mistletoe: From Mythology to Evidence-Based Medicine. Transl Res Biomed. 2015: 1–10.

Ramm H, Urech K, Scheibler M, Grazi G: Cultivation and development of Viscum album L. In: Büssing A (Ed.): Mistletoe: The Genus Viscum. Taylor & Francis. 2004: 75–94.

Valter Paes de Almeida[1], Irailson Thierry Monchak[1], João Vitor da Costa Batista[2], Mirio Grazi[2], Dr. Hartmut Ramm[2], Vijayasankar Raman[3], Prof. Dr. Stephan Baumgartner[2,4], Prof. Dr. Carla Holandino[2,5], Prof. Dr. Jane Manfron[1]

[1] Universidade de Ponta Grossa, 84017-220, Paraná, Brazil

[2] Society for Cancer Research, Hiscia Institute, 4144 Arlesheim, Switzerland

[3] National Identification Services, USDA-APHIS-PPQ, Beltsville, MD 20705, USA

[4] Institute of Complementary and Integrative Medicine, University of Bern, 3010 Bern, Switzerland

[5] Laboratório Multidisciplinar de Ciências Farmacêuticas, Faculdade de Farmácia, Universidade Federal do Rio de Janeiro, 21941-902 Rio de Janeiro, Brazil)

Corresponding authors:

janemanfron@hotmail.com

st.baumgartner@vfk.ch

cholandino@gmail.com

In welchen Phasen ihrer Entwicklung bildet *Viscum album* L. Statolithenstärke?

In Which Phases of its Development Does *Viscum album* L. Form Statolithic Starch?

Angelika Heinze, Anton Berg, Gero Leneweit

Zusammenfassung
Die Weißbeerige Mistel, *Viscum album* L., hat 3 verschiedene Wachstumsphasen, in denen sie aufrecht wächst, also der Erdenschwere entgegengesetzt: als ganze Pflanze in ihrer Jugendphase, nach der Blühreife mit den neuen einjährigen Trieben vor deren Einordung in den Kugelbusch und mit den Hypokotylen während der Keimung, wenn durch negativ heliotropes Wachstum keine feste Unterlage erreicht werden konnte.
Anfang des letzten Jahrhunderts wurde gezeigt, dass es sich bei dem aufrechten Wachstum von Hypokotylen um negativ gravitropes Wachstum handelt. Zum Vorkommen von Statolithenstärke, die als Grundlage gravitropen Pflanzenwachstums gilt, wurde andererseits berichtet, dass der Mistel Statolithenstärke fehlt.
Wir haben in aufrecht wachsenden Mistelhypokotylen Stärkekörnchen nachgewiesen, die wir aufgrund mehrerer Merkmale für Statolithenstärke halten. Der Nachweis, dass es sich tatsächlich um Statolithen handelt, soll in weiteren Versuchen erbracht werden. Auch in den anderen Phasen aufrechten Wachstums der Mistel soll das Vorkommen von Statolithenstärke untersucht werden.
Schlüsselwörter: *Viscum album* L., Weißbeerige Mistel, Statolithenstärke, Gravitropismus

Summary
The European mistletoe, *Viscum album* L., has 3 different growth phases in which it grows upright, i.e. opposite to the earth's gravity: 1. as a whole plant in its juvenile phase, 2. with the new shoots before they are arranged in the spherical bush after a phase of nutation movements and 3. with the hypocotyls during germination, when no solid base could be reached by negative heliotropic growth.

At the beginning of the last century, it was shown that the upright growth of hypocotyls is negative gravitropic. The occurrence of statolithic starch is regarded as the basis of gravitropic plant growth. On the other hand, it was reported that mistletoe lacks statolithic starch.
We have detected starch granules in upright growing mistletoe hypocotyls, which we believe to be statolithic starch based on several characteristics. Further experiments will be carried out to prove that these are indeed statoliths. The occurrence of statolithic starch in the other phases of upright mistletoe growth will also be investigated.
Keywords: *Viscum album* L., European mistletoe, statolithic starch, gravitropism

Einleitung

Die charakteristische Wuchsform von *Viscum album* L., der Weißbeerigen Mistel, ist ihr Kugelbusch. Er zeichnet sich dadurch aus, dass – ausgehend von dem Ansatzpunkt der Mistel am Wirtsbaum – die Zweige radiär in alle Richtungen wachsen.

In der Jugendphase wächst die Mistel noch pflanzentypisch aufrecht. Die Ausbildung des Kugelbusches beginnt erst, wenn sie nach ca. 3-4 Jahren blühreif ist. Auch dann wachsen alle neuen Triebe, die nun nach nur einem Internodium mit 2 Laubblättern in einem terminalen Blütenstand enden, zunächst noch aufrecht. Nach einer Phase von Nutationsbewegungen nehmen sie solche Positionen ein, die nicht mehr entgegen der Schwerkraftrichtung orientiert sind, sondern sich auf die Ansatzstelle am Baum als eigenen Mittelpunkt beziehen (Göbel, Dorka 1986). Das wiederholt sich Jahr für Jahr und führt schließlich zu dem mistelspezifischen Kugelbusch.

Außer bei der jungen Mistel und beim jährlichen Zuwachs der blühreifen Mistel kann eine weitere Phase aufrechten Wachstums während der Keimung auftreten. In der Regel gelangen die Samen der Mistel auf die Oberseite der Wirtsbaumzweige und die austreibenden Hypokotyle erreichen durch negativ heliotropes Wachstum auf kürzestem Weg die Baumrinde (Abb. 1). Wenn das austreibende Hypokotyl durch diesen

Wachstumsmodus keinen Anschluss an eine feste Unterlage findet, ändert es seine Wachstumsrichtung und wächst aufrecht. Wenn auch das nicht zu einem Kontakt führt, folgen freie „Suchbewegungen". Diese Zusammenhänge hat Tubeuf untersucht und unter anderem nachgewiesen, indem er keimende Mistelsamen unter Lichtausschluss anzog (Abb. 2), dass es sich bei dem aufrechten Wachstum während der Keimung um negativ gravitropes Wachstum handelt (Tubeuf 1923).

Allerdings macht Tubeuf (1923) keine Angaben zum Vorkommen von Statolithenstärke, die seit der von Haberlandt und Němec unabhängig voneinander aufgestellten Statolithentheorie des Gravitropismus (damals Geotropismus genannt) als Voraussetzung gravitropen Wachstums gilt (Haberlandt 1900; Němec 1900). Haberlandt selbst berichtet später, dass die Mistel nicht oder nur kaum merklich negativ gravitrop ist, dass die in jungen, noch wachsenden Trieben der Mistel auftretenden kleinen Stärkekörner nicht der Erdenschwere unterliegen und eine Stärkescheide mit beweglichen Stärkekörnern nicht vorhanden ist (Haberlandt 1903).

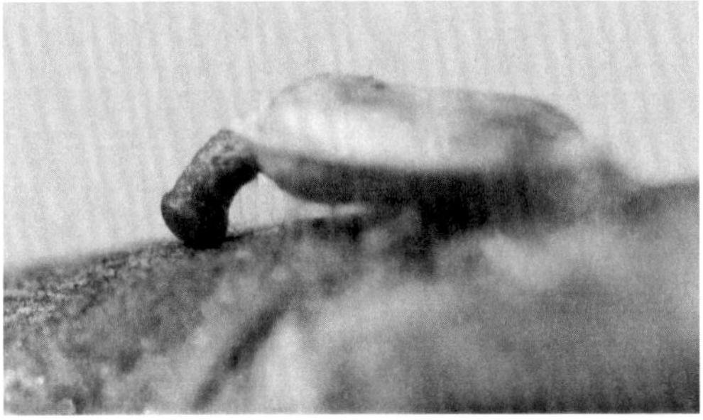

Abb. 1: Mistelsame mit auskeimendem Hypokotyl, das die Rinde des Wirtsbaumes erreicht hat

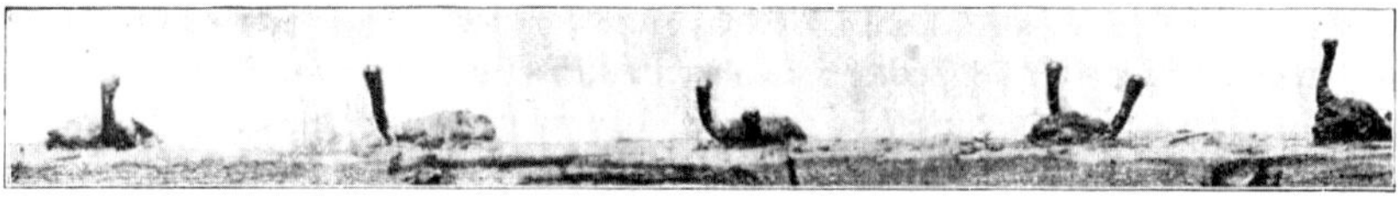

Abb. 2: Aufrechtes Wachstum von Mistelhypokotylen nach 7,5 Wochen im Licht-Dunkel-Wechsel und anschließender 12-wöchiger Verdunkelung (aus Tubeuf 1923)

Zur Charakterisierung der Mistel spricht auch Steiner mehrmals darüber, dass die Mistel keine Statolithenstärke ausbildet. Zum Beispiel sagt er 1910, dass „die Mistel nicht jene eigentümlichen Stärkezellen hat, welche die Pflanzen dahin bringen, nach dem Mittelpunkt der Erde zu zeigen“ (Steiner 1983). Er bezieht sich dabei sehr wahrscheinlich auf Haberlandt (1903), den er im selben Vortrag namentlich erwähnt. Und auch noch 1913 schreibt Jost in der 3. Auflage seiner „Vorlesungen über Pflanzenphysiologie“, dass der Mistel Statolithenstärke fehlt (Jost 1913). Diese Aussagen stehen im Widerspruch zu den beobachtbaren Phasen aufrechten Wachstums, insbesondere zu Tubeufs (1923) Dunkelversuchen mit Mistelkeimlingen.

Da bis heute unseres Wissens nicht untersucht wurde, ob die Mistel während der genannten Phasen Statolithenstärke aufweist, wollen wir dieser Frage nachgehen.

Versuchsdurchführung

Am 04.04.2023 wurden Beeren von der Mistel eines Apfelbaums geerntet. 40 Mistelsamen wurden am selben Tag aus der Beerenhaut befreit und einzeln auf Trägern befestigt. Um zu verhindern, dass die Hypokotyle in der heliotropen Anfangsphase der Keimung rasch eine feste Unterlage erreichen können, wurden die Samen so angebracht, dass die Austrittsstellen ihrer meist 2 Hypokotyle aus dem Endosperm nach oben gerichtet waren (Abb. 3). Der aushärtende, misteleigene Leim fixierte die Samen in dieser Position.

Die Mistelsamen wurden zunächst für 10 Tage in einem kühlen Raum ohne künstliche Beleuchtung unter einem Fenster aufgestellt. Am 14.04.2023 kamen sie dann in einem seitlich offenen Glasgefäß an einen hellen, vor direkter Sonneneinstrahlung geschützten Standort ins Freiland. Sie blieben so lange dem natürlichen Licht-Dunkel-Wechsel ausgesetzt, bis die Hypokotyle deutlich sichtbar zur Seite gewachsen waren und eine mehr oder weniger waagerechte Position erreicht hatten (Abb. 4). Danach, am 29.04.2023, wurden sie verdunkelt und waren nur zum Fotografieren und zur Protokollierung des Wachstums kurzzeitig dem Tageslicht ausgesetzt. Zum Vergleich wurden 10 Proben im Licht-Dunkel-Wechsel belassen.

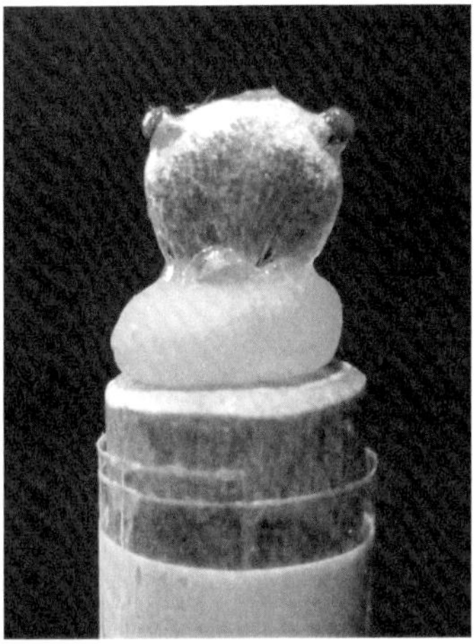

Abb. 3: Probe H24 am 12.04.2023, nach 8 Tagen unter Glas bei natürlichem Licht-Dunkel-Wechsel. Die keimenden Hypokotyle sind aus dem Nährgewebe des Samens herausgewachsen.
⌀ der hölzernen Träger: 0,8 cm

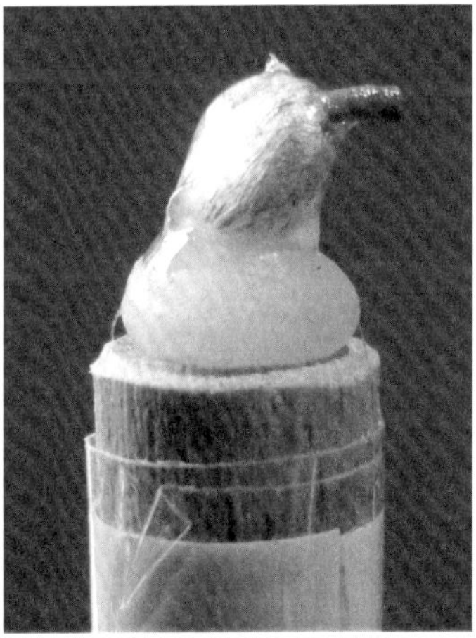

Abb. 4: Probe H24 am 29.04.2023, nach 17 Tagen im Freiland bei natürlichem Licht-Dunkel-Wechsel. Die Hypokotyle haben eine waagerechte Position erreicht.

Nachdem die Hypokotyle im Dunkeln ihre Wachstumsrichtung geändert hatten und aufrecht wuchsen (Abb. 5), wurden sie am 24.05.2023 an ihrer Austrittsstelle aus dem Endosperm mit einem Skalpell abgeschnitten und sofort zur Fixierung in AFE (Äthanol, Formaldehyd, Essigsäure) überführt.

Nach Einbettung in Paraffin wurden von den Hypokotylen 10 µm dünne, radiale Längsschnitte angefertigt und zum Stärkenachweis mit Lugolscher Lösung angefärbt.

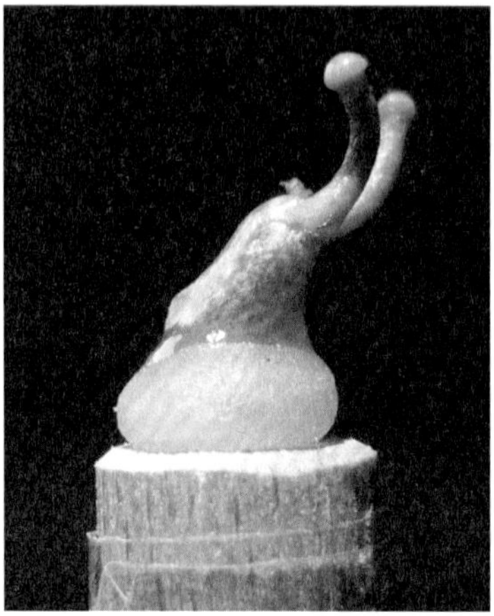

Abb. 5: Probe H24 am 24.05.2024, nach 25 Tagen im Dauerdunkel. Die Hypokotyle haben ihre Wachstumsrichtung geändert und wachsen aufrecht. Nach dem Fotografieren wurden sie abgenommen und sofort fixiert.

Ergebnisse

Im natürlichen Licht-Dunkel-Wechsel wuchsen die austreibenden Hypokotyle weder senkrecht nach oben noch ihrer Lage und der Austrittsstelle aus dem Endosperm entsprechend schräg aufwärts weiter, sondern krümmten sich zur Seite. Nach der in waagerechter Position der Hypokotyle erfolgten Verdunkelung änderte sich die Wachstumsrichtung. Die Hypokotyle richteten sich auf und wuchsen nach oben. Damit konnten die Ergebnisse von Tubeufs (1923) Dunkelversuch bestätigt werden.

Lichtmikroskopisch wurden in allen untersuchten Proben kugelige Stärkekörnchen von ca. 4–7 µm Durchmesser nachgewiesen. Der Schnitt durch das gesamte Hypokotyl zeigt, dass fast über die ganze Länge – zur Basis, dem endospermnahen, ältesten Teil des Hypokotyls zunehmend – solche kleinen Stärkekörnchen zu finden sind (Abb. 6). Innerhalb der Zellen liegen die Stärkekörnchen überwiegend auf derjenigen Seite, die an dem sich im Dunkeln aufgerichteten Hypokotyl nach unten orientiert war (Abb. 7 und 8).

Die im meristematischen, jüngsten Bereich an der Spitze des Hypokotyls zu sehenden großen Strukturen (Abb. 9) haben wir zunächst für Zellkerne gehalten. Ob es sich dabei eventuell ebenfalls um Stärke handelt, konnte derzeit noch nicht geklärt werden.

Fazit

Wir gehen davon aus, dass sich die keimende Mistel im Dunkeln an der Schwerkraft orientiert. Für negativ gravitropes Wachstum spricht, dass die Hypokotyle ihre Wuchsrichtung änderten und aus einer waagerechten Position zu aufrechtem Wachstum übergingen, nachdem durch die Verdunkelung der Keimlinge eine Orientierung am Licht ausgeschlossen war.

Weiterhin nehmen wir aufgrund der Größe, der Anzahl, der Verteilung im Hypokotyl und der Lage in den Zellen an, dass es sich bei den nachgewiesenen Stärkekörnchen um Statolithenstärke handelt.

Zukünftige Untersuchungen haben zum Ziel, diese Annahmen zu verifizieren und nachzuweisen, dass das aufrechte Wachstum des Mistelhypokotyls auf einer Schwerkraftwahrnehmung mittels Statolithenstärke beruht. Dazu sollen im Dunkeln aufrecht gewachsene Hypokotyle in eine andere Position gebracht werden – z. B. um 90 Grad gedreht –, um zu überprüfen, ob sich infolgedessen die Stärkekörner in Schwerkraftrichtung verlagern und ob eine entsprechende Änderung der Wachstumsrichtung eintritt. Außerdem soll geklärt werden, worum es sich bei den großen Strukturen in den Zellen des meristematischen Bereichs an der Spitze des Hypokotyls handelt.

Von Interesse sind auch die anderen Stadien der Keimung. Ist Statolithenstärke z. B. bereits in der heliotropen Wachstumsphase vorhanden und auch noch nach der Anheftung des Hypokotyls?

Die Untersuchungen sollen im Weiteren auf die beiden anderen Phasen aufrechten Wachstums ausgedehnt werden: auf die juvenile Mistel und auf verschiedene Stadien der einjährigen Triebe des Kugelbusches.

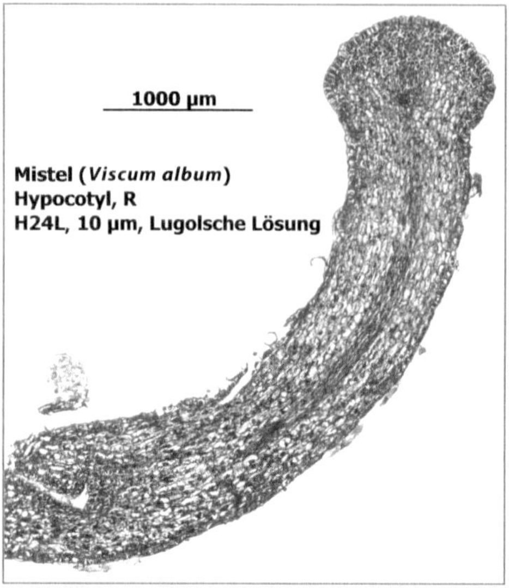

Abb. 6: Probe H24l, radialer Längsschnitt durch dasjenige Hypokotyl, das auf Abb. 3 links und auf Abb. 4 und 5 vorne zu sehen ist. Nach zunächst waagerechter Position im Licht-Dunkel-Wechsel war das Hypokotyl im Dauerdunkel aufrecht gewachsen.

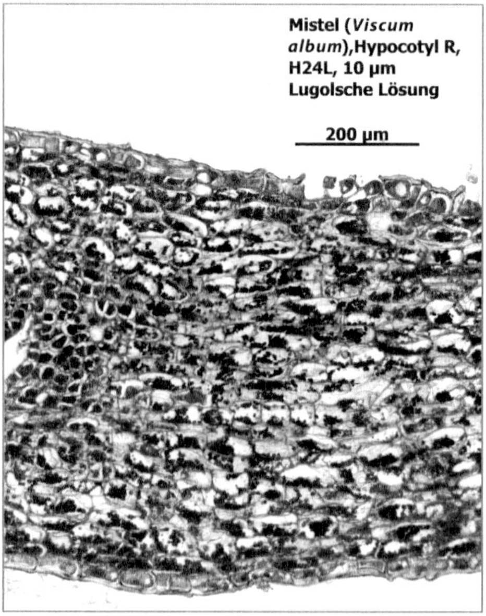

Abb. 7: Probe H24l, Ausschnitt aus dem unteren, gekrümmten Bereich des Hypokotyls

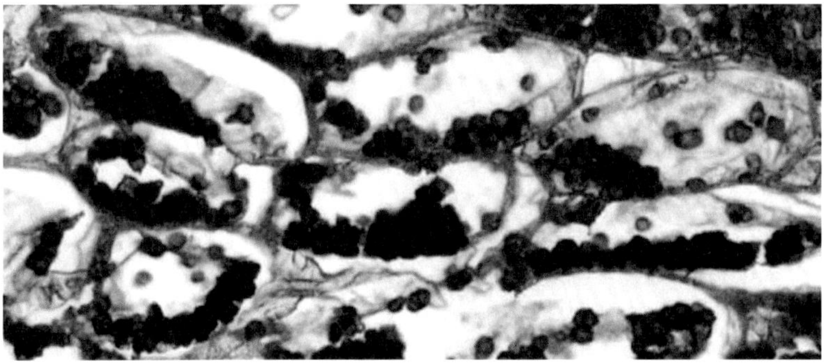

Abb. 8: Probe H24l, Detail aus Abb. 7, das die Ablagerung der Stärkekörnchen auf der Unterseite der Zellen zeigt

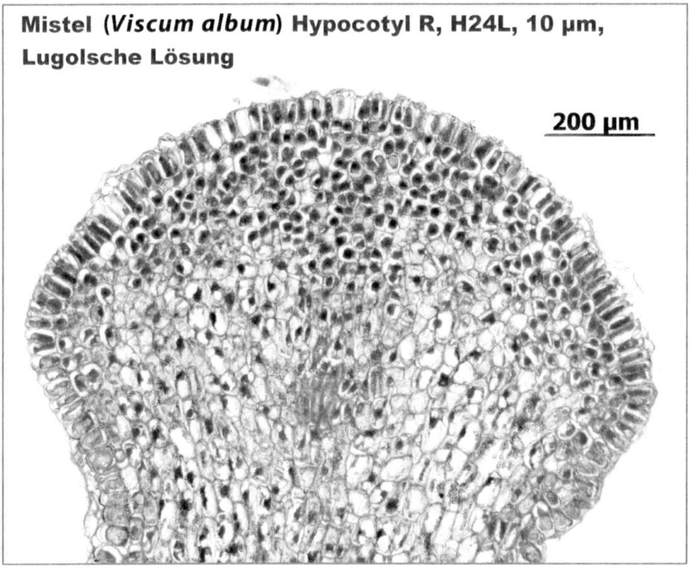

Abb. 9: Probe H24l, Wachstumszone an der Spitze des Hypokotyls

Interessenkonflikt

Die Autoren versichern, dass keine Interessenkonflikte bestehen.

Literatur

Göbel T, Dorka R: Zur Morphologie und Zeitgestalt der Mistel (Viscum album L.). Tycho de Brahe-Jahrbuch für Goetheanismus 1986. 1986; 167–193.

Haberlandt GJF: Zur Statolithentheorie des Geotropismus. Jahrbücher für wissenschaftliche Botanik. 1903; 38: 447–500

Haberlandt GJF: Ueber die Perception des geotropischen Reizes. Berichte der Deutschen Botanischen Gesellschaft. 1900; 18: 261–272.

Jost L: Vorlesungen über Pflanzenphysiologie. Jena: Fischer; 1913

Němec B: Ueber die Art der Wahrnehmung des Schwerkraftreizes bei den Pflanzen. Berichte der Deutschen Botanischen Gesellschaft. 1900; 18: 241–245

Steiner R: Der Geist im Pflanzenreich. In: GA 60, Vortrag vom 08.12.1910, Dornach, Rudolf Steiner Verlag; 1983: 157–185

Tubeuf K Freiherr von: Monographie der Mistel. München und Berlin: R. Oldenbourg; 1923

Angelika Heinze[1], PD Dr. Gero Leneweit[1], Anton Berg[2]

[1] Carl Gustav Carus-Institut, Niefern-Öschelbronn, Deutschland

[2] Mikroskopisches Kollegium Bonn, Deutschland

Korrespondenzadresse:

angelika.heinze@carus-institut.de

Liposomale Verkapselung von Mistelextrakten für die Therapie des Glioblastoms

Liposomal Encapsulation of Mistletoe Extracts for the Therapy of Glioblastoma

Josanna Kaufmann, Harden Rieger, Gero Leneweit

Zusammenfassung

Bei der Behandlung von Hirntumoren, insbesondere des *Glioblastoma multiforme*, sind Standardtherapien immer noch unzureichend. Die Blut-Hirn-Schranke (BHS) stellt bei der Entwicklung neuer Behandlungen eine schwer zu überwindende Barriere dar. Dies wird durch die infiltrative Natur des Tumors und durch die verstärkte Tendenz zur Ausbildung von Resistenzen gegen klassische Therapeutika weiter erschwert. Liposomen spielen bei der Entwicklung von Arzneimitteltransportsystemen eine zentrale Rolle, indem sie als multifunktionale Träger den Wirkstoff vor Degradation schützen und ihn zielgerichtet zum Wirkungsort transportieren. Verkapselte Arzneistoffe bieten den Vorteil einer höheren Wirksamkeit, einer Verringerung der toxischen Nebenwirkungen und einer längeren Zirkulationszeit im Blut. Wirkstoffe aus Mistelextrakten, insbesondere das zytotoxische und immunmodulatorische Mistellektin-1 (ML-1), wurden in Liposomen verkapselt, indem zunächst Nanoemulsionströpfchen in einer hydrophoben Phase hergestellt wurden, welche im Anschluss in Liposomen umgewandelt wurden. Das neuartige Arzneimitteltransportsystem wurde eingehend charakterisiert. Die Stabilität von ML-1 als Leitsubstanz der Mistelextrakte wurde während des Herstellungsprozesses evaluiert, um dessen antitumorale Aktivität nach der liposomalen Verkapselung zu gewährleisten. Die *in vitro* Zytotoxizität von liposomal verkapseltem ML-1 wurde auf Gliomzellen untersucht und mit freiem Wirkstoff verglichen, um dessen Anwendbarkeit als therapeutisches Wirkstofftransportsystem von Mistelextrakten zu bewerten.

Schlüsselwörter: Liposomen, Drug Delivery, Mistellektin, Wirkstoffstabilität, Einkapselung, Glioblastom, *in vitro* Zytotoxizität

Summary
Standard therapies are still inadequate for the treatment of brain tumours, especially *glioblastoma multiforme*. The blood-brain barrier (BBB) is a difficult obstacle to overcome in the development of new treatments against glioblastoma. This is further complicated by the infiltrative nature of the tumour and the increased tendency to develop resistance to classical therapeutics. Liposomes play a central role in the development of drug delivery systems by acting as multifunctional carriers that protect the active ingredient from degradation and transport it to the site of action in a targeted manner. Encapsulated drugs offer the advantage of greater efficacy, a reduction in toxic side effects and a longer circulation time in the blood. Active ingredients from mistletoe extracts, in particular the cytotoxic and immunomodulatory mistletoe lectin-1 (ML-1), were encapsulated in liposomes by first producing nanoemulsion droplets in a hydrophobic phase, which were then converted into liposomes. The novel drug delivery system was characterized in detail. The stability of ML-1 as the lead compound of mistletoe extracts was evaluated during the manufacturing process to ensure its antitumoural activity after liposomally encapsulation. The *in vitro* cytotoxicity of liposomal encapsulated ML-1 was studied on glioma cells and compared with free drug to evaluate its applicability as a therapeutic drug delivery system of mistletoe extracts.
Keywords: Liposomes, drug delivery, mistletoe lectin, drug stability, encapsulation, glioblastoma, *in vitro* cytotoxicity

Einleitung

Gliome sind die am häufigsten vorkommenden primären Hirntumoren mit einer durchschnittlichen jährlichen Inzidenz von sieben pro 100.000 Einwohnern, wobei circa die Hälfte der Fälle dem Glioblastom (*Glioblastoma multiforme*) zugeordnet werden kann (Schaff, Mellinghoff 2023). Seit 2005 haben sich die zwei-Jahres- und drei-Jahres-Überlebensraten auf 18 % bzw. 11 % verdoppelt, während die fünf-Jahres-Überlebensrate immer noch unter 5 % liegt (Poon *et al.* 2020). Durch die Tumorlokalisation ist sowohl die operative Entfernung als auch die systemische medikamentöse Zugänglichkeit aufgrund der Blut-Hirn-Schranke (BHS) stark eingeschränkt. Hinzu kommt die ausgeprägte Resistenzbildung gegen klassisch angewendete Therapeutika, wodurch sich die Krankheitsprognose weiter verschlechtert und die Notwendigkeit der Entwicklung effektiverer Therapien verdeutlicht wird. Innovative Arzneimitteltransportsysteme wie beispielsweise Liposomen sollen einen effizienten Transport des Wirkstoffs über die BHS ermöglichen. Bei der Verwendung von Liposomen mit funktionalisierter Peptid-Oberfläche konnte bereits eine erhöhte Permeabilitätsfähigkeit im *in vitro* BHS-Model und eine verbesserte Zellaufnahme in humane Glioblastomzellen gezeigt werden (Mellinger *et al.* 2023). Zusätzlich zur klassischen Therapie werden komplementärmedizinische Verfahren empfohlen, wie beispielsweise die Misteltherapie. Konventionell erhältliche Mistelpräparate mit hohem Gehalt an ML-1 zeigten in Glioblastom-Mausmodellen sowohl ein signifikant verzögertes Tumorwachstum (Podlech *et al.* 2012) als auch eine verstärkte antitumorale und immunologische Reaktion (Schötterl *et al.* 2018). Patienten, welche neben klassischen Therapien mit ML-1 behandelt wurden, zeigten eine signifikante Steigerung des Gesamtüberlebens im Vergleich zur Kontrollgruppe (Lenartz *et al.* 2000). Die Kombination aus liposomaler Formulierung und eingekapseltem ML-1 als Wirkstoff bietet daher großes Potenzial für eine neue zielgerichtete Behandlungsstrategie für das Glioblastom.

Material und Methoden

Behandlung von ML-1 bei verschiedenen liposomalen Prozessparametern

Für die Evaluierung der Stabilität von ML-1 während der Einkapselung in Liposomen wurde dieses zunächst als pure Proteinlösung (1 mL, 0,1 mg/mL) in Histidin/NaCl-Puffer (10 mM, 0,3 osmol/L, pH 7,4) verschiedenen physikalischen Einflüssen ausgesetzt. Hierbei wurde der zeitabhängige Einfluss auf die immunologische Nachweisbarkeit des Proteins mittels der ELISA Methode untersucht. Als Parameter wurde der Temperatureinfluss zwischen 40 °C und 70 °C, die Behandlung mit dem Ultraschallbad mit einer Intensität von 50 % (120 Watt) und 100 %

(240 Watt), sowie der Einfluss von Scherkräften mittels dem Emulgierwerkzeug T 25 digital Ultra-Turrax® (25.000 rpm, 500 Watt) betrachtet.

Herstellung der emulsionsbasierten Liposomen

Für die Herstellung der Liposomen wurden DMPC (1,2-dimyristoyl-sn-glycero-3-phosphocholine) und Cholesterol in einem Molverhältnis von 60:40 mit einer Gesamtkonzentration von 300 mM in Ethanol gelöst und das Lösungsmittel anschließend evaporiert. Der getrocknete Lipidfilm wurde mit ML-1 Lösung (1 mg/mL in Histidin/NaCl Puffer) mit Hilfe des Ultraschallbads (5 min, 120 Watt) resuspendiert. Bei den Kontroll-Liposomen wurde der entsprechende Lipidfilm mit Puffer ohne ML-1 resuspendiert. Die Herstellung der Liposomen erfolgte über eine hydrophobe Nanoemulsion als Intermediärprodukt, deren kontinuierliche Phase aus Perfluoroperhydrophenanthrene (PFP) bestand. Für die Herstellung der W/PFP-Emulsion (10 mL) wurden 1,5 % (v/v) der Lipidsuspension mittels des T 25 digital Ultra-Turrax® bei 25.000 rpm für 3 min emulgiert. Die Nanoemulsion wurde in einem Verhältnis von 1:1 mit Histidin/NaCl Puffer überschichtet und bei 4000 x *g* für 5 min bei Raumtemperatur zentrifugiert. Die Emulsionströpfchen mit Wirkstoff im wässrigen Innenraum steigen aufgrund des starken Dichteunterschieds zu der umgebenden PFP-Phase während der Zentrifugation auf und bilden eine Phospholipid-Doppelschicht an der PFP/Wasser-Grenzfläche aus. Anschließend erfolgt der vollständige Transfer der Liposomen in die obere Wasserphase. Die Liposomensuspension wurde anschließend bei 40 °C über track-etched Membranen mit definierter Porengröße extrudiert (2-fach bei 200 nm, 2-fach bei 100 nm). Für die Entfernung von freiem, nicht verkapseltem ML-1 wurden die Liposomen in einem 300-fachen Überschuss gegen Histidin/NaCl-Puffer nach dem Schema 2h/2h/24h dialysiert und abschließend sterilfiltriert (0,22 µm).

Dynamische Lichtstreuung und Quantifizierung der Lipid- und ML-1-Konzentration

Die dynamische Lichtstreuung (DLS) wurde zur Bestimmung der Größe (Z-Average) und des Polydispersitätsindex (PdI) der Liposomen verwendet. Die Quantifizierung des Lipidgehalts an DMPC erfolgte kolorimetrisch nach Stewart *et al.* (Stewart 1980). Die Wieder-findungsrate (WFR) an Gesamtlipid (DMPC und Cholesterol) wurde anhand des eingesetzten molaren Verhältnisses zu Cholesterol berechnet. Für die Quantifizierung der ML-1 Konzentration in den Liposomen wurde deren Struktur durch die Zugabe von 2 % (v/v) Triton X-100 aufgebrochen und anschließend ein kolorimetrischer ELISA-Nachweis basierend auf monoklonalen Antikörpern gegen ML-1 durchgeführt.

Zellviabilitätsassay

Der zytotoxische Effekt von freiem und verkapseltem ML-1 wurde anhand eines Resazurin-basierten Zellviabilitätsassay an Gliomzellen (F98) und cerebrale Endothelzellen (bEnd.3) getestet. Die Zellen wurden mit einer Dichte von 10^5 Zellen/mL in 96-Well Platten in supplementiertem Medium (DMEM) ausgesät und 24 h bei 37 °C und 5 % CO_2 inkubiert. Anschließend wurden 10 µL der Probe zugegeben und die Zellen weitere 24 h inkubiert. Es folgte die Zugabe von 10 µL Resazurin-Lösung (0,15 mg/mL) und die Absorptionsmessung nach circa 3 h bei 570 nm (Referenzwellenlänge 600 nm).

Ergebnisse

Stabilität von ML-1 bei verschiedenen Prozessbedingungen zur Herstellung von Liposomen

Die Verwendung von höheren Temperaturen (≥ 60 °C) führt zu einem zeitabhängigen steigenden Konzentrationsverlust beziehungsweise zur direkten Zerstörung von ML-1 (Abb. 1). Der T 25 digital Ultra-Turrax® als Werkzeug zur Herstellung der Nanoemulsion führt bei maximaler

Leistung (25.000 rpm) innerhalb der Behandlungsdauer zu keinem signifikanten Verlust von ML-1 (Abb. 2).

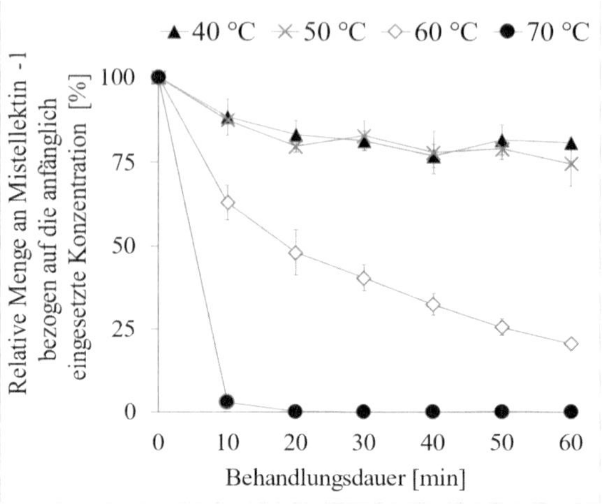

Abb. 1: Stabilität von ML-1 in Histidin/NaCl Puffer bei verschiedenen Temperaturen in Abhängigkeit der Behandlungsdauer; (n = 3)

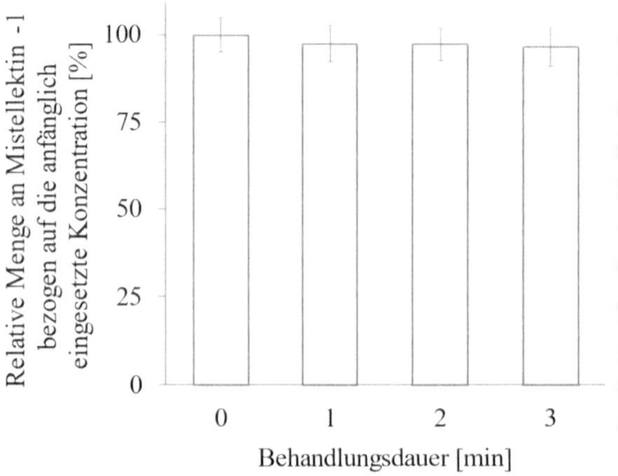

Abb. 2: Stabilität von ML-1 in Histidin/NaCl Puffer bei der Behandlung mittels T25 digital Ultra-Turrax® bei 25.000 rpm in Abhängigkeit der Behandlungsdauer; (n = 3)

Die Verwendung des Ultraschallbads zur Verbesserung der Rehydratisierung des Lipidfilms mit den Intensitäten 50 % (120 Watt) und 100 % (240 Watt) hat einen zeitabhängigen Einfluss auf die Nachweisbarkeit von ML-1 (Abb. 3). Während die Wiederfindungsrate direkt nach der Behandlung zwischen 50 % und 30 % bezogen auf die Anfangsmenge lag, kann nach 2 Wochen bei der erneuten Messung derselben Proben wieder eine Menge von 70 % bis 80 % bezogen auf die Anfangsmenge bestimmt werden (Abb. 3).

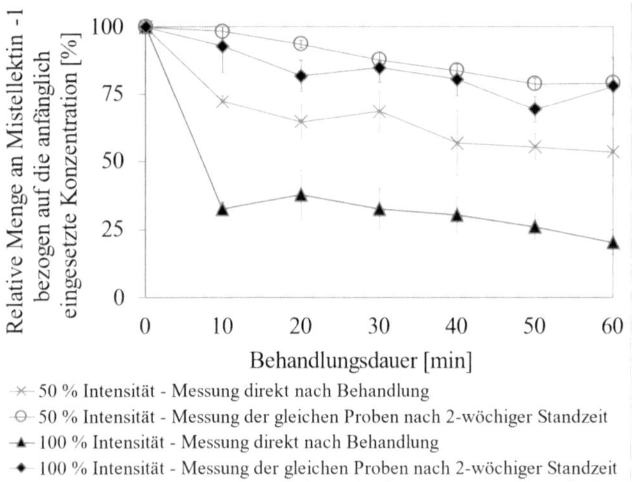

Abb. 3: Stabilität von ML-1 in Histidin/NaCl Puffer bei der Behandlung im Ultraschallbad bei 50 % (120 Watt) und 100 % (240 Watt) in Abhängigkeit der Behandlungsdauer und der Standzeit (bei 4 °C) der Proben; (n = 3)

Liposomale Charakterisierung

Die liposomalen Formulierungen mit und ohne ML-1 erreichten eine durchschnittliche Größe (Durchmesser) von < 150 nm mit einer einheitlichen Größenverteilung und geringem Polydispersitätsindex von < 0,3 (Tab. 1). Die Lipidwiederfindungsrate (WFR) betrug nach dem Herstellungsprozess und der Sterilfiltration 52 % bzw. 64 % (Tab. 1). Die Liposomen zeigten über vier Wochen bei 4 °C keine signifikanten Veränderungen hinsichtlich deren Größe und des Polydispersitätsindex.

Tab. 1: Liposomale Charakterisierung nach der Sterilfiltration (n = 3)

Zusammensetzung der liposomalen Formulierung	**Z-Average [nm]**	**PdI [/]**	**Lipid WFR [%]**
DMPC:Chol 60:40 mol%	138 ± 5	0,20 ± 0,05	64 ± 3
DMPC:Chol 60:40 mol% + ML-1	145 ± 10	0,26 ± 0,03	52 ± 4

Für die Entfernung von freiem, nicht verkapseltem ML-1 wurden die Liposomen nach dem Transfer aus der PFP-Phase in die Wasserphase dialysiert. Die Konzentration an ML-1 erfuhr durch die dialytische Aufreinigung keine signifikante Reduktion. Die finale Konzentration an ML-1 in den sterilfiltrierten Liposomen-Proben betrug 734 ± 22 ng/mL. Bezogen auf die initial eingesetzte Konzentration von ML-1 in der Nanoemulsion (15 µg/mL) entspricht dies einer Wiederfindungsrate von 4,9 ± 0,1 %.

In vitro Untersuchungen zu freiem und liposomal verkapseltem ML-1

Bei nicht verkapseltem ML-1 lag der IC_{50} für Gliomzellen (F98) bei 12 ng/mL und für cerebrale Endothelzellen (bEnd.3) bei 207 ng/mL. Dadurch wird die hohe Empfindlichkeit der Gliomzellen gegenüber ML-1 im Vergleich zu den Endothelzellen als Modellsystem für die BHS verdeutlicht. Die Behandlung der Gliomzellen mit der liposomalen aufgereinigten Formulierung mit verkapseltem ML-1 erreichte den IC_{50} bei einer 4-fach höheren ML-1 Konzentration von 50 ng/mL. Liposomen ohne ML-1 zeigten bei beiden Zelllinien keine zytotoxischen Effekte.

Diskussion und Ausblick

Die liposomalen Herstellungsparameter führen nicht zur Denaturierung und damit nicht zum Funktionsverlust von ML-1. Ultraschall zeigte einen temporären Einfluss auf die Nachweisbarkeit des Proteins. Die Verwendung und die Anwendungsdauer des Ultraschallbads innerhalb des liposomalen Herstellungsprozesses müssen weiter untersucht werden, um potenziell resultierende *in vitro* Aktivitätsverluste von ML-1 identifizieren zu können. Ultraschall kann die Sekundärstruktur von Proteinen beeinflussen und zur Reduktion der Disulfidbrücken bzw. zu einer fluktuierenden Menge an freien Thiolgruppen und Disulfid-brücken je nach Behandlungsdauer und Energieeintrag führen (Huang *et al.* 2008; Zhang *et al.* 2018).

Der liposomale Herstellungsprozess über eine W/PFP-Nano-emulsion führt zu kleinen homogenen Liposomen mit verkapseltem ML-1 und hoher zytotoxischer Aktivität gegen Gliomzellen. Innerhalb des Herstellungsprozesses wurde ein Verlust an ML-1 von 96,1 % festgestellt. Dieser wird hauptsächlich den Prozessschritten der Emulsionsherstellung (Homogenisierung und Zentrifugation) zu-geschrieben, da sich die Konzentration von ML-1 vor und nach der Dialyse der Liposomen nicht mehr signifikant reduziert hat. Das ML-1, welches sich in der Wasserphase nach der Zentrifugation befindet, ist somit in vollständiger Interaktion mit der liposomalen Struktur.

Die weitere Optimierung des Prozesses ist entscheidend, um sowohl den Verlust von ML-1 an den einzelnen Prozessschritten zu minimieren, als auch die Effizienz des Gesamtprozesses und der Verkapselung zu verbessern. Hinzukommend wird die Aufnahme- und Freisetzung von ML-1 aus den Liposomen untersucht, um eine optimale Lipidzusammen-setzung mit Funktionalisierung der Oberfläche zur effektiven Überwindung der BHS und zur Ausrichtung auf die spezifischen Gliomzellen zu erhalten.

Danksagung

Dieses Projekt (E! 113670) wurde durch das Eurostars-2 Programm unterstützt, mit Ko-Finanzierung durch das Programm Horizont 2020 und das Innovationsprogramm der Europäischen Union. Wir danken dem Bundesministerium für Bildung und Forschung für die Förderung (01QE2008A).

Interessenkonflikt

Im Zusammenhang mit dieser Veröffentlichung erklären alle Autoren, dass keine Interessenskonflikte bestehen.

Literatur

Huang H, Kwok KC, Liang HH: Inhibitory activity and conformation changes of soybean trypsin inhibitors induced by ultrasound. Ultrasonics sonochemistry. 2008; 15 (5): 724–730.

Lenartz D, Dott U, Menzel J et al.: Survival of glioma patients after complementary treatment with galactoside-specific lectin from mistletoe. Anticancer research. 2000; 20 (3B): 2073–2076.

Mellinger A, Lubitz LJ, Gazaille C et al.: The use of liposomes functionalized with the NFL-TBS.40–63 peptide as a targeting agent to cross the in vitro blood–brain barrier and target glioblastoma cells. International Journal of Pharmaceutics. 2023; 646: 123421.

Podlech O, Harter PN, Mittelbronn M et al.: Fermented Mistletoe Extract as a Multimodal Antitumoral Agent in Gliomas. Evid Based Complement Alternat Med. 2012; 2012:501796.

Poon MTC, Sudlow CLM, Figueroa JD et al.: Longer-term (≥ 2 years) survival in patients with glioblastoma in population-based studies pre- and post-2005; Scientific reports. 2020; 10 (1): 11622.

Schaff LR, Mellinghoff IK: Glioblastoma and Other Primary Brain Malignancies in Adults: A Review. JAMA. 2023; 329 (7): 574–587

Schötterl S, Huber SM, Lentzen H et al.: Adjuvant Therapy Using Mistletoe Containing Drugs Boosts the T-Cell-Mediated Killing of Glioma Cells and Prolongs the Survival of Glioma Bearing Mice. Evid Based Complement Alternat Med. 2018; 2018:3928572.
Stewart JC: Colorimetric determination of phospholipids with ammonium ferrothiocyanate. Analytical biochemistry. 2018; 104 (1): 10–14.
Zhang Y, Li Y, Li S, Zhang H et al.: In Situ Monitoring of the Effect of Ultrasound on the Sulfhydryl Groups and Disulfide Bonds of Wheat Gluten. Molecules. 2018; 23 (6):1376.

Josanna Kaufmann, Dr. Harden Rieger, Priv.-Doz. Dr. Gero Leneweit
Abnoba GmbH, Allmendstr. 55, Niefern-Öschelbronn,
75223 Niefern-Öschelbronn, Germany

Korrespondenzadresse:
kaufmann@abnoba.de

Novel Formulations of Mistletoe Extracts for Targeted Cancer Therapies

Neuartige Formulierungen von Mistelextrakten für zielgerichtete Krebstherapien

Gero Leneweit, Josanna Kaufmann, Larissa Lubitz, Harden Rieger

Summary

Since the beginning of mistletoe therapy for cancer, colloidal formulations of mistletoe extracts were considered as a way to reinforce the therapeutic capacities. Contemporary drug developments explore drug delivery systems, especially liposomes, which are similar to physiological archetypes like extracellular vesicles. The results achieved in the European collaborations RELIEF show the possibility to encapsulate macromolecular drugs in liposomes with high efficiencies. Current drug delivery widely employs surface coatings by polyethylene glycol to attenuate innate immune activation, but its significant disadvantages are well known, requiring alternative coatings. Heparin-coated liposomes were tested regarding their attenuation of the complement system. Ligands to improve liposomal uptake and potential tumour targeting were studied. Currently, pre-clinical research is in progress to evidence the feasibility of cancer treatments using liposomal formulations of mistletoe extracts.

Keywords: Mistletoe extracts, liposomes, immuno-protective coating, ligands

Zusammenfassung

Seit den Anfängen der Misteltherapie bei Krebs wurden kolloidale Formulierungen von Mistelextrakten zur Verstärkung der therapeutischen Fähigkeiten konzipiert. Heutige Arzneimittelentwicklungen erforschen Wirkstoff-Transportsysteme wie Liposomen, die physiologischen Vorbildern wie extrazellulären Vesikeln ähneln. Die in europäischen Kooperationen erzielten Ergebnisse zeigen die Möglichkeit, makromolekulare Arzneimittel mit hoher Effizienz in Liposomen einzukapseln. Bei Arzneimittel-Transport-systemen werden häufig Oberflächenbeschichtungen aus Polyethylenglykol verwendet, um die Aktivierung des angeborenen Immunsystems abzuschwächen.

Die erheblichen Nachteile dieser Beschichtung sind jedoch bekannt, sodass alternative Beschichtungen erforderlich sind. Heparin beschichtete Liposomen wurden auf ihre Abschwächung der Komplement-Reaktion getestet. Liganden auf Liposomen wurden zur Verbesserung des Tumor-Targetings und der Aufnahme in Tumorzellen erprobt. Derzeit werden präklinische Erfahrungen zur Durchführbarkeit von Krebsbehandlungen mit liposomalen Formulierungen von Mistelextrakten zu gewonnen.
Schlüsselwörter: Mistelextrakte, Liposomen, immunprotektive Beschichtungen, Liganden

Introduction

Modern cancer therapies are increasingly using or exploring drug delivery systems (DDS) with the goal of improving tumour targeting. Even the possibilities of using extracellular vesicles (EV) from suitable organisms are under study since EV are regarded as the natural and most universal delivery system for intra- and extracellular transport of relevant functional physiological molecules like proteins, DNA, RNA, etc. (Herrmann *et al.* 2021). Liposomes are the most widely used DDS showing similarity to EV and with currently 9 authorized anti-cancer drug formulations transporting well-known cytostatic agents (Gadekar *et al.* 2021) as active pharmaceutical ingredients (API). Liposomal formulations enable to reduce significantly the adverse effects like e.g. cardiotoxicity (O'Brien *et al.* 2004) in the case of doxorubicin, leading to a measurable increase in the quality of life (QoL). However, DDS-loaded therapeutics have not yet succeeded in enabling longer overall survival and progression-free survival in cancer therapy in comparison to the same drug being applied without a DDS in multi-armed clinical trials (Zhang *et al.* 2021). This is in contrary to the very strong effects on overall survival in animal tumour models. These discrepancies between slowly growing and often hypoxic and necrotic tumours in patients compared to fast growing tumours in animal models indicate several likely reasons: DDS so far only rely on the so-called 'Enhanced Permeability and Retention' (EPR effect) as "passive targeting" (Matsumura and Maeda 1986). EPR is built on the fact that leaky endothelia in fast growing tumours allow the diffusion of nanoparticles <200 nm from the blood stream into the tumour tissue and their accumulation there. In order to exploit the EPR effect it is assumed that the DDS needs to have a long half-life in blood circulation. Only recently it was discovered that long circulation is a necessary, but not sufficient condition to enable DDS accumulation in tumours. What is even more decisive is to unblock the perfusion rates in hypoxic tumour areas (Islam *et al.* 2021).

In order to develop the full potential of DDS, it is a helpful strategy to learn from the specific characteristics of EV and their long-circulating properties for optimized tumour accumulation. EV have specific functional features such as a polymer surface coating composed of glycans to avoid immune activation and specific ligands to reach the target cells (Hallal *et al.* 2022). The focus of the current research is to implement these functional concepts by novel formulations for mistletoe extracts and to evaluate the specific advantages and progress achieved.

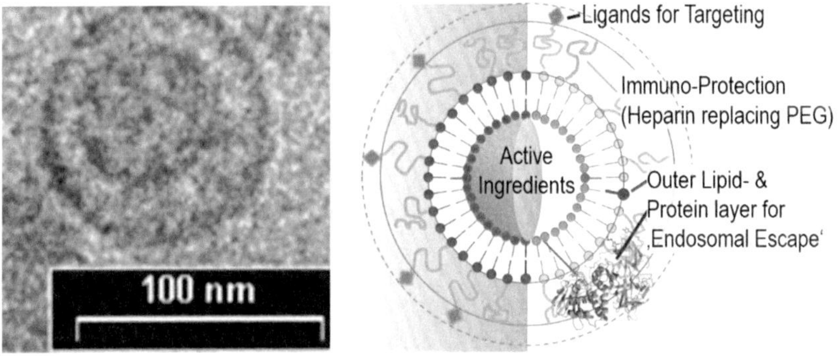

Fig. 1: Left: cryoTEM image of a mistletoe-membrane vesicle isolated from an ampoule of abnobaVISCUM® (Winkler *et al.* 2005)
Right: Schematic concept showing the functional demands of liposomal formulations of mistletoe extracts by a pharmaceutical flow process

Figure 1 (left) shows membrane vesicles in the authorized mistletoe drug abnobaVISCUM® as a DDS with high similarity to EV (Winkler *et al.* 2005). Membrane vesicles are generated by proprietary high-pressure homogenization, allowing the complete extraction of the cellular membranes as drug components. Figure 1 (right) presents the concept of a DDS to be produced by a pharmaceutical flow process under development, enabling the encapsulation of mistletoe extracts as active pharmaceutical ingredients inside the liposomal membrane. The concept of this pharmaceutical processing is inspired by Rudolf Steiner's research results on cancer therapy using mistletoe extracts to be treated by a flow process (Steiner 1923). This process is conceived to enable the formation of novel colloidal structures for the improvement of the therapeutic qualities.

To establish the physiological functionality of a colloidal DDS, several issues can be learned from EV, such as the protection of this DDS, preventing both innate and acquired immune activations. This is studied using heparin as a genuine human glycosaminoglycan to replace the frequently used polyethylene glycol (PEG) because of its many disadvantages. Specific ligands are explored to enable active targeting of specific tumour receptors. After liposomal uptake in tumour cells, specific components inside or outside the liposomal membrane can support the escape from endosomes to avoid the lysosomes where most drugs end without becoming effective in cancer therapy.

Materials and methods

As this publication provides an overview of recent results, interprets them and opens an outlook on ongoing work and future perspectives, the materials and methods can be read in the respective (open access) publications cited.

Results

Encapsulation of macromolecular biological API in liposomes

A centrifugal flow process was designed, using a dispersion of the aqueous drug in a hydrophobic excipient fluid, forming nano-emulsion droplets (Ullmann *et al.* 2023), emulsified by a layer of phospholipids as shown in Fig. 2 (Ullmann *et al.* 2021). These droplets are less dense than their surrounding hydrophobic phase, being driven by buoyancy to cross a phase boundary covered by a second phospholipid monolayer which then transforms an emulsion droplet into a liposome in aqueous environment. The experimental verification of the sketched flow process used an aqueous dye (fluorescein-Na) to determine the encapsulation efficiency. Figure 2 shows the results of different formulations with varying osmotic concentrations inside and outside the liposomal membrane in order to detect the influence of osmotic gradients during the formation of the liposomes. As can be seen, highest encapsulation efficiencies (EE) of around 95 % can be reached in salt-free deionized water or in case of a high osmotic excess concentration inside, leading to an influx of water which avoids the API (or the dye as API surrogate) to diffuse outward. On the contrary, opposite conditions of an excess of salt in the surrounding or equally high salt concentrations inside and outside lead to a much stronger loss of the dye with EE of 67 and 83 %, respectively. This confirms expectations in the sense that an osmosis-driven water flow out of the liposomal core into the surrounding is partially transporting also API out during the process of bilayer formation. In the opposite case of a water influx during bilayer formation and closure of the liposomal membrane, the diffusion of API out of the forming liposome is hindered by a counter flow of water inside. Encapsulation of mistletoe lectins in liposomes was described by Kaufmann *et al.* (2024).

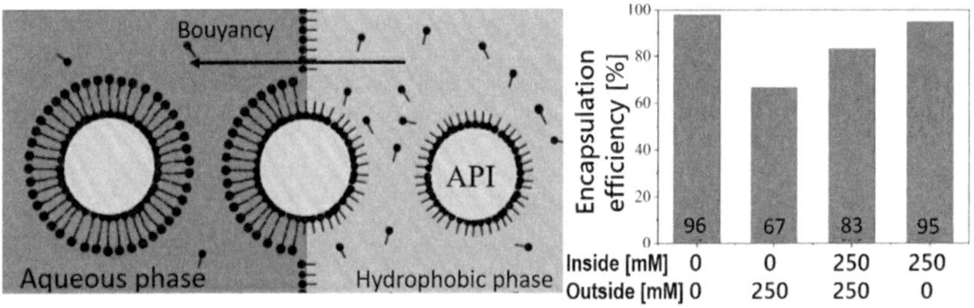

Fig. 2: Left: Schematic overview of the pharmaceutical flow process for high encapsulation efficiency of active pharmaceutical ingredients (API)
Right: Quantitative evaluation of encapsulation of an aqueous dye (Fluorescein-Na) in liposomes (Ullmann *et al.* 2021)

Surface Coating of Liposomes with Fragmented Heparin

Figure 3 shows an innovative coating method of liposomes using fragmented heparin (fHep) as a protection against the activation of innate immunity, specifically the complement system (Adler *et al.* 2023). Although heparin-coated liposomes have been studied already before (e.g. Han *et al.* 2006), the innovative aspect of our current work is that heparin was fragmented in lengths of 5-15 kDa by nitric acid and conjugated by its singular aldehyde group to lysine (K) attached in varying number n (with n = 0, 1, 2, 4, 8), bound to a terminal cysteine forming a peptide (KnC). This arrangement leads to a very structured surface due to the electrostatic repulsion of heparin, forming a "brush-like" glycosaminoglycan polymer coating. Prior preparations of heparin-coated liposomes used electrostatic or carboxyl bonds with the disadvantage of liposomal aggregation of liposomes because of multiple binding sites per heparin molecule which impedes long-circulation and leads to rapid blood clearance instead of tumour targeting. Figure 3 demonstrates that an increasing surface density of fHep leads to a strongly enhanced binding of factor H to the liposomal surfaces.

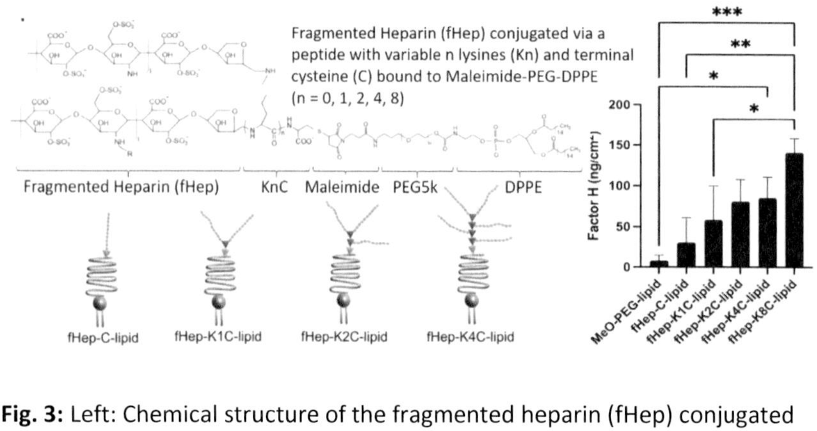

Fig. 3: Left: Chemical structure of the fragmented heparin (fHep) conjugated to a PEG-lipid anchor (Mal-PEG-DPPE) via an aldehyde group bound to n lysines (Kn) of a peptide (KnC)
Right: Attachment of factor H to the fHep-coated liposomes (Adler *et al.* 2023)

Factor H is an important regulator of innate immunity, enabling self-tolerance. Factor H is shown to be bound between 4-fold (with single fHep chain per DPPE) up to 30-fold with 8 fHep chains per DPPE (Adler *et al.* 2023).

Cellular uptake of liposomes with the ligand NFL-TBS.40-63

The uptake of liposomes by the human glioblastoma cell line U-87 MG and the murine endothelial cell line bEnd.3 was tested for different coating conditions (Mellinger *et al.* 2023). Figure 4 shows, that control liposomes (consisting of 60 mol-% DPPC and 40 mol-% cholesterol) had a roughly linear increase in cellular uptake with increasing liposomal concentration in the surrounding cell medium. Coating liposomes with PEG (5 mol-% of PEG-2000 Da) lead to an almost 10-fold drop in uptake for both cell lines (U-87 MG and bEnd.3) compared to control liposomes. Adding the peptide ligand NFL to the surface resulted in a 4-fold increase in uptake compared to the control liposomes and a 40-fold increased uptake compared to the PEG-coated liposomes. The ligand used for these tests is a peptide fraction of the 'Neurofilament Light Chain', using the amino acids 40-63 (abbreviated NFL-TBS.40-63) which has proven cell-penetrating properties.

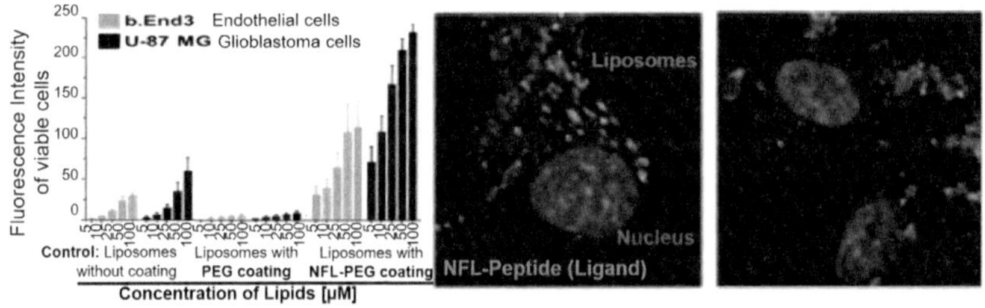

Fig. 4: Left: Flow cytometric quantification of cellular uptake of liposomes in endothelial cells (bEnd.3) and glioblastoma cells (U-87 MG)
Right: Confocal imaging of liposomal uptake using fluorescent labels for liposomes and the ligand NFL-TBS.40-63 (Mellinger *et al.* 2023, please see the colour version of the images there)

Conclusions and outlook

Ongoing research shows the possibility to encapsulate macromolecular API in liposomal DDS. The achievements are a clear step beyond the state of the art in liposomal production methods which can only encapsulate API of low molecular weight. Further developments are needed to establish production technologies for a liposomal formulation of mistletoe extracts as an Investigational Medicinal Product. The presented results give clear indications of the research demand in order to accomplish novel encapsulation technologies, immuno-protective coatings and ligands for active targeting. The envisioned cancer treatment by an actively targeting DDS goes beyond both the current treatments possibilities for cancer therapeutics and pharmaceutical production capabilities. This enables co-developments for both mistletoe extracts and other biologics for future integrative oncology. First steps in transfer from *in vitro* to *in vivo* research are currently in progress to provide more pre-clinical evidence about the feasibility of the treatment concepts.

Acknowledgments

The European project collaboration RELIEF (funding number E! 113670) has received funding from the Eurostars-2 programme with co-funding from the European Union's research and innovation programme Horizon 2020. The German consortium partner ABNOBA GmbH has received funding from the Federal Ministry of Education and Research (BMBF, funding number (01QE2008A). The authors sincerely thank the European collaborators from the universities of Angers/France, Uppsala/Sweden, and Utrecht/Netherlands.

Conflict of interest

The authors declare no competing interests.

Literature

Adler A, Fritsch M, Fromell K et al.: Regulation of the innate immune system by fragmented heparin-conjugated lipids on lipid bilayered membranes in vitro. J Mater Chem B. 2023; 11: 11121.

Gadekar V, Borade Y, Kannaujia S. et al.: Nanomedicines accessible in the market for clinical interventions. J Contr Rel. 2021; 330: 372–397.

Hallal S, Tüzesi A, Grau G et al.: Understanding the extracellular vesicle surface for clinical molecular biology. J Extracell. Vesicles. 2022; 11: e12260.

Han A, Lee A, Song C et al.: In vivo distribution and antitumor activity of heparin-stabilized doxorubicin-loaded liposomes. Int J Pharm. 2006; 313: 181–188.

Herrmann IK, Wood MJA, Fuhrmann G: Extracellular vesicles as a next-generation drug delivery platform. Nat. Nanotechn. 2021; 16: 748–759.

Islam R, Maeda H, Fanga J: Factors affecting the dynamics and heterogeneity of the EPR effect: pathophysiological and pathoanatomic features, drug formulations and physicochemical factors. Expert Opinion Drug Del. 2021; DOI: 10.1080/17425247.2021.1874916

Kaufmann J, Rieger H, Leneweit G: Liposomale Verkapselung von Mistelextrakten für die Therapie des Glioblastoms. In: Scheer R, Alban S, Klein R (Hrsg.): Die Mistel in der Tumortherapie 6. Essen: KVC; 2024: 67–77.

Matsumura Y, Maeda H: A New Concept for Macromolecular Therapeutics in Cancer Chemotherapy: Mechanism of Tumoritropic Accumulation of Proteins and the Antitumor Agent Smancs. Cancer Res. 1986; 46: 6387–6392.

Mellinger A, Lubitz L, Gazaille C et al.: The use of liposomes functionalized with the NFL-TBS.40–63 peptide as a targeting agent to cross the in vitro blood–brain barrier and target glioblastoma cells. Int J Pharm. 2023; 646: 123421

O'Brien M, Wigler N, Inbar M et al.: Reduced cardiotoxicity and comparable efficacy in a phase III trial of pegylated liposomal doxorubicin HCl (CAELYX™/Doxil®) versus conventional doxorubicin for first-line treatment of metastatic breast cancer. Annals Oncol. 2004; 15: 440–449.

Steiner R: Anthroposophical Knowledge of Man and Medicine, lecture in London, 03.09.1923. Complete Edition, Volume 319, Steiner Books 2000.

Ullmann K, Leneweit G, Nirschl H: How to Achieve High Encapsulation Efficiencies for Macromolecular and Sensitive APIs in Liposomes. Pharmaceutics. 2021; 13: 691.

Ullmann K. Fachet L, Nirschl H et al.: Monolayer/Bilayer Equilibrium of Phospholipids in Gel or Liquid States: Interfacial Adsorption via Monomer or Liposome Diffusion? Gels. 2023; 9: 803.

Winkler K, Leneweit G, Schubert R: Characterization of membrane vesicles in plant extracts. Colloids Surf. B: 2005; 45: 57–65.

Zhang KP, Fang X, Zhang Y et al.: The prognosis of cancer patients undergoing liposomal doxorubicin-based chemotherapy: a systematic review and meta-analysis. Medicine. 2021; 100:34(e26690).

PD Dr. Gero Leneweit[1, 2, 3], Josanna Kaufmann[1, 2, 3], Larissa Lubitz[1, 2, 3], Dr. Harden Rieger[1, 2]

[1] Carl Gustav Carus-Institute, Niefern-Öschelbronn, Germany

[2] ABNOBA GmbH, Niefern-Öschelbronn, Germany

[3] Karlsruhe Institute of Technology (KIT), Karlsruhe, Germany

Corresponding author:

gero.leneweit@carus-institut.de

II. Präklinik: Immunologie, Zytologie, *in vitro*- und *in vivo*-Untersuchungen

II. Preclinic: Immunology, Cytology, *In Vitro* and *In Vivo* Studies

Inhibition of Colorectal Cancer Cell Line Growth by Mistletoe Extracts

Hemmung des Wachstums von Kolorektalkarzinomzelllinien durch Mistelextrakte

Sebastian Wolfshöfer, Martina Gast, Friedemann Schad, Hedwig Lammert, Michael Hummel, Sebastian Stintzing, Patricia Grabowski

Summary

Background: Colorectal carcinomas are among the most frequent malignant tumors diagnosed in Germany. As metastasis is common after surgical removal of primary tumors, adjuvant chemotherapy is considered standard treatment for patients. However, many patients develop resistance to chemotherapy or progress during the disease. Extracts produced of mistletoe (*Viscum album*) are often administered in combination with chemotherapeutic agents to improve quality of life for patients, by reducing side effects, such as fatigue. Mistletoe extracts can differ substantially in their composition, depending on the host tree species and the harvesting time. Mistletoe extracts show immunomodulating properties that may improve effectivity of tumor therapy. Moreover, *in vitro* experiments suggest a direct effect on growth and proliferation of colorectal cancer cell lines. However, the involved intracellular pathways and the capacity of the anti-tumorigenic potential are not well characterized, yet.

Methods: We used MTT-assay to analyze the effects of two mistletoe extracts, Helixor A® (host: fir) and Helixor M® (host: apple tree), on cell viability in different colorectal cancer cell lines (Caco2, HT-29, SW48, SW480, HCT116, p53 deficient HCT116) and determined the half inhibitory concentration after 72 h of treatment. Cell cycle was analyzed by flow cytometry. In addition, we performed multiplex gene expression analyses to assess involved signaling pathways.

Results: Both mistletoe extracts reduced cell viability in a dose-dependent manner. Helixor A® extract was more potent than Helixor M® in all six cell lines. SW480 and Caco2 cells were most susceptible to both extracts.

Compared to 5 FU treated controls, the addition of mistletoe extract to 5-FU therapy reduced cell viability by approximately 50 % in SW480 cells and by 30 % in Caco2 cells, indicating an additive effect. Gene expression analysis revealed the involvement of Myc signaling. These results were validated by Western blot analysis.

Conclusions: These experiments demonstrate that mistletoe extracts can inhibit proliferation in colorectal cancer cells alone and in combination with 5-FU in vitro. Further validation of gene expression analysis results and additional combinatory treatment experiments may contribute to provide a rationale for investigation of mistletoe extracts as therapeutic agents in vivo and in clinical trials.

Keywords: *Viscum album*, chemotherapy, colorectal cancer, Myc signaling

Zusammenfassung

Hintergrund: Kolorektalkarzinome gehören zu den am häufigsten diagnostizierten Tumorerkrankungen in Deutschland. Adjuvante Behandlung mit Chemotherapeutika ist Standardtherapie, da auch nach operativer Entfernung des Primärtumors häufig Metastasen auftreten. Resistenzbildung gegenüber. Chemotherapie oder Progress ist jedoch häufig. Extrakte aus Mistelpflanzen (*Viscum album*) wurden zusätzlich zu Chemotherapeutika verabreicht, um Nebenwirkungen wie tumorbedingte Fatigue zu verringern und das allgemeine Wohlbefinden von Patienten zu verbessern. In Abhängigkeit von Wirtsbaum und Erntezeitpunkt unterscheiden sich Mistelextrakte substanziell in ihrer Zusammensetzung. Es konnte bereits gezeigt werden, dass Mistelextrakte immunmodulierend wirken und auf diese Weise die Effektivität von Tumortherapien verbessern könnten. Außerdem legen *in vitro* Experimente nahe, dass Mistelextrakte einen direkten Einfluss auf Wachstum und Proliferation von Kolorektalkarzinomzelllinien haben. Die daran beteiligten intrazellulären Signalwege und das Ausmaß der antitumorigenen Wirkung von Mistelextrakten sind jedoch bisher noch nicht detailliert beschrieben worden.

Methoden: Um den Einfluss von zwei verschiedenen Mistelextrakten, Helixor A® (Wirtsbaum: Tanne) und Helixor M® (Wirtsbaum: Apfel) auf die Zellviabilität von sechs verschiedenen Kolorektalkarzinomzelllinien (Caco2, HT-29, SW48, SW480, HCT116, p53-mutierte HCT116) zu untersuchen, wurde die mittlere inhibitorische Konzentration nach 72 Stunden Behandlung, mittels MTT-Assay bestimmt. Zellzyklusanalysen wurden mittels Durchflusszytometrie durchgeführt. Um die beteiligten Signalwege zu bestimmen, wurden Multiplex-Genexpressionsanalysen durchgeführt.

Ergebnisse: Beide verwendeten Mistelextrakte reduzierten die Zellviabilität von Kolorektalkarzinomzelllinien dosisabhängig. Helixor A® Extrakte waren in allen sechs untersuchten Zelllinien wirksamer als Helixor M® Extrakte. SW480 und Caco2 Zellen waren gegenüber beiden verwendeten Extrakten am anfälligsten. Im Vergleich mit 5-FU behandelten Zellen, konnte die Zellviabilität durch zusätzliche Behandlung mit Mistelextrakt von SW480 Zellen um ca. 50 % und von Caco2 Zellen um ca. 30 % verringert werden. Diese Ergebnisse weisen auf einen zusätzlichen, additiven Effekt des Mistelextrakts hin. In Genexpressionsanalysen wurde eine Beteiligung des Myc Signalwegs nachgewiesen. Diese Ergebnisse wurden mittels Western Blot Versuchen validiert.

Schlussfolgerungen: Unsere Experimente zeigen auf, dass Mistelextrakte allein, und in Kombination mit 5-FU das Wachstum von Kolorektalkarzinomzellen *in vitro* hemmen können. Weitere Validierung der Genexpressionsanalysen und zusätzliche kombinationstherapeutische Experimente können als Grundlage für *in vivo*-Untersuchungen und weiterführende klinische Studien zur Untersuchung von Mistelextrakten als therapeutische Substanzen dienen.

Schlüsselwörter: *Viscum album*, Chemotherapie, Kolorektalkarzinom, Myc Signalweg

Introduction

With approximately 60.000 new diagnoses per year, colorectal cancer is amongst the most frequent cancers in Germany representing the second most frequent cancerous disesase in women and the third most in men. Even after complete surgical resection of the primary tumor, metastasis is common. Therefore, adjuvant chemotherapy is often used as follow-up treatment to reduce the risk of relapse due to the potential presence of remaining cancer cells (Hofheinz *et al.* 2018). Adjuvant chemotherapy-induced resistance is possible and frequent in various cancers.

Recurrent side effects that occur during chemotherapy treatment include pain, fatigue, sickness and hair loss remain a challenge for patients. Therefore, an improvement of therapeutic options for patients with colorectal cancer is of great interest. Application of mistletoe extracts can reduce the aforementioned side effects of chemotherapy in the clinical practice (Evans *et al.* 2016).

For the treatment of colon cancer, FOLFOX (5-FU, leucovorin, and oxaliplatin) or CapeOx (capecitabine and oxaliplatin) regimens are used most often. Experimental studies with mistletoe extracts could show that additional therapy can improve quality-of-life and well-being of patients by reduction of side effects (Evans *et al.* 2016; Kienle, Kiene 2010). Furthermore, it could be shown that mistletoe extracts exhibit immunomodulating properties, which may contribute to the effectivity of anti-tumor therapy. In a recent study, additional mistletoe therapy was positively correlated with longer survival in patients with metastatic non-small cell lung cancer (Schad *et al.* 2018). However, the potential interactions with current state-of-the-art cancer therapies, like immune checkpoint inhibitors are not yet characterized.

Mistletoe extracts contain multiple pharmacologically active compounds. The underlying modes of action and intracellular effects are still not characterized completely. It has been proposed that the observed reduction of adverse effects is caused by direct cytotoxic activity of components of the mistletoe extracts, which have been observed in several tumor cell lines *in vitro* (Ribéreau-Gayon *et al.* 1986). This may lead to a reduction of tumor growth and contribute to an extension of survival time for patients. Furthermore, it was shown that treatment with mistletoe extracts can increase the number and activity of immune cells and leads to a higher release rate of pro-inflammatory cytokines (Kovacs 2000; Ribéreau-Gayon *et al.* 1996).

The composition of extracts of mistletoe varies considerably, depending on factors like production/extraction method and host tree. The main components are mistletoe lectins (ML) and viscotoxins. ML can modulate apoptosis of cancer cells in preclinical studies (Hostanska *et al.* 2003; Lyu *et al.* 2002). For instance, a combinational treatment of SW480 cells with ML and ionizing irradiation induces more apoptosis than irradiation treatment alone. The antiapoptotic oncogene Bcl-2 is one crucial component that is regulated by ML (Hostanska *et al.* 2003).

To investigate the effects and potential implications on apoptosis signaling of mistletoe extracts on colorectal cancer cell lines, we used the clinically approved mistletoe extracts Helixor A® and Helixor M® *in vitro*. The effects on growth rate and viability were analyzed by flow cytometry, western blot analysis and colorimetric viability assays.

The effects and modes of action, by which mistletoe extracts act on cancer cells directly, have not yet been characterized sufficiently. Therefore, we performed experiments to analyze involved intracellular signaling pathways and identify affected signaling components by multiplexed gene expression analysis.

Material and methods

The cell lines used were cultivated in RPMI (Caco2 and HT-29) or DMEM (SW48, SW480, HCT116, p53 deficient HCT116) medium containing 10 % fetal bovine serum, 100 µg/ml streptomycin and 100 U/ml penicillin at 37°C with 5 % CO_2. Aqueous mistletoe extracts Helixor A® (host: fir) and Helixor M® (host: apple tree) were diluted in cell culture medium. Cell Proliferation Kit I (MTT) from Roche® was used according to the manufacturer's protocol to measure cell viability and determine the half-inhibitory concentrations after 72 hours of treatment. Multiplexed gene expression analysis was conducted by Nanostring nCounter® analysis system.

Results

Half inhibitory concentrations (IC_{50}) of the commercially available mistletoe extracts Helixor A® and Helixor M® were determined after 72 hours of incubation followed by MTT assay (Table 1).

In all six CRC cell lines used, both mistletoe extracts were able to reduce the cell viability in a dose dependent manner. In all cell lines used, Helixor A® reduced cell growth and proliferation stronger than Helixor M®. Caco2 and SW480 cells were most susceptible for both mistletoe extracts.

Table 1: IC50 values of Helixor M® and Helixor A® in six different CRC lines.

	IC_{50} Helixor A (µg / ml)	IC_{50} Helixor M (µg / ml)
HCT116	371	557
HCT116 p53 -/-	496	690
HT-29	561	(> 2000)
Caco2	208	226
SW48	385	536
SW480	319	414

Mistletoe therapies are often used as complementary approaches in cancer treatment. Helixor M® is often used to improve quality of life of gastrointestinal cancer patients.

Therefore, we performed combinatory experiments with Helixor M® in combination with 5-fluorouracil (5-FU) chemotherapy. Addition of mistletoe extract Helixor M® to 5-FU therapy further reduced the cell viability in experiments with SW480 and Caco2 cells, indicating an additive effect (data not shown). The additional effect of Helixor M® co-treatment in SW480 cells was more pronounced than in Caco2 cells. However, we observed a significant reduction of cell viability in both cell lines at all measured time points.

In order to identify the involved pathways and quantify differentially expressed genes, we analyzed SW480 and Caco2 cells treated with or without Helixor M® by mRNA profiling.

In particular, genes involved in apoptosis / cytotoxicity and Myc signaling and NF-kB signaling were differentially expressed in response to treatment with the mistletoe extract (Fig. 1).

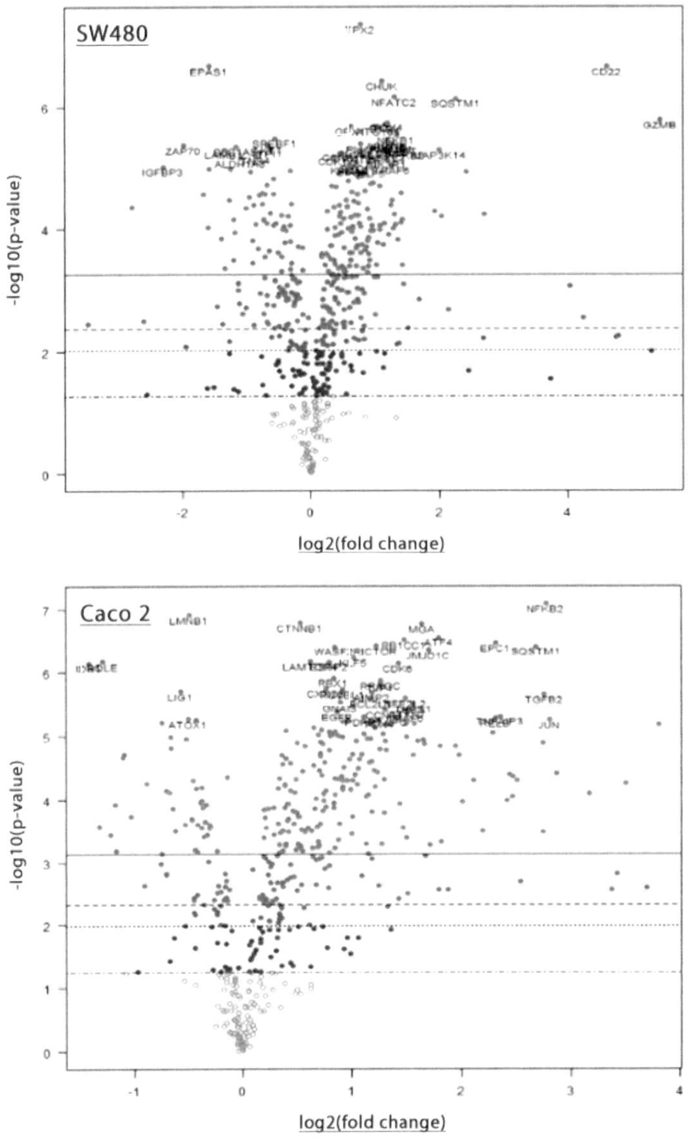

Fig. 1: Differential gene expression in SW480 and Caco2 cells following treatment with Helixor M

We assessed and validated these results on protein level (Fig. 2). A reduction of the proto-oncogene c-Myc could be observed in Helixor M® treated SW480 and Caco2 cells. We also detected reduced levels of the anti-apoptotic protein Bcl-2 in Helixor M® treated cells.

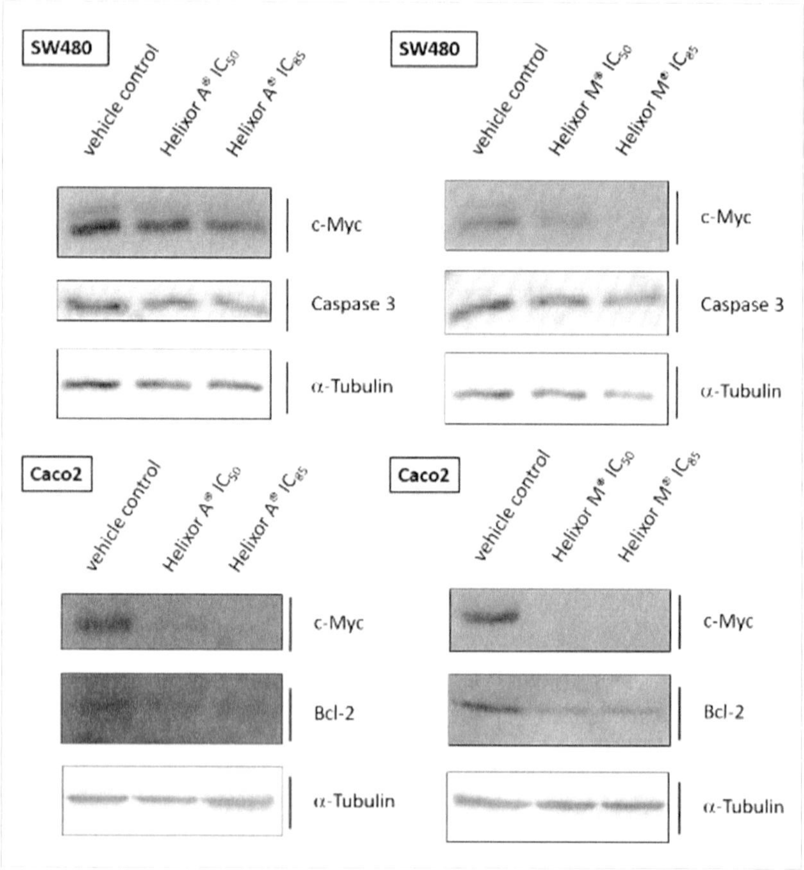

Fig. 2: Western blots displaying the influence of Helixor M® treatment on c-Myc and Bcl-2 protein levels in SW480 and Caco2 cell lines.

Discussion

Clinical use of extracts of *Viscum album* is well established as complementary therapy for gastrointestinal cancer patients who receive chemotherapy or radiation treatment to improve overall well-being and reduce certain adverse effects. *In vitro,* immunomodulatory effects have been shown for mistletoe extracts (Hajto *et al.* 1990). These immunological activities have mostly been attributed to the contained mistletoe lectins. Here, we demonstrated growth inhibitory effects of the commercially available mistletoe extracts Helixor A® and Helixor M® in different colorectal cancer cell lines. Mistletoe extracts and lectins can reduce the growth rate of various cancer cell lines (Kelter *et al.* 2007). However, the involved cellular mechanisms and the therapeutic potential have not been characterized well yet. In line with the results of our multiplexed gene expression analysis, experiments in hepatocellular carcinoma cells also indicate that mistletoe extracts act on the proto-oncogene c-Myc (Yang *et al.* 2019). The oncogene Myc is expressed constitutively in many different cancers and promotes cell proliferation by different mechanisms (Kalkat *et al.* 2017). Myc has been shown to interact with the anti-apoptotic protein Bcl-2 (Jin *et al.* 2004).

The suppression of anti-apoptotic c-Myc driven signals could help to improve the effects of conventional tumor therapies like chemotherapies and potentially have an influence more advanced therapeutics, like immune checkpoint inhibitors.

Additional combinatory experiments with other (chemo)therapeutic agents could elucidate the therapeutic potential of mistletoe extracts. This could justify further investigation of the effects of mistletoe extracts *in vivo* and in clinical trials.

Conflict of interest

This research was financially supported by Helixor Heilmittel GmbH, Rosenfeld Germany.

References

Evans M et al.: Cancer Patients' Experiences of Using Mistletoe (Viscum album): A Qualitative Systematic Review and Synthesis. Journal of alternative and complementary medicine. 2016; 22 (2): 134–144.

Hajto T et al.: Increased secretion of tumor necrosis factors alpha, interleukin 1, and interleukin 6 by human mononuclear cells exposed to beta-galactoside-specific lectin from clinically applied mistletoe extract. Cancer research. 1990; 50 (11): 3322–3326.

Hofheinz R-D, Arnold D, Borner M et al.: Kolonkarzinom. Oktober 2018: onkopedia leitlinien. https://www.onkopedia.com/de/onkopedia/guidelines/kolonkarzinom/@@guideline/html/index.html.

Hostanska K et al.: Recombinant mistletoe lectin induces p53-independent apoptosis in tumour cells and cooperates with ionising radiation. British journal of cancer. 2003; 88 (11): 1785–1792.

Jin Z, Gao F, Flagg et al.: Tobacco-specific nitrosamine 4 (methylnitrosamino)-1-(3-pyridyl)-1-butanone promotes functional cooperation of Bcl2 and c-Myc through phosphorylation in regulating cell survival and proliferation. J Biol Chem. 2004; 279 (38): 40209-19.

Kalkat M, De Melo J, Hickman KA et al.: MYC Deregulation in Primary Human Cancers. Genes (Basel). 2017; 8 (6):151.

Kelter G, Schierholz JM, Fischer IU, Fiebig HH: Cytotoxic activity and absence of tumor growth stimulation of standardized mistletoe extracts in human tumor models in vitro. Anticancer Res. 2007; 27 (1A): 223–233. PMID: 17352237.

Kienle GS, Kiene H: Review article: Influence of Viscum album L. (European mistletoe) extracts on quality of life in cancer patients: a systematic review of controlled clinical studies. Integr Cancer Ther. 2010; 9 (2): 142–157.

Kovacs E.: Serum levels of IL-12 and the production of IFN-gamma, IL-2 and IL-4 by peripheral blood mononuclear cells (PBMC) in cancer patients treated with Viscum album extract. Biomedicine & Pharmacotherapy. 2000; 54 (6): 305–310.

Lyu SY, Choi SH, Park WB: Korean mistletoe lectin-induced apoptosis in hepatocarcinoma cells is associated with inhibition of telomerase via mitochondrial controlled pathway independent of p53. Arch Pharm Res. 2002; 25 (1): 93–101.

Ribéreau-Gayon G et al.: Mistletoe lectins I, II and III induce the production of cytokines by cultured human monocytes. Cancer Letters. 1996; 109 (1–2): 33–38.

Ribéreau-Gayon G et al.: Effects of mistletoe (Viscum album L.) extracts on cultured tumor cells. Experientia. 1986; 42 (6): 594–599.

Schad F et al.: Overall survival of stage IV non-small cell lung cancer patients treated with Viscum album L. in addition to chemotherapy, a real-world observational multicenter analysis. PLoS One. 2018; 13 (8):e0203058.

Yang P, Jiang Y, Pan Y et al: Mistletoe extract Fraxini inhibits the proliferation of liver cancer by down-regulating c-Myc expression. Sci Rep. 2019; 9 (1): 6428.

Dr. Sebastian Wolfshöfer[1], Martina Gast[1],
Prof. Dr. med. Sebastian Stintzing[1], PD Dr. med. Friedemann Schad[2],
PD Dr. Patricia Grabowski[1, 2], Hedwig Lammert[3],
Prof. Dr. med. Michael Hummel[3]

[1] Charité – Universitätsmedizin Berlin, Medizinische Klinik m.S. Hämatologie, Onkologie und Tumorimmunologie – CC14, Berlin, Germany

[2] Gemeinschaftskrankenhaus Havelhöhe, Integrative Onkologie und Palliativmedizin, Berlin, Germany

[3] Charité – Universitätsmedizin Berlin, Institut für Pathologie, Berlin

Corresponding author:
patricia.grabowski@charite.de

Viscum album Mother Tinctures Interrupted the Warburg Effect in Breast Cancer Cells: Metabolite Profile and Antitumoral *In Vitro* Mechanisms

Michelle Nonato de Oliveira Melo, Alan Clavelland Ochioni, Patricia Zancan, Adriana Passos Oliveira, Mirio Grazi, Rafael Garrett, Carla Holandino, Stephan Baumgartner

This contribution is a summary of the publication of Melo *et al.* in *Frontiers in Pharmacology* 13:1027931. doi: 10.3389/fphar.2022.1027931

Summary

Aqueous *V. album* extracts have been used for over one hundred years in complementary cancer therapy. On the counterpart, ethanolic extracts, such as mother tinctures, permit better solubilization of phenolic compounds, and also have been shown antitumoral activity. To increase the scientific information about the chemical differences related to the host trees and to clarify the seasonal influences, in this study, the chemical composition of 50 *V. album* mother tinctures from three subspecies was evaluated using summer and winter plant harvests. The *in vitro* cytotoxic activities were investigated in breast cancer cells and human keratinocytes. The summer *V. album* mother tinctures presented higher cytotoxic activity than winter ones. Among the summer samples, those prepared with *V. album* subsp. *album* were more cytotoxic than those from *V. album* subsp. *abietis* and subsp. *austriacum*. The mother tinctures of *V. album* from *Quercus petraea* and *Abies alba* inhibited the key-glycolytic enzymes: hexokinase (HK), phosphofructokinase (PFK), pyruvate kinase (PK). The untargeted metabolomic approach was able to discriminate the mother tinctures according to respective botanical classification and host trees. Our study shows the interruption of the Warburg effect as a novel antitumoral mechanism triggered by *V. album* mother tinctures, which is related to their metabolite profile.

Keywords: *Viscum album*; mistletoe; metabolome; multivariate analysis; glycolytic enzymes; anticancer, *in vitro*

Introduction

Mistletoe aqueous extracts represent an important medical intervention in cancer treatment due to its cytotoxic and immunomodulatory effects (Tröger *et al.* 2013) promoted mainly by the presence of lectins, viscotoxins and polysaccharides (Büssing *et al.* 1996). However, *V. album* alcoholic extracts also have shown cytotoxicity suggesting the presence of other compounds that may have antitumor activities.

Alcoholic extracts of the *V. album*, known as mother tinctures (MT), according to homeopathic pharmacopoeias, have been widely used in folk medicine. The main use of this preparation is linked to blood pressure reduction (European Medicines Agency 2011). However, despite this traditional use of *V. album* MT for hypertension treatment, a study also demonstrated antitumor activity of alcoholic extracts in an *in vivo* Ehrlich ascite carcinoma (Stan *et al.* 2013).

It is known that cancer cells have a different metabolism to promote growth, proliferation, and long-term maintenance. The increased glucose uptake and fermentation of glucose to lactate is the most common feature of cancer metabolism.

Regarding the promising anticancer activity of *V. album* MT, and the lack of evidence about their action in the glycolytic metabolism, this study evaluated the anticancer effect of these preparations by the evaluation of enzymatic kinetics of hexokinase, phosphofructokinase, pyruvate kinase and glucose-6-phosphate dehydrogenase in a human breast cancer cell line. Additionally, liquid chromatography coupled with high-resolution mass spectrometry, followed by a multivariate statistical analysis was applied to show the influence of host trees on the chemical composition of these MT.

Materials and methods

Plant material and mother tinctures Preparation

All harvests followed the same pattern as previously described by Holandino *et al.* (2020). Fifty mother tinctures (MT) were prepared using three subspecies of *V. album* (*album*, *austriacum* and *abietis*) from five host trees harvested in Switzerland, in summer (MT code S) and winter (MT code W) (Melo *et al.* 2022).

Cytotoxic assay, glucose consumption and lactate production

MDA-MB-231 (triple negative human breast cancer cell line) and HaCaT (immortalized human keratinocyte) were used for the cytotoxic assay that was assessed by MTT method after 48 h of treatment with MT (0.5 to 3.0 % v/v). MDA-MB-231 glucose consumption was performed assessing the glucose content that remained in the culture media using an enzymatic system containing glucose oxidase. Lactate production was evaluated as described assessing the lactate released in the culture media. All methods were extensively described by Melo *et al.* (2022).

Spectrophotometric assay for enzyme activity

All the conditions for glycolytic enzyme activities of the Hexokinase (HK), pyruvate kinase (PK), phosphofructokinase (PFK-1) and glucose-6-phosphate dehydrogenase (G6PDH) of the MDA-MB-231 cells were detailed by Melo *et al.* (2022).

Quantification of viscotoxins in *Viscum album* mother tinctures by high performance liquid chromatography

The total viscotoxin content in (μg/mL) and mg/g of fresh material (FM) were calculated as the sum of each viscotoxin isoform as described before (Melo *et al.* 2022).

Viscum album MT analysis by liquid chromatography coupled to high-resolution mass spectrometry

The analysis was performed in a DionexUltiMate 3000 liquid Chromatography coupled to a hybrid Quadrupole-Orbitrap high-resolution mass spectrometer (Thermo Q-Exactive Plus) equipped with an electrospray ionization source (ESI). Pooled quality control samples (QC) containing

10 μL of each MT were also prepared. All the chromatographic and mass conditions were described by Melo *et al*. (2022).

Data pre-processing, multivariate data analysis and metabolite annotation

The raw data files were submitted to peak detection, deconvolution, normalization, and alignment processes using the freely available MZmine 2.35 software. Compound annotation was performed by MSDial 4.70 comparing the aligned *m/z* ions and their deconvoluted MS/MS spectra to those uploaded to the different mass banks. All parameters were detailed by Melo *et al*. (2022).

Results

Cell cytotoxicity and glycolytic enzymatic activity triggered by *Viscum album* mother tinctures

The summer MTs at 48 h had greater activity than winter MTs (Fig. 1A–B). The cytotoxicity evaluated in MDA-MB-231 (Fig. 1A–B) and in HaCat (Fig. 1C) cell lines was dose and time-dependent for A-S, M-S, Q-S, and U-S. *V. album* subsp. *album* was the most cytotoxic MT for MDA-MB-231 and HaCat (Fig. 1A, C). However, the lowest cytotoxic activity was related to MT P-S (Fig. 1A, C). Mother tincture A-S at 2.0 % v/v reduced approximately 50 % of the glucose uptake after 48 h of treatment, with more significant effects after 72 h of sample incubation (Fig. 1D). The MT Q-S at 1.0 % v/v inhibited approximately 20 % of the glucose uptake in both incubation times analyzed. A similar result was observed on Q-S 0.5 % after 72h. A significant reduction ($p < 0.05$) in extracellular lactate levels was observed, especially after 72 h of incubation with Q-S 0.5 %, Q-S 1.0 %, and A-S 2.0 % v/v (Fig. 1E). HK activity was significantly inhibited by MT (A-S 2.0 %, Q-S 0.5 %, and Q-S 1.0 % v/v) after 72h of incubation (Fig. 1D). Additionally, PFK-1 activity was dramatically impaired at 48 h, and at 72 h it was not possible to detect enzymatic activity.

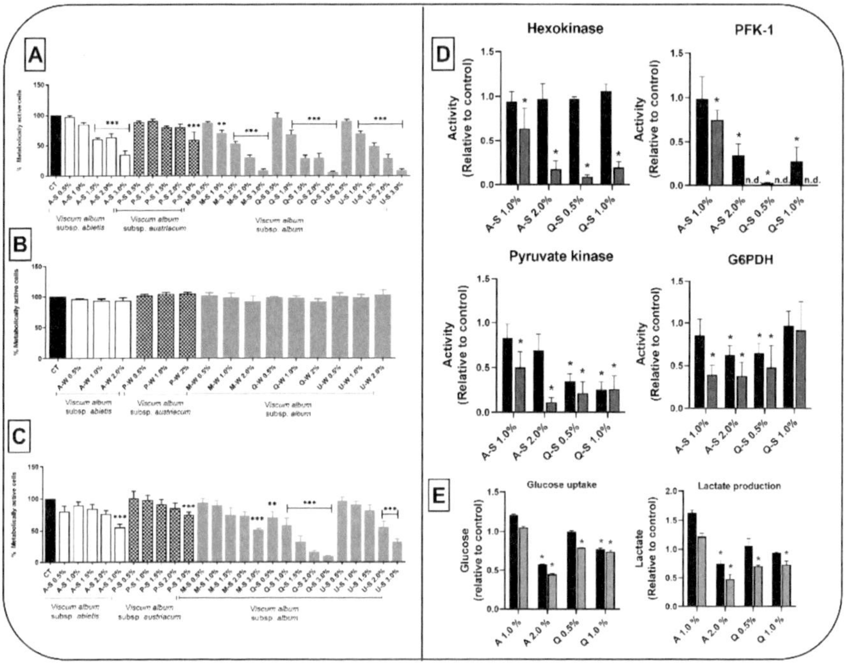

Fig. 1: (A) and (B) MDA-MB-231 summer and winter-dose effects after 48h of treatment with MTs, respectively; (C) HaCat summer-dose response effects after 24h of treatment with MTs; (D) Effect of *V. album* summer mother tinctures on the MDA-MB-231 glycolysis and pentose phosphate pathway enzymes. HK, PFK-1, PK (glycolytic enzymes), and G6PDH (Pentose Phosphate Pathway) analyzed after 48h (black bars) and 72h (grey bars) of the treatment with A-S (1.0 % and 2.0 % v/v) and Q-S (0.5 % and 1 % v/v); (E) Glucose uptake and lactate production by MDA-MB-231 cells treated with MT for 48h (black bars) and 72h (grey bars) of the treatment with A-S (1.0 % and 2.0 % v/v) and Q-S (0.5 % and 1 % v/v). Plotted values are relative to the control (ethanol vehicle) at the same concentration of the summer mother tinctures. *p < 0.05; **p < 0.001; ***p < 0.0001 obtained with one-way ANOVA/ Dunnet's post hoc test. Legend symbols: (CT) control untreated cells; (Alc) cells incubated with ethanol solvent; *V. album* subsp. *album* growing on *Malus domestica* (M-S/W), *Quercus petraea* (Q-S/W) and *Ulmus carpinifolia* (U-S/W); *V. album* subsp. *abietis* growing on *Abies alba* (A-S/W); and *V. album* subsp. *austriacum* growing on *Pinus sylvestris* (P-S/W). Samples were harvested in summer (S) and winter (W) seasons.

After 72 h, A-S incubation inhibited the enzymatic activity of the PK activity in a dose-dependent manner. Nevertheless, MT Q-S promoted a homogeneous and constant inhibition of this kinase for both concentrations and treatment times. The effects of MT on the pentose phosphate pathway (PPP) were analyzed by evaluating the activity of glucose-6-phosphate dehydrogenase (G6PDH). Figure 1D shows a great response variation, which does not suggest direct effects on this enzyme activity.

Chemical variability of the *Viscum album* mother tinctures

Mother tinctures and viscotoxin content

The viscotoxin (VT) contents were evaluated by HPLC-DAD according to the *V. album* subspecies, host tree, and season (Fig. 2). In general, subspecies of *V. album* harvested in summer had the highest amount of these proteins. Regarding deciduous trees, they were able to produce the highest concentration of viscotoxin in mg/g fresh material (FM), and this profile was mostly related to the cultivars Disli and Rösli (*Malus domestica*), and Rütti (*Quercus* sp.) harvesting sites (Fig. 2A–C). Additionally, *V. album* MT (*Malus domestica*) from Rösli produced the maximum VT amount detected, which was around 4 mg of VT/g FM (Fig. 2A). On the other hand, VT contents of MT from conifers were smaller than deciduous host trees (Fig. 2D, E). The analyses of VT from host trees at the same location (Rütti) showed summer season positive influence on this protein production, except for *V. album* MT from *Ulmus carpinifolia* (Fig. 2F).

Untargeted metabolome analysis focusing on host tree influence

Firstly, PCA plot was able to demonstrate the natural clustering of samples into 3 groups related to the botanical subspecies for both negative and positive electrospray ionization modes (Fig. 3A). The pooled QC samples were tightly clustered, showing a good reproducibility of the LC-HRMS system (Fig. 3A).

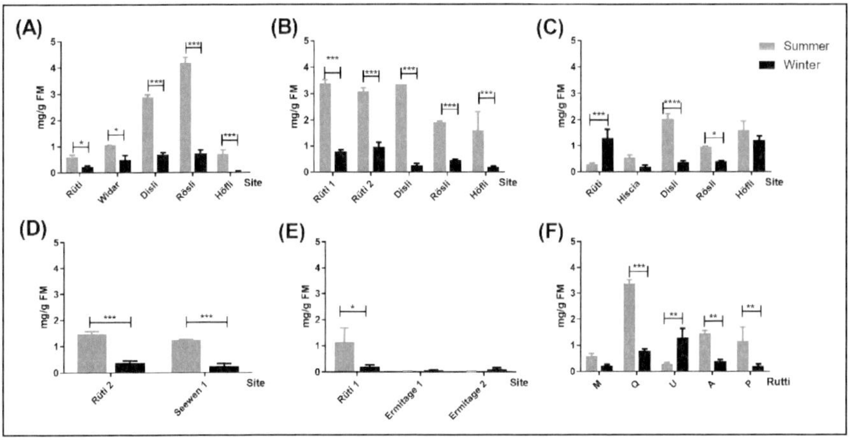

Fig. 2: Amount of viscotoxin in mg/g of fresh material (FM) of *V. album* mother tinctures prepared with plants harvested in summer (grey bars) and in winter (black bars), in the following locations: Rütti, Widar, Disli, Rösli, Höfli, Hiscia, Seewen, Ermitage. MTs were prepared with mistletoe collected from the following host trees: *Malus domestica* (A), *Quercus* sp. (B), *Ulmus carpinifolia* (C), *Abies alba* (D) and *Pinus sylvestris* (E). Comparison of the viscotoxin content from the different host trees in the same location, Rüti (F). The numbers added to Rütti and Ermitage locations represent *V. album* from different host-trees harvested in the same location. * $p \leq 0.05$; ***$p < 0.0001$.

In the PCA, the first principal component (PC1) explained 20.2 % of the total co-variance for both ionization modes, whereas the second principal component (PC2) accounted for 16.2 and 16.4 % (for negative and positive modes, respectively) of the total variability of the data set.

Then, PLS-DA was conducted considering the host tree groups. The 3D score plot showed a clear subspecies separation in three clusters (Fig. 3B).

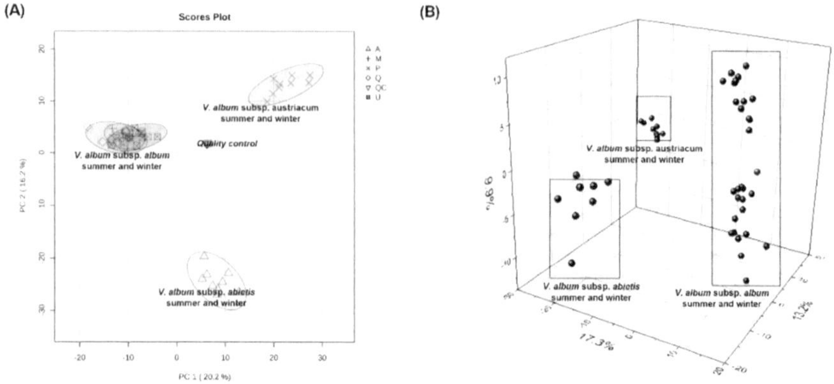

Fig. 3: Multivariate analysis from LC-HRMS data of *V. album* MT. (A) PCA 2D score plot of the negative ESI mode; (B) PLS-DA 3D score plot of the negative ESI mode.

Furthermore, it was possible to identify five different groups related to each host tree evaluated in this study. Then, the main compounds responsible for host tree discrimination were determined by variable important projection (VIP) in the negative and positive ionization modes. The R2/Q2 metrics for PLS-DA were > 0.8 for both modeling processes (Worley, Powers 2012). In the negative ionization mode, it was observed that there were increased levels of 4 molecules in the A group (*V. album* subsp. *abietis*) comprising three flavonoids and one terpene, respectively: flavanone-hexose-pentose; naringenin-pentose-hexose; 2-hydroxy-4-(6-hydroxy-5,7-dimethoxy-4-oxo-4H-chromen-3-yl) phenyl6-Ohexopyranosylhexopyranoside; 6′-O-β-D-apiofuranosylsweroside).

In parallel, the positive ionization mode showed four compounds that were important to group A discrimination, namely, one organic acid, two phenylpropanoids and one flavanone, respectively: (4-(β-D-glucopyranosyloxy) phenyl) acetic acid; Syringin; [5-hydroxy-6-[2-(4-hydroxy-3-methoxyphenyl) ethoxy]-2-(hydroxymethyl)-4-(3,4,5-trihydroxy-6-methyloxan-2-yl) oxyoxan-3-yl] (E)-3-(4-hydroxy-3-methoxyphenyl) prop-2-enoate; naringenin-pentose-hexose. Naringenin-pentose-hexose was a flavanone annotated with *m*/*z* 565 in negative, and *m*/*z* 567 in positive ionizations modes, which demonstrates its importance for the group A discrimination.

Discussion

It is known that *V. album* aqueous extracts have different cytotoxic activities related to their host tree. However, a recent study conducted by our group showed that ethanolic preparations of this plant also demonstrated subspecies and host tree-antitumoral dependence (Holandino *et al.* 2020). The researchers developed by our group have demonstrated the impact of harvest conditions and host tree influences on the chemical composition (Jäger *et al.* 2021) and biological activities of different *V. album* mother tinctures. New important findings related to tumor metabolism were introduced for the first time by glycolytic enzyme investigation conducted in the present study. Natural compounds that interact with components of glycolytic pathway can reduce the cancer cell's ability to synthesize nucleotides, proteins, or lipids (Schulze, Harris 2012). The reduction in the glucose uptake, glycolytic enzyme activities and the consequent lactate production is a very interesting effect of *V. album* MT, since this treatment probably interrupts the Warburg effect (Schulze, Harris 2012). By assessing glycolytic enzymes activities, we evaluated the metabolic profile of the cells by measuring the conversion of NAD+ to NADH or NADP+ to NADPH through light absorbance at 340 nm in a microplate reader, which could attribute the breast cancer cells death to the inhibition of glycolytic key enzymes (e.g., HK, PFK-1, and PK). This activity suggests a new antitumor mechanism triggered by *V. album* mother tinctures.

Some available research reports described the anticancer effects of natural products and their relation with the glycolytic enzymes' inhibition. Xu *et al.* (2017) demonstrated that a bioactive flavone (chrysin) from plant extracts promoted cell apoptosis through HK-2 suppression in hepatocellular carcinoma. Furthermore, significant inhibition in glucose uptake and lactate release was promoted by curcumin across the four cell lines: lung (H1299), breast (MCF-7), cervical (HeLa), and prostate (PC3). The authors conjectured that the Warburg effect inhibition was crucial for cell death, with the aid of pyruvate kinase (PKM2) down-regulation promoted by 20 μM of curcumin (Siddiqui *et al.* 2018).

Viscum album mother tinctures present different chemical profiles related to host subspecies

The content of plant primary and secondary metabolites is directly influenced by factors, such as location, season, and in the case of parasitic plants, the host tree. Viscotoxins are some of those that contribute to the antitumor potential of mistletoe preparations. In this sense, the present study has shown the influence of the season and host tree on viscotoxin and secondary metabolite contents, as well as their influence on anticancer activity. The highest VT content in summer *V. album* mother tinctures was a pattern also observed by Urech *et al.* (2006) in aqueous mistletoe samples. Moreover, considering the summer samples, MT of the *V. album* subsp. *album* presented higher VT than *V. album* subsp. *abietis* and *austriacum*. Schaller *et al.* (1998) also demonstrated that *V. album* subsp. *austriacum* presented the smallest content of viscotoxins in aqueous extracts, compared to other subspecies.

In addition to VT, our work suggested the influence of the secondary metabolites host tree-dependent in the cytotoxicity and glycolytic enzyme inhibition. So, an untargeted metabolome analysis was conducted to provide a better understanding of the chemical variability among *V. album* MT from different host trees. The PCA showed a clear separation related to the botanical subspecies in both ionization modes, which could explain the differences in cytotoxic activity as follows: *V. album* subsp. *album* > *V. album* subsp. *abietis* > *V. album* subsp. *austriacum*. The PLS-DA analysis showed increased levels of flavanone-hexose-pentose; naringenin-pentose-hexose; 2-hydroxy-4-(6-hydroxy-5,7-dimethoxy-4-oxo-4H-chromen-3-yl) phenyl6-Ohexopyranosylhexopyranoside; 6′-*O*-*β*-D-apiofuranosylsweroside) 4 in *V. album* subsp. *abietis* mother tinctures. These data support the previous findings that also demonstrated the presence of flavonoids in aqueous and alcoholic *V. album* extracts. Naringenin and derivatives have already been described in commercial *V. album* aqueous extracts (Iscador®) (Peñaloza *et al.* 2020) and alcoholic extracts (Jäger *et al.* 2021). On the other hand, we detected four compounds that were important to *V. album* subsp. *abietis* discrimination: (4-(β-D-glucopyranosyloxy) phenyl) acetic acid; Syringin; [5-hydroxy-6-[2-(4-hydroxy-3-methoxyphenyl) ethoxy]-2-(hydroxymethyl)-4-(3,4,5-trihydroxy-6-methyloxan-2-yl) oxyoxan-3-yl] (E)-3-(4-hydroxy-3-methoxyphenyl) prop-2-enoate; naringenin-pentose-hexose. Regarding these compounds, syringin is a phenylpropanoid known to occur in mistletoe species (Jäger *et al.* 2021), but its intensity related to *V. album* host trees is described for the first time in this work. Flavonoids can block glycolysis through regulation activity, expression, and glycolytic enzyme allosteric inhibition in many cancer cell lines (Samec *et al.* 2020). The present study provides basic information in which the LC-RHMS and multivariate statistical analysis can be useful in classifying *V. album* tinctures from different subspecies and host trees. Moreover, this work indicated some compounds that could be useful as biomarkers for the respective subspecies according to their host tree.

In conclusion, this study described for the first time the inhibition of the glycolytic enzymes HK, PFK-1, and PK in breast cancer cells by mother tinctures prepared from different subspecies of *V. album*. Summer MT promoted the highest cellular damage compared to winter preparations. It was possible to identify the promising antitumoral activity of *V. album* subsp. *album*, followed by *V. album* subsp. *abietis*. Concerning the *V. album* subsp. *album*, the mother tincture prepared with mistletoe from *Quercus petraea* presented better cytotoxic results. Higher contents of viscotoxins in the summer mother tinctures could also be responsible for this bioactivity. The multivariate statistical analyses using LC-HRMS data showed to be an efficient approach to screening and tracking chemical differences concerning *V. album* mother tinctures.

Acknowledgements

We are grateful to João Vitor da Costa Batista (Society for Cancer Research, Switzerland) for critical comments and inputs for this publication, and to Claudia Dalla Torre (ISCADOR AG, Switzerland) for the viscotoxins analysis. This study was supported by fellowships from Coordenação de Aperfeiçoamento de Pessoal de Nível Superior (CAPES) and Fundação de Amparo à Pesquisa do Estado do Rio de Janeiro (FAPERJ). The authors also thank to the Laboratório de Oncobiologia Molecular (LaboMol)-Universidade Federal do Rio de Janeiro for the enzymatic activity analysis.

This study was funded by Coordenação de Aperfeiçoamento de Pessoal de Nível Superior of Brasil (CAPES; Finance Code 001; 88887.569108/2020-00) and Fundação de Amparo à Pesquisa do Estado do Rio de Janeiro (FAPERJ; BPP 201.004/2022).

Conflict of interest

The authors declare that the research was conducted in the absence of any commercial or financial relationships that could be construed as a potential conflict of interest.

References

Büssing A, Suzart K, Bergmann J et al.: Induction of apoptosis in human lymphocytes treated with Viscum album L. is mediated by the mistletoe lectins. Cancer Letters. 1996; 99 (1): 59–72.

European Medicines Agency: Assessment report on Viscum album L., herba. 2011. https://www.ema.europa.eu/en/documents/herbal-report/final-assessment-report-viscum-album-l-herba_en.pdf.

Holandino C, Melo MNO, Oliveira AP et al.: Phytochemical analysis and in vitro anti-proliferative activity of Viscum album ethanolic extracts. BMC complementary medicine and therapies. 2020; 20 (1): 215–215.

Jäger T, Holandino C, Melo MNO et al.: Metabolomics by UHPLC-Q-TOF Reveals Host Tree-Dependent Phytochemical Variation in Viscum album L. Plants. 2021; 10 (8): 1726–1726.

Melo MNO, Ochioni AC, Zancan P et al.: Viscum album mother tinctures: Harvest conditions and host trees influence the plant metabolome and the glycolytic pathway of breast cancer cells. Front Pharmacol. 2022; 13: 1027931.

Peñaloza E, Holandino C, Scherr C et al.: Comprehensive Metabolome Analysis of Fermented Aqueous Extracts of Viscum album L. By Liquid Chromatography – High Resolution Tandem Mass Spectrometry. Molecules. 2020; 25 (17):4006. doi: 10.3390/molecules25174006.

Samec M, Liskova A, Koklesova L et al.: Flavonoids against the Warburg phenotype-concepts of predictive, preventive and personalized medicine to cut the Gordian knot of cancer cell metabolism. EPMA Journal. 2020; 11: 377–398.

Schaller G, Urech K, Grazi G, Giannattasio M: Viscotoxin composition of the three European subspecies of Viscum album. Planta Medica. 1998; 64 (7): 677–678.

Schulze A, Harris AL: How cancer metabolism is tuned for proliferation and vulnerable to disruption. Nature. 2012; 491 (7424): 364–373. doi: 10.1038/nature11706.

Siddiqui FA, Prakasam G, Chattopadhyay S et al.: Curcumin decreases Warburg effect in cancer cells by down-regulating pyruvate kinase M2 via mTOR-HIF1alpha inhibition. Sci Rep. 2018; 8 (1): 8323.

Stan R, Hangan A, Dican L et al.: Comparative study concerning mistletoe viscotoxins antitumor activity. Acta Biologica Hungarica. 2013; 64 (3): 279–288.

Tröger W, Galun D, Reif M et al.: Viscum album [L.] extract therapy in patients with locally advanced or metastatic pancreatic cancer: A randomised clinical trial on overall survival. Eur J Cancer. 2013; 49 (18): 3788–3797.

Urech K, Schaller G, Jäggy C: Viscotoxins, mistletoe lectins and their isoforms in mistletoe (Viscum album L.) extracts Iscador: Analytical results on pharmaceutical processing of mistletoe. Arzneimittel-Forschung/Drug Research. 2006; 56 (6 A): 428–434.

Xu D, Jin J, Yu H et al.: Chrysin inhibited tumor glycolysis and induced apoptosis in hepatocellular carcinoma by targeting hexokinase-2. J Exp Clin Cancer Res. 2017; 36 (1):44. doi: 10.1186/s13046-017-0514-4.

Michelle Nonato de Oliveira Melo[1], Alan Clavelland Ochioni[2], Patricia Zancan[2], Adriana Passos Oliveira[1], Mirio Grazi[3], Rafael Garrett[4], Prof. Dr. Carla Holandino[1,3], Prof. Dr. Stephan Baumgartner[3,5]

[1] Multidisciplinary Laboratory of Pharmaceutical Sciences, Universidade Federal do Rio de Janeiro, Rio de Janeiro, Brazil.

[2] Laboratório de Oncobiologia Molecular (LabOMol), Universidade Federal do Rio de Janeiro, Rio de Janeiro, Brazil.

[3] Hiscia Institute, Society for Cancer Research, Arlesheim, Switzerland.

[4] Metabolomics Laboratory, Chemistry Institute, Universidade Federal do Rio de Janeiro, Rio de Janeiro, Brazil.

[5] Institute of Integrative Medicine, University of Witten/Herdecke, Herdecke, Germany.

Corresponding authors:
st.baumgartner@vfk.ch
cholandino@gmail.com

In Vitro Mutagenicity Assessment of Aqueous *Viscum album* L. Preparations

Bewertung der *in vitro*-Mutagenität von wässrigen *Viscum album* L. Zubereitungen

Ilona Zilkowski, Claudia Turek, Nora Mörbt, Peter Vögele, Florian C. Stintzing

Summary

Background: *Viscum album* L. preparations obtained from different host trees, conifers as well as deciduous trees, are frequently used in complementary therapy to treat cancer patients. Genotoxic potential of herbal substances and preparations therefrom can be assessed *in vitro*, complementing already existing preclinical and clinical safety data. In the present study, test results of eight different *Viscum album* L. preparations produced according to the official method 38 of the German Homeopathic Pharmacopeia are presented.

Methods: *Viscum album* L. preparations were produced according to current pharmaceutical standards using mistletoe from eight different host trees. The preparations Iscucin® Abietis (fir), Crataegi (hawthorn), Mali (apple), Pini (pine), Populi (poplar), Salicis (willow) and Tiliae (lime) (all strength H, dilution 1:20, 50 mg/ml) and Iscucin® Quercus (oak) (strength F, dilution 1:8000, 0.125 mg/ml) (WALA Heilmittel GmbH, Bad Boll, Germany) were tested for their mutagenic potential in an *in vitro* bacterial reverse mutation assay, with and without exogenic metabolic activation, following current OECD standards.

Results: Under the experimental conditions reported, none of the preparations induced gene mutations by base pair changes or frameshifts in the genome of the bacterial strains used.

Conclusion: None of the tested *Viscum album L.* preparations caused gene mutations. Thus, all items were considered non-mutagenic in this official OECD assay. These new data contribute to a more differentiated preclinical safety assessment of the tested aqueous mistletoe extracts derived from different host trees.

Keywords: Mistletoe extracts, *Viscum album*, genotoxicity

Zusammenfassung

Hintergrund: Zubereitungen aus *Viscum album* L. werden häufig komplementärmedizinisch zur Behandlung von Krebspatienten eingesetzt. Hierzu werden Misteln verschiedener Wirtsbäume, sowohl Nadelbäume als auch Laubbäume, verarbeitet. Das genotoxische Potenzial von pflanzlichen Substanzen und Zubereitungen kann durch *in* vitro Tests bewertet werden und ergänzt die bereits vorhandenen präklinischen und klinischen Sicherheitsdaten. In der vorliegenden Studie werden Testergebnisse von acht verschiedenen Zubereitungen aus *Viscum album* L. vorgestellt, die nach der offiziellen Vorschrift 38 des Homöopathischen Arzneibuches (HAB) hergestellt wurden.

Methoden: Präparate aus *Viscum album* L. wurden nach den gängigen pharmazeutischen Standards aus Misteln von acht verschiedenen Wirtsbäumen hergestellt. Die Präparate Iscucin® Abietis (Tanne), Crataegi (Weißdorn), Mali (Apfel), Pini (Kiefer), Populi (Pappel), Salicis (Weide) und Tiliae (Linde) (alle Stärke H, Verdünnung 1:20, 50 mg/ml) und Iscucin® Quercus (Eiche) (Stärke F, Verdünnung 1:8000, 0.125 mg/ml) (WALA Heilmittel GmbH, Bad Boll, Deutschland) wurden auf ihr mutagenes Potential in einem bakteriellen *in vitro* Rückmutationstest mit und ohne exogene Stoffwechselaktivierung nach den aktuellen OECD-Standards getestet.

Ergebnisse: Unter den angegebenen Versuchsbedingungen induzierte keines der Präparate in den verwendeten Bakterienstämmen Genmutationen durch Basenaustausch oder Rasterverschiebungen.

Schlussfolgerung: Keines der getesteten *Viscum album* L. Präparate verursachte Genmutationen. Somit wurden alle Präparate in diesem offiziellen OECD-Test als nicht mutagen eingestuft. Diese neuen Daten tragen zu einer differenzierteren präklinischen Sicherheitsbewertung der getesteten wässrigen Mistelextrakte aus verschiedenen Wirtsbäumen bei.

Schlüsselwörter: Mistelextrakte, *Viscum album*, Genotoxizität

Introduction

Mistletoe preparations are frequently used in complementary therapy of cancer patients. For the production of mistletoe preparations, *Viscum album* L. from various host trees is used, which can be divided into conifers and deciduous trees. Since the ingredient profile of each mistletoe extract is dependent on the respective host tree (Rostock *et al.* 2020) also the safety profiles of the resulting mistletoe preparations require individual evaluation. In addition to clinical safety data (e. g. Huber *et al.* 2011), preclinical safety data (e.g., genotoxicity testing) are fundamental for overall safety assessment. This article presents *in vitro* test results regarding the mutagenic potential of eight *Viscum album* L. preparations based on eight host trees. The preparations were manufactured according to current pharmaceutical standards. Analysis and evaluation were performed according to up-to-date guidelines of the Committee on Herbal Medicinal Products (HMPC) of the European Medicines Agency (EMA) (HMPC 2008).

Materials and methods

Medicinal products

The test items, authorized anthroposophic medicinal products named Iscucin® Abietis (fir), Crataegi (hawthorn), Mali (apple), Pini (pine), Populi (poplar), Salicis (willow) and Tiliae (lime) (all strength H, dilution 1:20, 50 mg/ml) and Iscucin® Quercus (oak) (strength F, dilution 1:8000, 0.125 mg/l) (WALA Heilmittel GmbH, Bad Boll, Germany), were produced according to current pharmaceutical standards (HAB 38) using aqueous extracts of *Viscum album* L. from the eight indicated host trees.

Reverse mutation assay

Using the plate-incorporation and the pre-incubation method, a reverse mutation assay with *Salmonella typhimurium* (*S. typhimurium*) strains TA98, TA100, TA1535, TA1537 and either TA 102 or *Escherichia coli* (*E. coli*) strain WP2 uvrA was performed in two independent experiments by ICCR-Roßdorf GmbH (Rossdorf, Germany) / BSL Bioservice Scientific Laboratories GmbH (Planegg, Germany) in accordance with good laboratory practice (GLP) and the respective OECD guideline (OECD 2020). Each assay was conducted with and without metabolic activation (S9-mix) and performed in triplicate using positive and negative controls. Several dosing levels up to the recommended maximum test item concentration were applied.

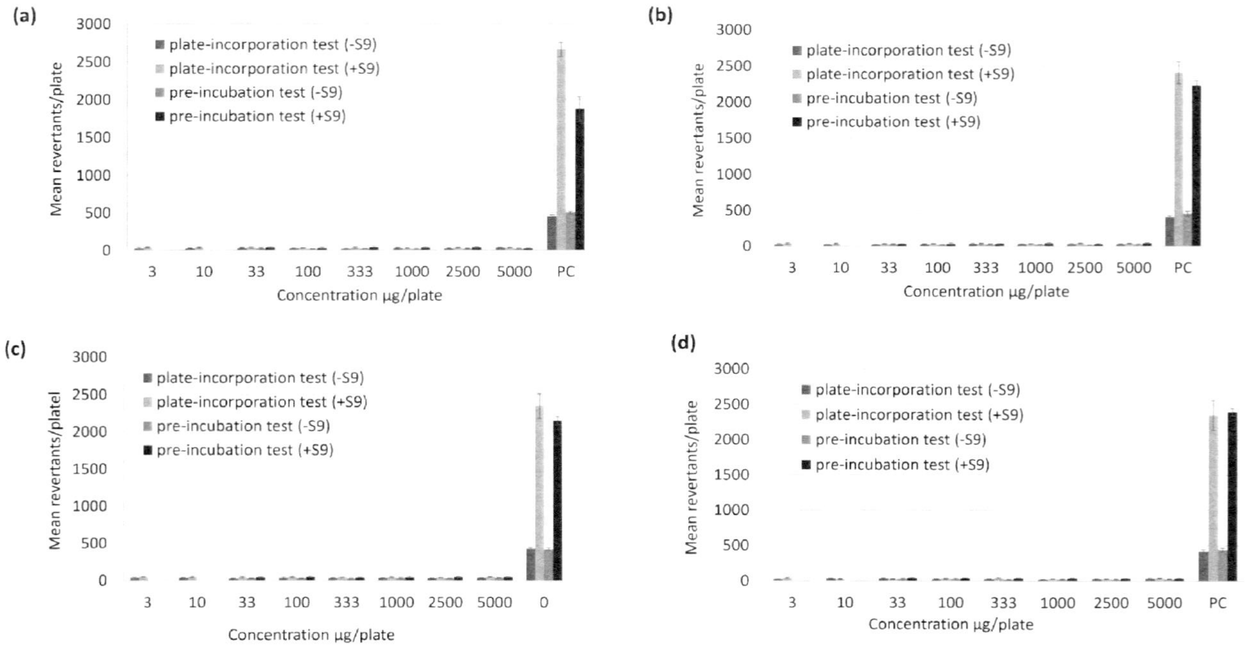

Fig. 1a: Results obtained from the reverse mutation assay with *S. typhimurium* TA98 on Iscucin® Abietis (a), Crataegi (b), Mali (c) and Pini (d) preparations with and without metabolic activation (S9) applying the pre-incubation and plate-incorporation method. PC: positive control (4-nitro-o-phenylene-diamine and 2-aminoanthracene).

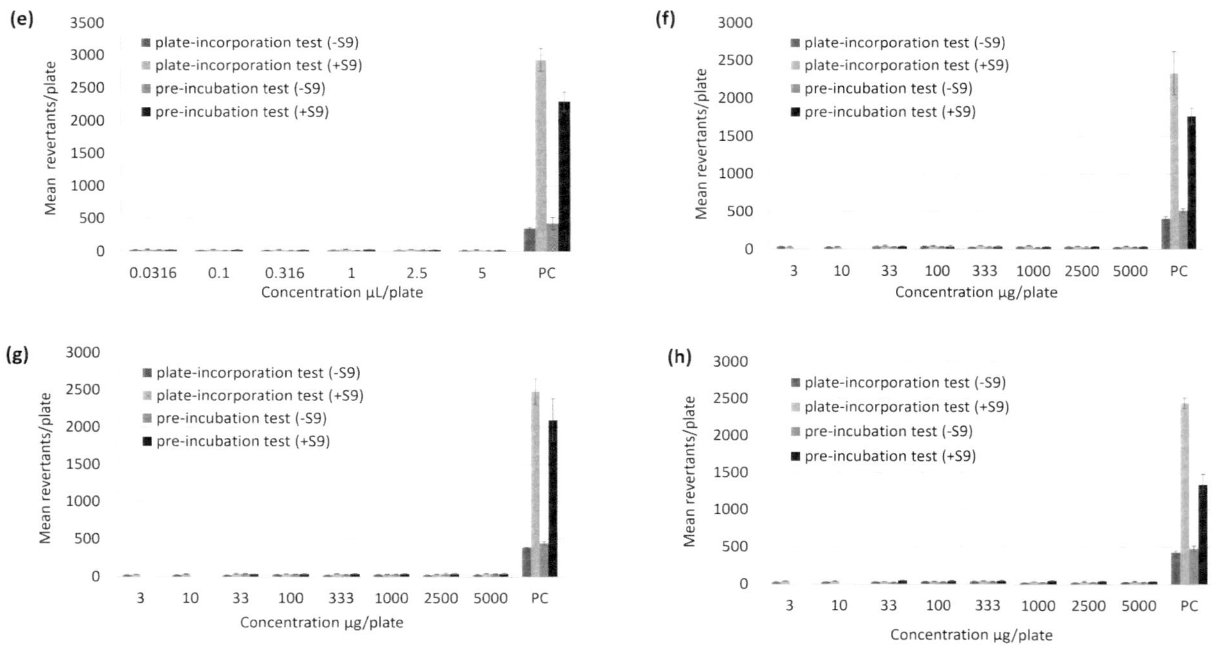

Fig. 1b: Results obtained from the reverse mutation assay with *S. typhimurium* TA98 on Iscucin® Populi (e), Salicis (f), Tiliae (g) and Quercus (h) preparations with and without metabolic activation (S9) applying the pre-incubation and plate-incorporation method. PC: positive control (4-nitro-o-phenylene-diamine and 2-aminoanthracene).).

Results

Under the experimental conditions reported, none of the test items induced gene mutations by base pair changes or frameshifts in the *genome* of the bacterial strains used.

The mutagenic potential of the selected aqueous *Viscum album* L. extracts was evaluated in a plate-incorporation and pre-incubation test on different *S. typhimurium* strains and a *Escherichia coli* strain in order to differentiate between base pair (TA100, TA1535, TA102 or WP2 uvrA) and frame shift (TA98, TA1537) mutations. The tested concentrations of the extracts did not cause any of the mutations mentioned above. Metabolic activation by the addition of mammalian S9 liver microsome fraction did not reveal any mutagenic potential. Furthermore, no toxic effects were observed under the experimental conditions. As an example, the results derived from tester strain TA98 for all extracts are shown in Figure 1.

Discussion and conclusions

According to HMPC (HMPC 2008) recommendations the *in vitro* test system applied likely covers the majority of the relevant genetic changes resulting from interaction of herbal substances with DNA. Although not all genotoxic endpoints can be detected, this assay is considered a pragmatic first step in a multistep approach, taking into account the special characteristics of herbal substances. None of the tested *Viscum album* L. preparations caused gene mutations in this official OECD assay. Following the stepwise approach, no further genotoxicity testing is required. Thus, all preparations are considered non-mutagenic. These new data contribute to a more differentiated preclinical safety assessment of the tested aqueous mistletoe extracts derived from different host trees.

Conflict of interest

Ilona Zilkowski, Nora Mörbt, Peter Vögele and Florian C. Stintzing are employed by WALA Heilmittel GmbH. Claudia Turek has been employed by WALA Heilmittel GmbH at the time of data generation and analysis.

Literature

Huber R, Lüdtke H, Wieber J et al.: Safety and effects of two mistletoe preparations on production of interleukin-6 and other immune parameters – a placebo controlled clinical trial in healthy subjects. BMC Complement Altern Med. 2011; 11: 116. doi: 10.1186/1472-6882-11-116.

HMPC: Guideline on the assessment of genotoxicity of herbal substances/preparations. 2008. https://www.ema.europa.eu/en/documents/scientific-guideline/guideline-assessment-genotoxicity-herbal-substancespreparations_en.pdf.

OECD: Test No. 471: Bacterial Reverse Mutation Test, OECD Guidelines for the Testing of Chemicals. Sektion 4. Paris: OECD Publishing; 2020. --11.

Rostock M: Die Misteltherapie in der Behandlung von Patienten mit einer Krebserkrankung. Bundesgesundheitsbl. 2020; 63: 535–540.

Ilona Zilkowski, Dr. Claudia Turek, Dr. Nora Mörbt, Peter Vögele, Prof. Dr. Florian C. Stintzing
WALA Heilmittel GmbH, Bad Boll/Eckwälden, Germany

Corresponding author:
ilona.zilkowski@wala.de

A Fermented Mistletoe Extract Elicits Endoplasmic Reticulum Stress Driven Immunogenic Cell Death in Breast Cancer and Melanoma Cells

Ein fermentierter Mistelextrakt induziert einen durch Stress im Endoplasmatischen Retikulum hervorgerufenen immunogenen Zelltod in Brustkrebs- und Melanomzellen

Ulrike Weissenstein, Bettina Leonhard, Stephan Baumgartner

Summary

Introduction and objective: Tumors prevent a patient's immune system from recognizing and eliminating them through various escape mechanisms. Immunogenic cancer cell death (ICD) is an important step for the initiation of a specific anti-cancer T-cell response. Triggering ICD can make an existing tumor recognizable and attackable for the immune system. An ideal ICD inducer activates different pathways such as apoptotic cell death, endoplasmic reticulum (ER) stress response and the induction of reactive oxygen species (ROS). An activation of these pathways leads to the cellular expression of damage-associated molecular patterns (DAMPs).

Cancer patients often get extracts from European mistletoe (*Viscum album* L.) as supportive therapy, frequently together with classical oncological treatment procedures. The aim of our in vitro study was to investigate whether mistletoe extracts are able to induce immunogenic tumor cell death.

Methods: Three human breast carcinoma cell lines and one murine melanoma cell line (SKBR3, MDA-MB-231, MCF-7 and B16F10) were treated with an aqueous, fermented *Viscum album* extract (VAE: Iscador Q spez.), Paclitaxel and Tunicamycin (ICD/ER stress inducer positive controls), respectively. Cell surface exposure of DAMPs (Calreticulin, heat shock proteins hsp70 and hsp90) and apoptosis were assessed by flow cytometry. To investigate whether VAE induces ribotoxic stress, we measured the ER stress regulators p-eIF2a, ATF4, and CHOP in the cancer cells by Western blot.

Results: Treatment with either VAE, paclitaxel or tunicamycin induced a cell line and concentration dependent cell surface exposition of DAMPs, which significantly correlated with early apoptosis in all cell lines except MCF-7. Phosphorylation of EIF2α was induced by VAE and tunicamycin. The ER stress inducer tunicamycin also stimulated the expression of ATF4 and CHOP. VAE induced an incomplete ER stress response in all cancer cell lines.
Conclusions: In this *in vitro* study, we demonstrated the potential of mistletoe extracts to induce immunogenic cell death for the first time. This could be of clinical interest especially for a potential application of intratumorally applied mistletoe extracts in combination with systemic cancer immunotherapy.
Keywords: Mistletoe (*Viscum album* L.), mistletoe therapy, immunogenic cell death, oncological immunotherapy

Zusammenfassung
Einleitung und Zielsetzung: Tumoren können Mechanismen entwickeln, die das Immunsystem von Patientinnen und Patienten daran hindern, sie zu erkennen und zu eliminieren. Der immunogene Zelltod (immunogenic cell death, ICD) ist ein wichtiger Schritt für die Auslösung einer spezifischen T-Zell-Antwort gegen Krebszellen. Die Auslösung des ICD kann einen vorhandenen Tumor für das Immunsystem erkennbar und angreifbar machen. Durch Medikamente, die einen ICD induzieren, werden verschiedene Signalwege wie der apoptotische Zelltod, die Stressreaktion des endoplasmatischen Retikulums (ER) und die Induktion reaktiver Sauerstoffspezies (ROS) aktiviert. Das führt zur zellulären Expression von schadensassoziierten molekularen Mustern (damage-associated molecular patterns, DAMPs).
Krebspatienten erhalten oft Präparate aus der Europäischen Mistel (*Viscum album* L.) als unterstützende Therapie, häufig zusammen mit klassischen onkologischen Behandlungsverfahren. Ziel unserer *in vitro*-Studie war es zu untersuchen, ob Mistelextrakte in der Lage sind, einen immunogenen Tumorzelltod zu induzieren.
Methoden: Drei humane Brustkrebs- und eine murine Melanomzelllinie (SKBR3, MDA-MB-231, MCF-7 und B16F10) wurden mit einem wässrigen, fermentierten *Viscum album*-Extrakt (VAE: Iscador Q spez.), Paclitaxel bzw. Tunicamycin (ICD/ER-Stressinduktor-Positivkontrollen) behandelt. Die Exposition der DAMPs Calreticulin, Hitzeschockprotein 70 (hsp70) und Hitzeschockprotein 90 (hsp90) auf der Zelloberfläche und die Apoptose wurden mittels Durchflusszytometrie analysiert.

Um zu untersuchen, ob VAE ribotoxischen Stress auslöst, haben wir die ER-Stressregulatoren p-eIF2a, ATF4 und CHOP in den Tumorzellen mittels Western Blot gemessen.
Ergebnisse: Die Behandlung mit VAE, Paclitaxel oder Tunicamycin induzierte eine zelllinien- und konzentrationsabhängige Exposition der DAMPs an der Zelloberfläche, die bei allen Zelllinien außer MCF-7 signifikant mit einem frühen Stadium der Apoptose korrelierte. Die Phosphorylierung von EIF2α wurde sowohl durch VAE und Tunicamycin induziert. Der ER-Stress-Induktor Tunicamycin aber nicht VAE stimulierte außerdem die Expression von ATF4 und CHOP. VAE induzierte demzufolge eine unvollständige ER-Stressreaktion in den Tumorzellen.
Schlussfolgerungen: In dieser *in vitro*-Studie konnten wir erstmals das Potenzial von Mistelextrakten zur Induktion eines immunogenen Zelltodes nachweisen. Dies könnte von klinischem Interesse sein, insbesondere für eine mögliche Anwendung von intratumoral applizierten Mistelextrakten in Kombination mit einer systemischen onkologischen Immuntherapie.
Schlüsselwörter: Mistel (*Viscum album* L.), Misteltherapie, immunogener Zelltod, onkologische Immuntherapie

Conflict of interest

The Society for Cancer Research holds a minority share in stocks of the manufacturer (Iscador AG, Arlesheim, Switzerland) of the mistletoe extracts investigated. S. Baumgartner is part-time employee of Iscador AG.

Dr. Ulrike Weissenstein[1], Bettina Leonhard[1],
Prof. Dr. Stephan Baumgartner[1, 2]
[1] Verein für Krebsforschung, Arlesheim, Schweiz
[2] Iscador AG, Arlesheim, Schweiz

Corresponding author:
u.weissenstein@vfk.ch

Einfluss eines Mistelextrakts in Kombination mit einer Checkpoint-Inhibitor-Therapie auf die Aktivität der natürlichen Killerzellen gegen Brustkrebsspheroide

Effect of Mistletoe Extract on the Activity of Natural Killer Cells in Combination With Checkpoint Inhibitor Therapy Against Breast Cancer Spheroids

Michael Schink, Eugenia Violeta Díez García de Olalla, Alexander Sebastian Franzén, Martin J. Raftery, Sabine Rieger, Gabriele Pecher

Zusammenfassung

Hintergrund: Helixor® A ist ein Mistelextrakt, der in der integrativen Medizin häufig verwendet wird, unter anderem zur supportiven Krebsbehandlung von Brustkrebspatientinnen mit aggressiven Tumoren. Da Checkpoint-Inhibitoren wie Atezolizumab (PD-L1 Blocker) und Pembrolizumab (PD-1 Blocker) ebenfalls immer häufiger zur Behandlung dieser Patientengruppe zum Einsatz kommen, ist es wichtig, mögliche Interaktionen von Helixor® A mit diesen blockierenden Antikörpern zu untersuchen.

Methoden: Die 2D-Zellkultur-Experimente wurden mit den Mammakarzinom (MK)-Zelllinien HCC1937 und T47D durchgeführt. Mit diesen Zelllinien wurden auch Spheroide für weitere Experimente gebildet. Die MK-Zelllinien dienten zusammen mit K562 Zellen als Targets für die Bestimmung der NK-Zellaktivität. Hierzu wurden alle drei Zelllinien so modifiziert, dass sie Nano-Luciferase zur Verwendung im NK-Zellaktivitätstest in stabiler Form exprimierten. Die Isolierung der NK-Zellen erfolgte aus Blut/Buffy coats gesunder menschlicher Spender mittels Standardverfahren. Die Effekte von Helixor® A, Pembrolizumab und Atezolizumab auf die NK-Zellaktivität wurden einzeln oder in Kombination in Konzentrationen von 1 µg/ml und 10 µg/ml geprüft. Die Bestimmung der Expressionsdichte der Oberflächenmarker CD63, EpCAM, PD-L1 und CEACAM5 auf den MK-Zellen erfolgte durchflusszytometrisch.

Ergebnisse: Helixor® A zeigte unter den gewählten Bedingungen keine Effekte auf die NK-Zellaktivität, d. h. das Präparat schien die Targetzelllyse der PD-1 negativen oder PD-1 schwach exprimierenden NK-Zellen gesunder Spender weder zu beeinträchtigen, noch zu fördern. Desweiteren hatte Helixor® A auch keinen signifikanten Einfluss auf die Effekte von Atezolizumab oder Pembrolizumab auf die NK-Zellaktivität. Es konnte dagegen gezeigt werden, dass Helixor® A die PD-L1-Expression speziell in den 3D-Spheroiden signifikant reduzieren kann.

Schlussfolgerung: Diese Ergebnisse verdeutlichen, dass die Effekte potenzieller Krebstherapien eher in 3D-Spheroidmodellen als in 2D-Zellkulturen untersucht werden sollten. So war die Expressionsdichte von PD-L1 auf den Brustkrebszellen in den beiden Modellen unterschiedlich und Helixor® A konnte diesen Marker ausschließlich unter 3D-Bedingungen signifikant reduzieren. Auch im Hinblick auf die Zytotoxizitätstests und die Effekte von Helixor® A auf die NK-Zellaktivität konnten Unterschiede zwischen den beiden Kulturmodellen beobachtet werden.

Schlüsselwörter: Triple-negativer Brustkrebs, Mistel, Spheroide, PD-L1, Checkpoint Inhibitoren, natürliche Killerzellen, Antikörpertherapie

Summary

Background: Helixor® A is a mistletoe extract widely used in integrative medicine as a supplementary cancer therapy, including breast cancer patients with aggressive tumors. Since checkpoint inhibitors, like Atezolizumab (PD-L1 blocker) and Pembrolizumab (PD-1 blocker), are becoming more widely used to treat such patients, it is important to research the interactions of Helixor® A, and these antibody blockers.

Methods: 2D cell culture experiments were carried out with the cell lines HCC1937 and T47D. These cell lines were also used to form spheroids for further experiments. The BC cell lines and K562 cells were used as target cells for NK cell cytotoxicity testing. For this, all three cell lines were modified to express NanoLuciferase in a stable manner to be used to carry out NK cell cytotoxicity assays. The NK cells were isolated from healthy human donor blood/buffy coats according to standard procedures. The effect of Helixor® A, Pembrolizumab and Atezolizumab were tested alone and in combination at concentrations of 1 µg/ml and 10 µg/ml, respectively on NK cell cytotoxicity. Surface marker expression (CD63, EpCAM, PD-L1, and CEACAM5) on BC cells was analyzed by use of a flow cytometer.

Results: There was no effect of Helixor® A on NK cell cytotoxicity under the conditions tested. It seems that Helixor® A doesn't hinder nor aid the target cell lysis with PD-1 negative or PD-1 low expressing NK cells from healthy donors. Moreover, Helixor® A did not significantly affect the effect of Atezolizumab or Pembrolizumab on NK cell cytotoxicity. On the other hand, it was found that in BC spheroids, Helixor® A significantly reduced PD-L1 expression.
Conclusion: These findings highlight the importance of studying potential cancer therapies in spheroid models rather than in a 2D cell culture model. Not only were PD-L1 expression levels different, but also the effect of Helixor® A on this marker was only significantly observed under 3D conditions. Furthermore, in regard to the cytotoxicity assays and the effect of Helixor® A on NK cell cytotoxicity, a different effect on NK cytotoxicity was seen when comparing the two culture conditions.
Keywords: Triple-negative breast cancer, mistletoe, spheroids, PD-L1, checkpoint inhibitors, natural killer cells, antibody therapy

Interessenkonflikt

Die Autoren erklären, dass die Forschung in Abwesenheit jeglicher kommerzieller oder finanzieller Beziehungen durchgeführt wurde, die als potenzieller Interessenkonflikt ausgelegt werden könnten. MS und SR sind Mitarbeiter des Sponsors. Der Sponsor hatte keinen Einfluss auf die Konzeption, Planung, Durchführung oder Analyse der Untersuchungen.

Dr. Michael Schink[1], Eugenia Violeta Díez García de Olalla[2], Alexander Sebastian Franzén[2], Dr. Martin J. Raftery[2], Sabine Rieger[1], Prof. Dr. med. Gabriele Pecher[2]
[1] Helixor Heilmittel GmbH, Rosenfeld, Deutschland
[2] Kompetenzzentrum Immunonkologie und Translationale Zelltherapie (KITZ), Medizinische Klinik m.S. Hämatologie, Onkologie und Tumorimmunologie, CCM, Charité-Universitätsmedizin Berlin, Deutschland

Korrespondenzadresse:
mschink@helixor.de

III. Klinische Anwendung

a) Studien, Fallberichte, klinische Erfahrung

III. Clinical Application

a) Studies, Case Reports, Clinical Experience

Improvement of Quality of Life in Lung Cancer Patients Receiving Targeted Oncological Treatment in Combination With *Viscum album* L.

Verbesserung der Lebensqualität von Lungenkrebspatienten unter zielgerichteter onkologischer Therapie in Kombination mit *Viscum album* L.

Shiao Li Oei, Anja Thronicke, Hannah Wüstefeld, Christian Grah, Friedemann Schad

Summary

Background: Lung cancer (LC) is associated with high mortality and poor quality of life (QoL), but advances in diagnosis and targeted oncology are improving patient prognosis and survival. In previous evaluations, we have reported that combined systemic oncological treatment with *Viscum album* L. (VA) extracts is feasible and the aim of this study was to analyze the self-reported QoL of LC patients.

Methods: The real-world-data study was conducted using data from an oncological registry accredited by the German Cancer Society (DRKS00013335). Self-reported QoL of LC patients was assessed by evaluation of the European Organization of Research and Treatment Health-Related Quality of Life Core Questionnaire scale (EORTC QLQ-C30). Factors associated with QoL changes were analyzed with adjusted multivariate linear regression analyses using R software.

Results: A total of 112 primary all-stage LC patients (median age 70 years) answered QoL questionnaires at diagnosis and 12 months later. In addition to standard systemic oncological treatments 53 (47 %) patients received VA applications. Targeted treatments including immune checkpoint inhibitors were given to 47 (42 %) patients, 36 of them in combination with VA applications. Twelve months after diagnosis, significant improvements in global health, symptoms of fatigue and constipation were observed in patients receiving combined targeting/VA therapy.

Conclusions: The addition of VA therapy appears to be associated with improved self-reported QoL in LC patients 12 months after diagnosis.
Keywords: Immune checkpoint inhibitors, lung cancer, quality of life, *Viscum album* L.

Zusammenfassung

Hintergrund: Lungenkrebs (LK) ist mit einer hohen Sterblichkeitsrate und einer schlechten Lebensqualität verbunden, aber dank der Fortschritte bei der Diagnose und Behandlung mit zielgerichteten Onkologika verbessern sich Prognose und Überleben von LK-Patienten zunehmend. In früheren Auswertungen berichteten wir, dass eine kombinierte systemische onkologische Behandlung mit Extrakten aus *Viscum album* L. (VA) durchführbar ist, und das Ziel dieser Studie war es, die selbstberichtete Lebensqualität der behandelten Patienten zu evaluieren.

Methoden: Diese Real-World Data-Studie wurde mit Daten aus einem von der Deutschen Krebsgesellschaft akkreditierten onkologischen Register durchgeführt (DRKS00013335). Die selbstberichtete Lebensqualität wurde durch Auswertung der European Organization of Research and Treatment Health-Related Quality of Life Core Questionnaire Skala (EORTC QLQ-C30) erfasst. Die Assoziationsfaktoren der Lebensqualitätsänderungen wurden durch adjustierte multivariate lineare Regressionsanalysen unter Verwendung der Software R analysiert.

Ergebnisse: Insgesamt 112 primäre LK-Patienten in allen Stadien (Medianalter 70 Jahre) beantworteten Fragebögen zur Lebensqualität bei der Diagnose und 12 Monate später. Zusätzlich zu den standardmäßigen systemischen onkologischen Behandlungen erhielten 53 (47 %) Patienten VA-Anwendungen. Zielgerichtete Therapien einschließlich Immun-Checkpoint-Inhibitoren wurden 47 (42 %) Patienten verabreicht, 36 davon in Kombination mit VA-Anwendungen. Zwölf Monate nach der Diagnose wurden bei den Patienten, die eine Kombinationstherapie aus zielgerichteter Therapie und VA erhielten, signifikante Verbesserungen des allgemeinen Gesundheitszustands, der Erschöpfung und der Verstopfung beobachtet.

Schlussfolgerungen: Eine zusätzliche VA-Therapie scheint bei LK-Patientinnen und -patienten 12 Monate nach der Diagnose mit einer Verbesserung der selbst eingeschätzten Lebensqualität verbunden zu sein.
Schlüsselwörter: Immun-Checkpoint-Inhibitoren, Lebensqualität, Lungenkrebs, *Viscum album* L.

Introduction

Lung cancer (LC) remains the leading cause of cancer deaths worldwide (Siegel *et al.* 2022) and is also associated with poor quality of life (QoL). For LC patients in particular, impairments are reported in the emotional, physical, social, and cognitive domains, as well as in activities of daily living (Bennett *et al.* 2017). Biomarker-directed targeted therapies (tt) currently are endorsed by several clinical oncology guidelines, and in clinical practice, these advances in recent years have led to significant improvements in overall survival (Cameron *et al.* 2022). Since 2011, kinase inhibitor therapies with ceri-, crizo-, erlo-, and afatinib have been approved and in addition a meta-analysis found that treatments with immune checkpoint inhibitors were associated with better QoL and longer time to clinical worsening compared with chemotherapy (Boutros *et al.* 2021). However, despite the obvious benefits of ICIs, these drugs may affect multiple organ systems, and their use can be associated with severe adverse effects, which requires appropriate long-term management (Brahmer *et al.* 2018). *Viscum album* L. (VA)-extracts have effectively been utilized as an add-on therapy of cancer treatment in Europe, with the goal to reduce disease- and treatment-related symptoms and to improve QoL (Loef, Walach 2020). In previous studies, we reported that combined therapies of tt and VA extracts are feasible and safe in cancer patients (Thronicke *et al.* 2018; Thronicke *et al.* 2017). Patient-reported outcome measures (PROs) are commonly included in LC clinical trials, but few publications have systematically addressed self-reported QoL in LC patients (Wood *et al.* 2019) and only little is known about combined treatments with VA extracts with respect to QoL in patients with LC (Bar-Sela *et al.* 2013; Piao *et al.* 2004). In a real-world data (RWD) study, our group has shown that LC patients, especially younger LC patients report increased pain, low mood and financial difficulties at diagnosis before treatment (Thronicke *et al.* 2020). The present longitudinal RWD study investigated changes in self-reported QoL in LC patients and its associations with applied VA treatment alone or in combination with targeted treatment.

Methods

Study design and patients

We conducted a longitudinal RWD study by extracting and analyzing demographic data, information on diagnosis, histology, as well as integrative oncological treatment data from the oncological registry Network Oncology (NO) (Schad *et al.* 2013).

Ethics approval

The study complies with the principles laid down in the Declaration of Helsinki and has been approved by the ethics committee of the Medical Association Berlin (Berlin – Ethik-Kommission der Ärztekammer Berlin). The reference number is Eth-27/10, it has been retrospectively registered at the WHO-approved registry German Registry for Clinical Trials (Deutsches Register Klinischer Studien, DRKS), trial registration number DRKS00013335 on 27/11/2017. Written informed consent has been obtained from all patients prior to study enrollment.

Data collection

Patients with a histologically proven primary diagnosis of LC, seen and treated at the certified German Lung Cancer Center (GKH, Berlin, Germany) between 2013 and 2021, were screened. Patients were enrolled in the study from which assessable QoL data sets at least for T0 (diagnosis) and T1 (12 months after diagnosis) were available. The details of tumor stage, received surgery, radiation, and all treatment regimens were retrieved from the NO registry. All data reported here are based on retrievable data from the NO registry at cut-off date of July 15, 2021. Surveys were conducted using the European Organization of Research and Treatment Health-Related Quality of Life Core Questionnaire (EORTC QLQ-C30) (Aaronson *et al.* 1993).

Statistical analysis

Demographic and diagnostic variables were collected at T0. Continuous variables were described as median with interquartile range (IQR); categorical variables were summarized as frequencies and percentages. Multivariable regression analyses were performed to identify influencing factors and to address potential sources of bias and confounders. For various treatments regimen rank-ordered variables were assigned. Zero was allocated for no treatment, 1 was allocated when a treatment occurred within the observation period of 12 months. p-values < 0.05 were considered to be significant. All statistical analyses were performed using the software R (R Version 3.1.2 (2014)).

Results

Patients' characteristics

A total of 112 LC patients, diagnosed and treated between 2013 and 2021 in the certified German LC center, answered the EORTCT QLQ-C30 questionnaires at first diagnosis (T0) and 12 months later (T1). For longitudinal analyses of treatment regimens, the 112 patients were allocated to four different groups according to the therapies they received within the twelve months. 48 patients receiving neither tt nor VA served as reference group, 17 patients receiving VA applications without tt were allocated to the VA group, 11 patients receiving tt without VA were allocated to the tt group, and 36 patients received combined tt and VA were allocated to the ttVA group. In Table 1, the main characteristics of analyzed patients are given for the entire study cohort and the groups separately. Major differences in age, gender, histology, and tumor stages were found between the groups.

Table 1: Baseline characteristics of lung cancer patients

	total n = 112 (100 %)	reference n = 48 (43 %)	VA n = 17 (15 %)	tt n = 11 (10 %)	ttVA n = 36 (32 %)
Sex: Men n (%)	50 (45)	26 (54)	7 (41)	6 (55)	11 (31)
Women n (%)	62 (55)	22 (46)	10 (59)	5 (45)	25 (69)
			p = 0.52	p = 1	p = 0.053
Age, years, median (IQR)	70 (63–75)	70 (63–75)	67 (59–74)	73 (71–77)	66 (66–75)
			p = 0.396	p = 0.125	p = 0.116
Histology					
Non-small cell LC (NSCLC)	103 (92)	45 (94)	16 (94)	11 (100)	31 (86)
Small cell LC (SCLC)	6 (5)	1 (2)	1 (6)	0	4 (11)
Other[#]	3 (3)	2 (4)	0	0	1 (3)
			p = 0.523	p = 0.70	p = 0.217
UICC tumor stage:					
I	23 (21)	21 (44)	2 (12)	0	0
II	13 (12)	10 (21)	2 (12)	1 (16)	0
III	30 (27)	12 (25)	6 (35)	4 (31)	8 (22)
IV	46 (41)	5 (10)	7 (41)	6 (22)	28 (78)
			p = 0.011*	**p = 0.002***	**p < 0.001***

IQR, Interquartile Range; significant p-values are indicated: *: p-value < 0.05. [#]Other: One spindle cell carcinoid, two carcinoids without further specification

In Table 2, the treatments received within the observation period of 12 months are listed. 47 (42 %) patients received tt, of which 33 (70 %) ICIs and 15 (32 %) patients kinase inhibitors. In addition to standard guideline oncological systemic therapy, 53 (47 %) patients received VA applications.

Table 2: Treatments of lung cancer patients

n = 112 (100 %)	N (%)
Surgery	**62 (100 %)**
Radiation (Rad)	**56 (100 %)**
Chemotherapy (Ctx)	**69 (100 %)**
Targeted (tt)	**47 (42 %)**
kinase inhibitors	15 (13 %)
immune checkpoint inhibitors	33 (29 %)
***Viscum album L.* (VA)**	**53 (47 %)**
subcutaneous	49 (44 %)
intravenous	35 (31 %)
intra-tumoural/-pleural	3 (3 %)

The numbers in rows and columns of treatments applied to patients do not necessarily add to one hundred percent as patients may have received various combinations of preparations. N, numbers.

Evaluation of longitudinal EORTC QLQ-C30 changes

For 112 patients completed EORTC QLQ-C30 questionnaires at T0 and T1 were available, analyzed, and longitudinal changes from T0 to T1 for all 15 EORTC QLQ-C30 scale scores were calculated. All EORTC QLQ-C30 scores at T0 were within the range of formerly published EORTC QLQ-C30 reference values for LC patients and similar as published previously (Thronicke *et al.* 2020). Adjusted multivariate regression analyses were performed with classification into VA, tt, and ttVA groups and patients receiving neither tt nor VA as the reference group (Table 3). Improvements on functional scales are indicated by positive estimates, while symptoms are indicated by negative estimates.

Table 3: Association factors for combined treatments and changes of QoL

n = 112 Functional	**QL**	**PF**	**RF**	**EF**		**CF**		**SF**	
Reference no tt no VA (n = 48)									
tt, n = 11	3.81	-8.35	-13.46	-1.47		-8.11		-15.07	
VA, n = 17	-0.40	9.35	6.59	0.17		9.88		10.11	
ttVA, n = 36	**14.01***	7.65	2.92	7.68		9.84		1.85	
Symptoms	**FA**	**NV**	**PA**	**DY**	**SL**	**AP**	**CO**	**DI**	**FI**
Reference no tt no VA (n = 48)									
tt, n = 11	1.98	12.55	4.89	9.12	4.02	17.23	5.94	12.61	5.18
VA, n = 17	-5.72	-6.11	-12.21	-6.55	-4.92	-9.55	-9.98	3.45	3.11
ttVA, n = 36	**-11.88***	-5.33	-10.91	-11.53	-8.67	-9.09	**-19.20***	1.46	7.50

Multivariate linear regression analyses, adjusted for gender, age, date of first diagnosis, and the respective QoL-values at T0, were performed for EORTC QLQ-C30 scale changes (T0→T1) and oncological treatments. Improvements > 10 are highlighted in dark grey and deteriorations > 10 in pale grey. *Significant p-values are indicated. tt, targeted; VA, *Viscum album* L.; ttVA, combined tt and VA treatment; QL, global health status; functional scales: PF, physical; RF, role; EF, emotional; CF, cognitive; SF, social; symptoms: FA, fatigue; NV, nausea/ vomiting; PA, pain; DY, dyspnea; SL, insomnia; AP, appetite loss; CO, constipation; DI, diarrhea; FI, financial difficulties.

Functional scales and symptoms worsened in the tt group but improved in the VA groups. Significant improvements for changes of global health (estimate β = 14.01; p = 0.011), symptoms fatigue (estimate β = -11.88; p = 0.047), and constipation (estimate β = -19.2; p = 0.013) were found for ttVA combined treated patients (Table 3).

Discussion

This study is the first to systematically assess targeted treatments in combination with VA applications and QoL for a larger number of cases. The results of the present RWD study demonstrate that significant improvements in self-reported QoL were observed in LC patients receiving VA therapy, particularly in combination with targeted therapy.

In several high-quality clinical trials PROs are integrated but are not primary outcome measures, and significant improvements on QoL measures have never been reported (Malone *et al.* 2021). In a longitudinal study of 32 advanced LC patients, was found that adverse skin toxicities were associated with targeted treatments, caused discomfort and affected QoL (Chan *et al.* 2019). A large population-based study found that patients who were prescribed kinase inhibitors shortly before death had a significantly higher need for acute care interventions, such as multiple emergency department visits, hospitalizations, or admissions to intensive care units (Tsai *et al.* 2018). A meta-analysis of ICIs in SCLS patients found that ICIs resulted in immune-related toxicities, but neither study reported a clinically meaningful change in QoL scores over the course of the study (Korde *et al.* 2022). The relevance of results from controlled clinical trials is somewhat limited because not all patients are represented due to inclusion and exclusion criteria, e.g., multiple comorbidities, etc. This may explain why an LC registry-based study of PROs and ICIs reported a higher rate of adverse events than previously reported in clinical trials (Jim *et al.* 2020). A recently published observational study of 162 ICI-treated patients with myeloma or NSCLC found that the most commonly reported clinically relevant symptoms were: inactivity, fatigue, pain, cough, and sleep disturbance, which affect patients' well-being (Koldenhof *et al.* 2022). In the present RWD study, associations between VA receipt and longitudinal QoL changes in LC patients after 12 months of treatment were evaluated. Consistent with our findings in LC patients, a randomized trial of 72 inoperable LC patients found significant QoL benefits for the VA group (Bar-Sela *et al.* 2013), and another controlled randomized trial of 223 cancer patients, 94 of whom were diagnosed with LC, reported improvements in fatigue, insomnia, appetite, nausea, and pain with concomitant VA therapy (Piao *et al.* 2004). Notably, significant improvements in changes in global health, fatigue, and constipation, as well as considerable reductions in pain and dyspnea, were observed in patients treated with combined ttVA (Table 3).

Limitations of our study include the nonrandomized, noncontrolled, and unblinded nature of the study design, which is prone to various biases, including selection bias. As the NO registry was not population-based, the participants in the current study should not be considered representative of the larger population of LC patients. In addition, it is unknown whether patients who did not respond to these questionnaires would have reported similar QoL scores to those who did provide data. However, we attempted to reduce confounding bias by performing adjusted multivariate linear regression analyses. Nevertheless, this RWD study provides implications for the clinical efficacy of concomitant VA treatment in LC patients that are consistent with published data in LC patients and for other cancer entities. Unwanted biases may have been introduced into the analyses, e.g., physicians may have inadvertently selected patients with a better prognosis for VA therapy. The strengths of our study include the presentation of real-world data, longitudinal data collection, and that confounding was reduced by conducting adjusted multivariate regression analyses.

Conclusions

Our results suggest that LC patients receiving VA therapy are supported in several parameters of their QoL, in particular significant benefits in self-reported global health, fatigue and constipation appear to be associated with combined ttVA treatment. This highlights the importance of considering and evaluating combined oncologic treatments with VA in future concepts to improve clinical outcomes in patients with LC.

Conflict of interest

CG reports grants from grants from Iscador AG, outside the submitted work. FS reports grants from Helixor Heilmittel GmbH (travel costs and honoraria for speaking), grants from AstraZeneca (travel costs and honoraria for speaking), grants from Abnoba GmbH, and grants from Iscador

AG, outside the submitted work. The other authors have declared that no competing interests exist.

References

Aaronson NK et al.: The European Organization for Research and Treatment of Cancer QLQ-C30: a quality-of-life instrument for use in international clinical trials in oncology. J Natl Cancer Inst. 1993; 85 (5): 365–376.

Bar-Sela G, Wollner M, Hammer L et al.: Mistletoe as complementary treatment in patients with advanced non-small-cell lung cancer treated with carboplatin-based combinations: a randomised phase II study. Eur J Cancer. 2013; 49 (5): 1058–1064. doi:10.1016/j.ejca.2012.11.007.

Bennett BM, Wells JR, Panter C, Yuan Y, Penrod JR: The Humanistic Burden of Small Cell Lung Cancer (SCLC): A Systematic Review of Health-Related Quality of Life (HRQoL) Literature. Front Pharmacol. 2017; 8:339. doi:10.3389/fphar.2017.00339.

Boutros A et al.: Health-related quality of life in cancer patients treated with immune checkpoint inhibitors in randomised controlled trials: A systematic review and meta-analysis. Eur J Cancer. 2021; 159: 154–166. doi:10.1016/j.ejca.2021.10.005.

Brahmer JR et al.: Management of Immune-Related Adverse Events in Patients Treated With Immune Checkpoint Inhibitor Therapy: American Society of Clinical Oncology Clinical Practice Guideline. J Clin Oncol. 2018; 36 (17): 1714–1768. doi:10.1200/jco.2017.77.6385.

Cameron LB, Hitchen N, Chandran E et al.: Targeted therapy for advanced anaplastic lymphoma kinase (<I>ALK</I>)-rearranged non-small cell lung cancer. Cochrane Database Syst Rev. 2022; 1 (1): CD013453. doi:10.1002/14651858.CD013453.pub2.

Chan JC, Lee YH, Liu CY et al.: A Correlational Study of Skin Toxicity and Quality of Life in Patients With Advanced Lung Cancer Receiving Targeted Therapy. J Nurs Res. 2019; 27 (6): e51. doi:10.1097/jnr.0000000000000339.

Jim HSL, Eisel SL, Hoogland AI et al.: Use of a Cancer Registry to Evaluate Patient-Reported Outcomes of Immune Checkpoint Inhibitors. Cancers (Basel). 2020; 13 (1): 103. doi:10.3390/cancers13010103.

Koldenhof JJ et al.: Patient-Reported Outcomes During Checkpoint Inhibition: Insight into Symptom Burden in Daily Clinical Practice. J Pain Symptom Manage. 2022; 63 (6): 997–1005. doi:10.1016/j.jpainsym-man.2022.02.013.

Korde R, Veluswamy R, Allaire JC, Barnes G: Small cell lung cancer patients treated with immune checkpoint inhibitor: a systematic literature review of treatment efficacy, safety, and quality of life. Curr Med Res Opin. 2022; 38 (8): 1361–1368. doi:10.1080/03007995.2022.2078101.

Loef M, Walach H: Quality of life in cancer patients treated with mistletoe: a systematic review and meta-analysis. BMC Complement Med Ther. 2020; 20 (1): 227. doi:10.1186/s12906-020-03013-3.

Malone E, Barua R, Meti N et al.: Quality of patient-reported outcomes in oncology clinical trials using immune checkpoint inhibitors: A systematic review. Cancer Medicine. 2021; 10: 5031–5040. doi:10.1002/cam4.4086.

Piao BK, Wang YX, Xie GR et al.: Impact of complementary mistletoe extract treatment on quality of life in breast, ovarian and non-small cell lung cancer patients. A prospective randomized controlled clinical trial. Anticancer Res. 2004; 24 (1): 303–309.

Schad F et al.: Network Oncology (NO) – a clinical cancer register for health services research and the evaluation of integrative therapeutic interventions in anthroposophic medicine. Forsch Komplementmed. 2013; 20 (5): 353–360. doi: 10.1159/000356204.

Siegel RL, Miller KD, Fuchs HE, Jemal A: Cancer statistics, 2022. CA Cancer J Clin. 2022; 72 (1): 7–33. doi:10.3322/caac.21708.

Thronicke A, Oei SL, Merkle A et al.: Clinical Safety of Combined Targeted and Viscum album L. Therapy in Oncological Patients. Medicines (Basel). 2018; 5 (3): 100. doi:10.3390/medicines5030100.

Thronicke A, Steele ML, Grah C et al.: Clinical safety of combined therapy of immune checkpoint inhibitors and Viscum album L. therapy

in patients with advanced or metastatic cancer. BMC Complement Altern Med. 2017; 17 (1): 534. doi:10.1186/s12906-017-2045-0.
Thronicke A, von Trott P, Kröz M et al.: Health-Related Quality of Life in Patients with Lung Cancer Applying Integrative Oncology Concepts in a Certified Cancer Centre. Evid Based Complement Alternat Med. 2020; 5917382. doi:10.1155/2020/5917382.
Tsai HY, Chung KP, Kuo RN: Impact of Targeted Therapy on the Quality of End-of-Life Care for Patients With Non-Small-Cell Lung Cancer: A Population-Based Study in Taiwan. J Pain Symptom Manage. 2018; 55 (3): 798–807. e794. doi:10.1016/j.jpainsymman.2017.10.009.
Wood R, Taylor-Stokes G, Smith F, Chaib C: The humanistic burden of advanced non-small cell lung cancer (NSCLC) in Europe: a real-world survey linking patient clinical factors to patient and caregiver burden. Quality of Life Research. 2019; 28: 1849–1861. doi:10.1007/s11136-019-02152-6.

Dr. Shiao Li Oei[1], Dr. Anja Thronicke[1], Dr. Christian Grah[2], Dr. Hannah Wüstefeld[2], PD Dr. Friedemann Schad[1, 3]
[1] Forschungsinstitut Havelhöhe, Berlin, Germany
[2] Pneumologie, Gemeinschaftskrankenhaus Havelhöhe Berlin, Germany
[3] Onkologisches Zentrum, Gemeinschaftskrankenhaus Havelhöhe, Berlin, Germany

Corresponding author:
shiaoli.oei@havelhoehe.de

Verbesserung der Lebensqualität von Lungenkrebspatienten nach Bestrahlung und additiver *Viscum album* L. Therapie: Eine Real-World Data-Studie

Improvement of Quality of Life in Lung Cancer Patients Receiving Radiotherapy in Combination With *Viscum album* L.: A Real-World Data Study

Friedemann Schad, Diana Steinmann, Anja Thronicke, Christian Grah, Shiao Li Oei

Zusammenfassung

Hintergrund: Lungenkrebs (LK) ist mit sehr ungünstigen Prognosen und einer deutlich eingeschränkten Lebensqualität verbunden. Es hat sich gezeigt, dass eine additive Therapie mit Extrakten aus *Viscum album* L. (Weißbeerige Europäische Mistel, VA) in der Anwendung sicher ist, im Allgemeinen nur leichte Nebenwirkungen auftreten und die Lebensqualität von Krebspatienten verbessern kann. Ziel dieser Studie war es, die Veränderungen der selbstberichteten Lebensqualität von LK-Patienten zu evaluieren, die zusätzlich zur Standard-Strahlentherapie mit Mistelpräparaten behandelt wurden.

Methoden: Diese Real-World Data-Studie wurde mit Daten aus einem von der Deutschen Krebsgesellschaft akkreditierten onkologischen Register durchgeführt (DRKS00013335). Die selbst eingeschätzte Lebensqualität wurde durch Auswertung der European Organization of Research and Treatment Health-Related Quality of Life Core Questionnaire Skala (EORTC QLQ-C30) erfasst. Die Assoziationsfaktoren der Lebensqualitätsänderungen wurden durch adjustierte multivariate lineare Regressionsanalysen unter Verwendung der Software R analysiert.

Ergebnisse: Insgesamt 112 primäre LK-Patienten (Medianalter 70 Jahre, 45 % männlich, 41 % UICC-Stadium IV) beantworteten Fragebögen zur Lebensqualität bei der Diagnose und 12 Monate später.

Die Evaluation der Lebensqualität Veränderungen nach 12 Monaten ergab bei den Patienten, die eine Kombination aus radioonkologischer Bestrahlung und VA-Therapie erhielten, eine signifikante Verbesserung von 27 Punkten für Schmerzen (p = 0,006) und 17 Punkten für Übelkeit und Erbrechen (p = 0,005). Darüber hinaus wurden Verbesserungen von 15 bis 21 Punkten für die Rollenfunktion (p = 0,03), die physische (p = 0,02), kognitive (p = 0,04) und die soziale Funktionsfähigkeit (p = 0,04) bei den mit Standardtherapie ohne Bestrahlung behandelten Patienten, die eine additive VA-Therapie erhielten, festgestellt.

Schlussfolgerungen: Die additive VA-Therapie hat einen positiven Einfluss auf die Lebensqualität von LK-Patienten. In Kombination mit einer radioonkologischen Bestrahlung wurde insbesondere eine signifikante Reduktion von Schmerzen und Übelkeit/Erbrechen beobachtet.

Schlüsselwörter: Radiotherapie, Lebensqualität, Lungenkrebs, *Viscum album* L.

Summary

Background: Lung cancer (LC) is associated with a unfavorable prognosis and a significantly reduced quality of life. It has been shown that an additive therapy with extracts of *Viscum album* L. (mistletoe, VA) is safe to use, generally causes only mild side effects and can improve the quality of life of cancer patients. The aim of this study was to evaluate the changes in self-reported quality of life of LK patients treated with mistletoe preparations in addition to standard radiotherapy.

Methods: The real-world-data study was conducted using data from an oncological registry accredited by the German Cancer Society (DRKS00013335). Self-reported quality of life of LC patients was assessed by evaluation of the European Organization of Research and Treatment Health-Related Quality of Life Core Questionnaire scale (EORTC QLQ-C30). Factors associated with quality of life changes were analyzed with adjusted multivariate linear regression analyses using R software.

Results: A total of 112 primary LC patients (median age 70 years, 45 % male, 41 % UICC stage IV) completed questionnaires on quality of life at diagnosis and 12 months later. The evaluation of quality of life changes after 12 months showed a significant improvement of 27 points for pain (p = 0.006) and 17 points for nausea and vomiting (p = 0.005) in patients who received a combination of radiooncologic radiation and VA therapy.

In addition, improvements of 15 to 21 points were seen for role functioning ($p = 0.03$), physical functioning ($p = 0.02$), cognitive functioning ($p = 0.04$) and social functioning ($p = 0.04$) in patients treated with standard therapy without radiation who received additive VA therapy.
Conclusions: Additive VA therapy has a positive impact on the quality of life of lung cancer patients. In combination with radiation therapy, a significant reduction in pain and nausea/vomiting was observed.
Keywords: Radiotherapy, lung cancer, quality of life, *Viscum album* L.

Einleitung

Die Diagnose Lungenkrebs (LK) ist nach wie vor die häufigste Krebstodesursache weltweit (Siegel *et al.* 2022) und ist häufig mit einer schlechten Lebensqualität verbunden. Aufgrund der Fortschritte bei den Behandlungsmöglichkeiten für LK-Patienten wächst die Zahl der Langzeitüberlebenden und ihre Lebensqualität gewinnt zunehmend an Bedeutung. Krankheitsbedingte Beeinträchtigungen der Lebensqualität betreffen emotionale, körperliche, soziale und kognitive Bereiche sowie die Aktivitäten des täglichen Lebens von Krebspatienten (Bennett *et al.* 2017). Es wurde festgestellt, dass die Verschlechterung der körperlichen Funktionsfähigkeit häufig über zwei Jahre nach der Diagnose von LK andauert, wobei Schmerzen, Müdigkeit, Atemnot und Husten die häufigsten und belastendsten Symptome sind (Poghosyan *et al.* 2013). Die radioonkologische Bestrahlung kann in allen Stadien der LK zum Einsatz kommen (S3-Leitlinie 2022). In Abhängigkeit von den befallenen Lymphknoten, der Leistungsfähigkeit der Patienten mit LK und ihren Begleiterkrankungen oder bei Inoperabilität kann eine neoadjuvante oder definitive Radiochemotherapie mit anschließender Resektion empfohlen werden. Im Stadium IV kann die Strahlentherapie zur Linderung von tumorbedingten Symptomen oder zur Behandlung von Hirnmetastasen eingesetzt werden. Die Evaluierung von Patienten mit verschiedenen Krebsarten, die mit einer palliativen Strahlentherapie für Hirnmetastasen behandelt wurden, ergab eine Verschlechterung der Lebensqualität drei Monate nach der Bestrahlung (Steinmann *et al.* 2012). Ziel der integrativen Krebstherapie ist es, die onkologischen Standardtherapien wie Operation, Chemotherapie oder Bestrahlung durch eine Linderung der Nebenwirkungen zu ergänzen und damit auch die Lebensqualität zu verbessern. *Viscum album L.* (VA)- Extrakte werden in Europa wirksam als Zusatztherapie bei der Krebsbehandlung eingesetzt, mit dem Ziel, krankheits- und behandlungsbedingte Symptome zu lindern und die Lebensqualität zu verbessern (Loef, Walach 2020). In einer früheren Real-World Data-Studie (RWD) hatten wir festgestellt, dass das Sterberisiko bei LK-Patienten im Tumorstadium IV, die mit einer Kombination aus Chemotherapie und VA behandelt wurden, im Vergleich zur alleinigen Chemotherapie reduziert war (Schad *et al.* 2018). Mit der selbstberichteten Lebensqualität von LK-Patienten haben sich bisher nur wenige Publikationen befasst (Wood *et al.* 2019). Im Hinblick auf integrative Behandlungen, wie z. B. mit VA-Extrakten, ist wenig über die selbstberichtete Lebensqualität von LK-Patienten bekannt, und in den meisten klinischen LK-Studien wird die Lebensqualität nur als sekundärer Parameter verfolgt (Bar-Sela *et al.* 2013; Piao *et al.* 2004) In einer weiteren RWD-Studie konnten wir zeigen, dass die finanzielle Sorge von LK-Patienten bei Diagnose im fortgeschrittenem Tumorstadium verstärkt jüngere Patienten betraf und in früheren Tumorstadien signifikant mit Schmerzen assoziiert war (Thronicke *et al.* 2020). Die vorliegende RWD-Längsschnittstudie evaluiert die selbstberichtete Lebensqualität von leitliniengerecht behandelten LK-Patienten im Zusammenhang mit zusätzlichen VA-Behandlungen, die allein oder in Kombination mit radioonkologischer Bestrahlung durchgeführt wurden.

Methoden

Studiendesign und Patienten

Wir führten eine monozentrische longitudinale RWD-Studie durch, in der wir demographische Daten, Informationen zur Diagnose, Histologie, Daten zur integrativen onkologischen Behandlung und Daten zur Lebensqualität aus dem onkologischen Register Netzwerk Onkologie (NO) (Schad *et al.* 2013) extrahierten und analysierten.

Ethik-Zulassung

Die Studie entspricht den Prinzipien der Deklaration von Helsinki und wurde von der Ethikkommission der Ärztekammer Berlin unter der Referenznummer Eth-27/10 genehmigt und beim WHO-anerkannten Deutschen Register Klinischer Studien (DRKS) unter der Studienregistriernummer DRKS00013335 registriert. Vor Einschluss in die Studie wurde von allen Patienten eine schriftliche Einverständniserklärung eingeholt.

Datenerhebung

Eingeschlossen wurden Patienten mit histologisch gesicherter Primärdiagnose eines Lungenkarzinoms, die zwischen 2013 und 2021 im zertifizierten deutschen Lungenkrebszentrum (GKH, Berlin, Deutschland) untersucht und behandelt wurden. Es wurden Patienten in die Studie eingeschlossen, von denen auswertbare Lebensqualitätsfragebögen mindestens für T0 (Erstdiagnose) und T1 (12 Monate nach Diagnosestellung) vorlagen. Alle hier berichteten Daten basieren auf den verfügbaren Daten des NO-Registers zum Stichtag 15. Juli 2021. Für die explorative Evaluation der selbstberichteten Lebensqualität wurde der EORTC-QLQ-C30-Fragebogen verwendet und analysiert, der Bewertungen des globalen Gesundheitszustands, der Funktionsfähigkeit und Symptomskalen enthält (Aaronson *et al.* 1993).

Statistische Auswertung

Demographische und diagnostische Variablen wurden zum Zeitpunkt der Primärdiagnose (T0) erhoben. Kontinuierliche Variablen wurden durch Median und Interquartilbereich (IQR) beschrieben; kategoriale Variablen wurden durch Häufigkeiten und Prozentsätze zusammengefasst. Zur Ermittlung von Unterschieden wurden Students t-Tests durchgeführt; p-Werte $< 0,05$ galten als signifikant. Multivariate lineare Regressionsanalysen wurden durchgeführt, um Einflussfaktoren zu identifizieren und mögliche Quellen von Verzerrungen und Störvariablen zu berücksichtigen. Um zuverlässige Modelle zu erhalten, wurden schrittweise Regressionen durchgeführt und Modelle mit hohem korrigiertem

R^2 ausgewählt. Nach der Interpretation von Cohen (1992) weisen R-Werte zwischen 0,13 und 0,25 auf mittlere und R^2-Werte von 0,26 oder mehr auf hohe Effektstärken hin. p-Werte < 0,05 wurden als signifikant angesehen. Alle statistischen Analysen wurden mit dem Programm R Version 3.1.2 (2014) durchgeführt.

Ergebnisse

Charakteristika der Patienten

Insgesamt 112 Patientinnen und Patienten mit Lungenkrebs, die zwischen 2013 und 2021 in einem zertifizierten Lungenzentrum diagnostiziert und behandelt wurden, beantworteten den EORTCT QLQ-C30-Fragebogen bei Erstdiagnose (T0) und 12 Monate später (T1). Zusätzlich zur leitliniengerechten onkologischen systemischen Standardtherapie erhielten 53 (47 %) Patienten VA-Anwendungen, die im Median 43 Tage (ICR: 23–74 Tage) nach der Erstdiagnose verabreicht wurden. Für die Longitudinalanalysen wurden die 112 Patienten entsprechend der innerhalb von 12 Monaten erhaltenen Therapien in vier verschiedene Gruppen eingeteilt. 27 Patienten, die weder Bestrahlung noch VA erhielten, dienten als Referenzgruppe, 29 Patienten, die VA-Anwendungen ohne Bestrahlung erhielten, wurden der VA-Gruppe zugeordnet, 32 Patienten, die Bestrahlung ohne VA erhielten, wurden der Rad-Gruppe zugeordnet und 24 Patienten, die Bestrahlung und VA erhielten, wurden der kombinierten RadVA-Gruppe zugeordnet. Tabelle 1 zeigt die wichtigsten Charakteristika der untersuchten Patienten für die gesamte Studienkohorte und für jede Gruppe. Hinsichtlich Alter, Geschlecht, Histologie und UICC-Stadien zeigten sich Unterschiede zwischen den Gruppen.

Tab. 1: Charakteristika der Lungenkrebspatienten

	Total n = 112 (100 %)	**Referenz n = 27 (24 %)**	**VA n = 29 (26 %)**	**Rad n = 32 (29 %)**	**RadVA n = 24 (21 %)**
Geschlecht:					
Mann, n (%)	50 (45)	15 (56)	6 (21)	17 (53)	12 (50)
			p = 0.02*	**p = 1**	p = 0.9
Alter:					
Jahre, median (IQR)	70 (63–75)	71 (64–76)	65 (58–74)	72 (67–76)	68 (62–75)
			p = 0.12	p = 0.66	p = 0.36
Histologie:					
Nichtkleinzelliger LK (NSCLC)	103 (92)	25 (93)	29 (100)	31 (97)	18 (75)
Kleinzelliger LK (SCLC)	6 (5)	0	0	1 (3)	5 (21)
Sonstige#	3 (3)	2 (7)	0	0	1 (4)
			p = 0.33	p = 0.20	**p = 0.04***
UICC Tumor Stadien:					
I	23 (21)	11 (41)	2 (7)	10 (31)	0
II	13 (12)	6 (22)	2 (7)	5 (16)	0
III	30 (27)	6 (22)	6 (21)	10 (31)	8 (33)
IV	46 (41)	4 (15)	19 (66)	7 (22)	6 (67)
			p = 0.0004*	p = 0.67	**p = 0.002***

UICC, Union for International Cancer Care; IQR, Interquartilsbereich; Signifikante p-Werte sind angegeben: *: p-Wert < 0,05. #Sonstige: Ein spindelzelliges Karzinoid, zwei Karzinoide ohne weitere Spezifikation.

Alle Patienten wurden gemäß den Empfehlungen eines interdisziplinären Tumorboards leitliniengerecht behandelt. Tabelle 2 listet für die gesamte Studienkohorte alle Behandlungen auf, die im Beobachtungszeitraum von 12 Monaten durchgeführt wurden.

Tab. 2: Therapien von Lungenkrebspatienten

n = 112 (100 %)	**n (%)**
Operation	**62 (55)**
Bestrahlung (Rad)	**56 (50)**
Thorax	45 (40)
Gehirn	14 (13)
Skeleton	7 (6)
Chemotherapy (Ctx)	**69 (62)**
Zielgerichtete Therapien (tt)	**47 (42)**
***Viscum album* L. (VA)**	**53 (47)**
subkutan	49 (44)
intravenös	35 (31)
intra-tumoral/-pleural	3 (3)

Die Zahlen in den Spalten für die Behandlungen, die den Patienten verabreicht wurden, addieren sich nicht unbedingt zu 100 %, da die Patienten verschiedene Kombinationen von Präparaten erhalten haben können; n = Anzahl.

Evaluierung der EORTC QLQ-C30 Änderungen

Die ausgefüllten EORTC QLQ-C30 Fragebögen wurden für die gesamte Studienkohorte zu den Zeitpunkten T0 und T1 ausgewertet und analysiert. Alle EORTC QLQ-C30-Werte zu T0 lagen im Bereich der zuvor publizierten EORTC QLQ-C30-Referenzwerte für LK-Patienten (Scott *et al.* 2008). Multivariate lineare Regressionsanalysen wurden für alle longitudinalen Veränderungen der EORTC-QLQ-C30-Skalenwerte durchgeführt, wobei für Alter, Geschlecht, Jahr der Krebsdiagnose, jeweiligen T0-Wert und erhaltene zielgerichtete Therapien adjustiert wurde.

Bei den Patienten, die eine VA-Behandlung ohne Bestrahlung erhielten, wurden erhebliche Verbesserungen in vier Funktions- und acht Symptomskalen festgestellt (Tab. 3). Diese Patienten erreichten signifikante und klinisch relevante Verbesserungen der physischen (estimate $\beta = 16{,}1 \pm 6{,}9$; $p = 0{,}02$), rollen (estimate $\beta = 21{,}2 \pm 9{,}6$; $p=0{,}03$), kognitiven (estimate $\beta= 15{,}7 \pm 7{,}6$; $p=0{,}04$) und sozialen (estimate $\beta = 17{,}0 \pm 8{,}4$; $p = 0{,}04$) Funktionsfähigkeit. Für die kombinierten RadVA-Patienten wurden in multivariaten Analysen mit starken Effektgrößen (adjustiertes $R^2 > 0{,}30$) signifikante und klinisch relevante Verringerungen von Schmerzen (estimate $\beta = -27{,}9 \pm 10{,}0$; $p = 0{,}006$) und Übelkeit/Erbrechen (estimate $\beta = -17{,}1 \pm 6{,}0$; $p = 0{,}005$) festgestellt (Tab. 3).

Tab. 3: Assoziationsfaktoren zwischen Bestrahlung (Rad), *Viscum album* Behandlung (VA) und Veränderungen der Lebensqualität

n = 112 Funktions-skalen	**QL**	**PF**	**RF**	**EF**		**CF**		**SF**	
Referenz: ohne Rad ohne VA (n = 27)									
VA, n = 29	1.1	**16.1***	**21.2***	6.9		**15.7***		**17.0***	
Rad, n = 32	-4.8	0.9	10.2	6.2		3.4		-0.9	
RadVA, n = 24	1.2	8.7	10.5	7.3		**14.0^{+}**		6.2	
Symptome	**FA**	**NV**	**PA**	**DY**	**SL**	**AP**	**CO**	**DI**	**FI**
Referenz: ohne Rad ohne VA (n = 27)									
VA	**-13.5^{+}**	**-11.5^{+}**	-12.7	-10.4	-14.6	**-18.0^{+}**	-10.7	-10.3	7.2
Rad	-8.3	-6.2	-9.9	3.0	-11.5	-0.4	4.3	-10.6	0.6
RadVA	**-13.6^{+}**	**-17.1****	**-27.9****	-8.6	-12.5	-14.6	-15.9	-5.7	-1.5

Multivariate lineare Regressionsanalysen, adjustiert für Geschlecht, Alter, Jahr der Erstdiagnose, erhaltene zielgerichtete Therapien und die jeweiligen EORTC QLQ-C30 Scores zu T0, wurden für EORTC QLQ-C30 Skalenänderungen (T0→T12) und Rad- und VA-Behandlungen durchgeführt. Verbesserungen der Funktionsskalen werden durch positive, Symptome durch negative estimate β angezeigt. Signifikante substantielle Verbesserungen sind grau hervorgehoben. Signifikante p-Werte sind gekennzeichnet:
**: p-Wert < 0,01; *: p-Wert < 0,05, +: p-Wert < 0,1.
QL: globaler Gesundheitszustand;
Funktionsskalen: PF: physisch, RF: rollen, EF: emotional, CF: kognitiv, SF: sozial,
Symptome: FA: Fatigue, NV: Übelkeit/Erbrechen, PA: Schmerzen, DY: Dyspnoe, SL: Schlaflosigkeit, AP: Appetitlosigkeit, CO: Verstopfung, DI: Diarrhöe, FI: finanzielle Schwierigkeiten.

Diskussion

Die Befunde der vorliegenden RWD-Studie zeigen signifikante Verbesserungen der selbstberichteten Lebensqualität bei LK-Patienten, die eine VA-Therapie allein oder zusätzlich zur Strahlentherapie erhielten. Klinische Daten zur Radiochemotherapie mit zusätzlichen VA-Extrakten wurden bislang für Patienten mit kolorektalem Karzinom im Tumorstadium I-III (Friedel *et al.* 2009) oder für Patienten mit lokal fortgeschrittenem Rektumkarzinom in der neoadjuvanten Therapie (Baek *et al.* 2021) publiziert. Beide Arbeiten zeigten jeweils für die Kombinationsgruppe einen Überlebensvorteil bzw. ein besseres pathologisches Komplettansprechen. Die hier vorgestellten Ergebnisse stehen im Einklang mit einer randomisierten, kontrollierten Studie an 223 Krebspatienten, von denen 94 an LK erkrankt waren, in der über Verbesserungen der selbstberichteten Fatigue, Schlaflosigkeit, Appetitlosigkeit, Übelkeit und Schmerzen sowie Verringerungen der chemotherapiebedingten Nebenwirkungen im Zusammenhang mit der begleitenden VA-Therapie berichtet wurden (Piao *et al.* 2004). In der vorliegenden RWD-Studie wurden bei Patienten, die eine VA-Therapie ohne Bestrahlung erhielten, auf allen Symptomskalen mit Ausnahme der finanziellen Schwierigkeiten deutliche, wenn auch nicht signifikante Reduktionen (negative Estimate β zwischen 10 und 18 Punkten) beobachtet (Tab. 3). Da sich die Begrenzung des Schweregrads der Krankheitssymptome als entscheidend für die Verbesserung der Lebensqualität von LK-Patienten erwiesen hat (Polanski *et al.* 2016), könnte dies erklären, warum der hier beobachtete Trend der Symptomreduktion mit signifikant günstigen Assoziationen für die körperliche, funktionale, kognitive und soziale Funktion korreliert zu sein scheint.

Eine Metaanalyse zur Lebensqualität von LK-Patienten ergab, dass insbesondere die körperliche Aktivität mit einem besseren allgemeinen Gesundheitszustand und einer geringeren Symptombelastung assoziiert waren (Teba *et al.* 2022). Da bei Patienten, die eine VA-Behandlung erhielten, signifikante funktionelle Verbesserungen gemessen werden konnten (Tab. 3), kann sich dies möglicherweise auch positiv auf die körperliche Aktivität und damit auf die allgemeine Lebensqualität dieser Patienten auswirken.

Zu den Limitationen der vorliegenden Studie gehört das nichtrandomisierte, nichtkontrollierte und nichtverblindete Studiendesign, welches anfällig für verschiedene Verzerrungen sein kann, insbesondere für Selektionsverzerrungen. Eine weitere Limitation ergibt sich aus der Tatsache, dass der Beobachtungszeitraum 12 Monate betrug und daher keine Rückschlüsse auf die Lebensqualität von Patienten gezogen werden können, die nach 12 Monaten nicht mehr antworten konnten oder wollten oder die bereits verstorben waren. Wir haben jedoch versucht, das Verzerrungsrisiko durch die Durchführung adjustierter multivariater linearer Regressionsanalysen zu verringern. So liefert diese RWD-Studie Hinweise auf die klinische Wirksamkeit einer begleitenden VA-Behandlung bei LK-Patienten, die mit publizierten Daten von LK-Patienten und anderen Krebsarten übereinstimmen. Zu den Stärken unserer Studie gehört die Präsentation von versorgungsnahen Behandlungsdaten von LK-Patienten aus einem zertifizierten Lungenkrebszentrum.

Schlussfolgerungen

Unsere Ergebnisse deuten darauf hin, dass bei Lungenkrebspatienten, die eine Misteltherapie erhielten, noch nach 12 Monaten nach der primären Diagnose die selbst eingeschätzte Lebensqualität verbessert war. Bei Patienten, die eine Misteltherapie ohne Bestrahlung erhielten, wurden signifikant positive Assoziationen für körperliche, rollenbezogene, kognitive und soziale Funktionen beobachtet. Ein bemerkenswerter Vorteil in Bezug auf selbstberichtete Schmerzen und Übelkeit/ Erbrechen scheint in dieser Kohorte mit einer kombinierten Strahlen- und Misteltherapie verbunden zu sein. Dies unterstreicht die Bedeutung der Berücksichtigung und Bewertung kombinierter onkologischer Behandlungen mit Mistelpräparaten in zukünftigen Konzepten zur Verbesserung der Lebensqualität von Lungenkrebspatienten.

Interessenkonflikte

FS berichtet über Zuwendungen von Helixor Heilmittel GmbH (Reisekosten und Vortragshonorare), Zuwendungen von AstraZeneca (Reisekosten und Vortragshonorare), Zuwendungen von Abnoba GmbH und Zuwendungen von Iscador AG, die nicht im Zusammenhang mit der eingereichten Arbeit stehen. CG berichtet über Zuwendungen von Iscador AG, die nicht im Zusammenhang mit der eingereichten Arbeit stehen. Die anderen Autoren haben erklärt, dass keine Interessenkonflikte bestehen.

Literatur

Aaronson NK et al.: The European Organization for Research and Treatment of Cancer QLQ-C30: a quality-of-life instrument for use in international clinical trials in oncology. J Natl Cancer Inst. 1993; 85 (5): 365–376.

Baek J-H, Jeon Y, Han K-W et al.: Effect of mistletoe extract on tumor response in neoadjuvant chemoradiotherapy for rectal cancer: a cohort study. World J Surg Oncol. 2021; 19: 178. doi:10.1186/s12957-021-02293-4

Bar-Sela G, Wollner M, Hammer L et al.: Mistletoe as complementary treatment in patients with advanced non-small-cell lung cancer treated with carboplatin-based combinations: a randomised phase II study. Eur J Cancer. 2013; 49 (5): 1058–1064. doi:10.1016/j.ejca.2012.11.007.

Bennett BM, Wells JR, Panter C, Yuan Y, Penrod JR: The Humanistic Burden of Small Cell Lung Cancer (SCLC): A Systematic Review of Health-Related Quality of Life (HRQoL) Literature. Front Pharmacol. 2017; 8:339. doi:10.3389/fphar.2017.00339.

Cohen J: A power primer Psychological bulletin. 1992; 112: 155–159. doi:10.1037//0033-2909.112.1.155

Friedel WE, Matthes H, Bock PR, Zänker KS: Systematic evaluation of the clinical effects of supportive mistletoe treatment within chemo- and/or radiotherapy protocols and long-term mistletoe application in nonmetastatic colorectal carcinoma: multicenter, controlled, observational cohort study. J Soc Integr Oncol. 2009; 7: 137–145.

Loef M, Walach H: Quality of life in cancer patients treated with mistletoe: a systematic review and meta-analysis. BMC Complement Med Ther. 2020; 20 (1): 227. doi:10.1186/s12906-020-03013-3.

Piao BK, Wang YX, Xie GR et al.: Impact of complementary mistletoe extract treatment on quality of life in breast, ovarian and non-small cell lung cancer patients. A prospective randomized controlled clinical trial. Anticancer Res. 2004; 24 (1): 303–309.

Poghosyan H, Sheldon LK, Leveille SG, Cooley ME: Health-related quality of life after surgical treatment in patients with non-small cell lung cancer: a systematic review. Lung Cancer (Amsterdam). 2013; 81: 11–26. doi:10.1016/j.lungcan.2013.03.013.

Polanski J, Jankowska-Polanska B, Rosinczuk J et al.: Quality of life of patients with lung cancer. Onco Targets Ther. 2016; 9: 1023–1028. doi:10.2147/ott.s100685.

S3-Leitlinie Prävention, Diagnostik, Therapie und Nachsorge des Lungenkarzinoms. Leitlinienprogramm Onkologie https://www.leitlinienprogramm-onkologie.de/fileadmin/user_upload/Downloads/Leitlinien/Lungenkarzinom/Version_2/LL_Lungenkarzinom_Langversion_2.1.pdf; 2022.

Schad F, Thronicke A, Steele ML et al.: Overall survival of stage IV non-small cell lung cancer patients treated with Viscum album L. in addition to chemotherapy, a real-world observational multicenter analysis. PloS one. 2018; 13:e0203058. doi:10.1371/journal.pone.0203058.

Schad F et al.: Network Oncology (NO) – a clinical cancer register for health services research and the evaluation of integrative therapeutic interventions in anthroposophic medicine. Forsch Komplementmed. 2013; 20 (5): 353–360. doi: 10.1159/000356204.

Scott NW, Fayers PM, Aaronson NK et al. on behalf of the EORTC Quality of Life Group: EORTC-QLQ-C30 Reference Values. The EORTC Quality of Life Group. 2008. https://www.eortc.org/app/uploads/sites/2/2018/02/reference_values_manual2008.pdf (Stand: 20.07.2024).

Siegel RL, Miller KD, Fuchs HE, Jemal A: Cancer statistics, 2022. CA Cancer J Clin. 2022; 72 (1): 7–33. doi:10.3322/caac.21708.

Steinmann D et al.: Prospective evaluation of quality of life effects in patients undergoing palliative radiotherapy for brain metastases. BMC Cancer. 2012; 12: 283. doi:10.1186/1471-2407-12-283.

Teba PP, Esther MG, Raquel SG: Association between physical activity and patient-reported outcome measures in patients with lung cancer: a systematic review and meta-analysis. Qual Life Res. 2022; 31 (7): 1963–1976. doi: 10.1007/s11136-021-03053-3.

Thronicke A, von Trott P, Kröz M et al.: Health-Related Quality of Life in Patients with Lung Cancer Applying Integrative Oncology Concepts in a Certified Cancer Centre. Evid Based Complement Alternat Med. 2020; 5917382. doi:10.1155/2020/5917382.

Wood R, Taylor-Stokes G, Smith F, Chaib C: The humanistic burden of advanced non-small cell lung cancer (NSCLC) in Europe: a real-world survey linking patient clinical factors to patient and caregiver burden. Quality of Life Research. 2019; 28: 1849–1861. doi:10.1007/s11136-019-02152-6.

PD Dr. Friedemann Schad[1, 2], Prof. Dr. Diana Steinmann[3], Dr. Shiao Li Oei[1], Dr. Anja Thronicke[1], Dr. Christian Grah[4]

[1] Forschungsinstitut Havelhöhe, Berlin, Deutschland

[2] Onkologisches Zentrum, Gemeinschaftskrankenhaus Havelhöhe, Berlin, Deutschland

[3] Klinik für Strahlentherapie und Spezielle Onkologie, Medizinische Hochschule Hannover, Hannover, Deutschland

[4] Pneumologie, Gemeinschaftskrankenhaus Havelhöhe, Berlin, Deutschland

Korrespondenzadresse:
fschad@havelhoehe.de

Kombination von zielgerichteter Therapie und Helixor *Viscum album* L. bei Patientinnen mit Brust- oder anderen gynäkologischen Tumoren

Combination of Targeted Therapy and Helixor *Viscum album* L. in Breast and Gynecological Cancer Patients

Anja Thronicke, Shiao Li Oei, Patricia Grabowski, Friedemann Schad

Zusammenfassung

Die vorliegende Studie untersucht die Sicherheit der kombinierten Anwendung von zielgerichteter Therapie und Helixor VA (*Viscum album* L.) bei Patientinnen mit Brust- oder anderen gynäkologischen Tumoren. Zielgerichtete Therapie, bestehend aus kleinen Molekülen oder monoklonalen Antikörpern, beeinflusst das Wachstum von Krebszellen. Helixor VA wird zusätzlich zur Standard-Krebstherapie angewendet, um die Lebensqualität zu verbessern. In einer Real-World-Data Studie mit 242 Patientinnen wurde die Sicherheit der zielgerichteten Therapie mit und ohne Helixor VA analysiert. Die Ergebnisse weisen darauf hin, dass die zusätzliche Gabe von Helixor VA das Sicherheitsprofil der zielgerichteten Therapie nicht negativ beeinflusst. Weitere größere klinische Studien sind notwendig, um diese Ergebnisse zu bestätigen und die Anwendbarkeit auf verschiedene Krebsarten zu prüfen.

Schlüsselwörter: Zielgerichtete Therapie, *Viscum album* L., Immunotherapie, Misteltherapie, monoklonale Antikörper, Tyrosinkinaseinhibitoren, PARP-Inhibitoren, CDK 4/6-Inhibitoren.

Summary

The present study investigates the safety of the combined application of targeted therapy and Helixor VA (*Viscum album* L.) in breast and gynecological cancer patients. Targeted therapy, consisting of small molecules or monoclonal antibodies, affects the growth of cancer cells. Helixor VA is applied in addition to standard cancer therapy to improve the quality of life. In a real-world data study involving 242 patients, the safety of targeted therapy with and without Helixor VA was analyzed.

The results suggest that the additional administration of Helixor VA does not adversely affect the safety profile of targeted therapy. Further larger clinical studies are needed to confirm these results and assess their applicability to different types of cancer.
Key words: Targeted therapy, *Viscum album* L., mistletoe therapy, immunotherapy, monoclonal antibodies, tyrosinkinase inhibitors, PARP-inhibitors, CDK 4/6-inhibitors

Einleitung

Zielgerichtete Therapie bildet die Grundlage für die Präzisionsmedizin und umfasst kleine Moleküle oder monoklonale Antikörper, die das Wachstum, die Proliferation und/oder die Mobilität von Krebszellen beeinflussen (NCI 2022). Die zielgerichtete Therapie kann monoklonale Antikörper (mAB), Tyrosinkinaseinhibitoren (TKI), Poly(ADP-Ribose)-Polymerase-Inhibitoren (PARP-Inhibitoren oder PARPi) oder Cyclin-abhängige Kinase (CDK) 4/6-Inhibitoren (CDKi) umfassen (Chan *et al.* 2021; Braal *et al.* 2021). Extrakte von *Viscum album* L. (VA, Europäische Mistel) werden zusätzlich zur Standard-Krebstherapie angewendet, um die Lebensqualität zu verbessern (Bock *et al.* 2004; Bar-Sela *et al.* 2013; Büssing *et al.* 2006; Piao *et al.* 2004).

Helixor Mistelextrakte wurden in dieser Studie daraufhin untersucht, ob sie die Sicherheit der angewendeten zielgerichteten Therapie bei Patientinnen mit Brustkrebs oder anderen gynäkologischen Tumoren beeinträchtigen

Methoden

Studiendesign

Die Sicherheit der zielgerichteten Therapie mit oder ohne begleitende Helixor VA-Extrakte wurde in einer Real-World-Data Studie untersucht, die Daten aus dem onkologischen Register „Network Oncology" nutzte, welches neben demographischen Informationen, Diagnosen und Histologien auch Daten zu standardonkologischen und integrativen Therapien, Therapieanpassungen und unerwünschten Ereignissen sowie Daten zur Lebensqualität von Krebspatientinnen und Krebspatienten beinhaltet. Die Patientinnen der Studie erhielten Helixor VA-Therapie subkutan gemäß der Fachinformation. Die intravenöse Anwendung von Helixor VA wurde in Einzelfällen off-label durchgeführt.

Primäre und sekundäre Zielparameter

Das Hauptziel der Studie war die Untersuchung des Auftretens von unerwünschten Ereignissen (adverse events, AE) während einer zielgerichteten Therapie mit und ohne Helixor VA bei Patientinnen mit Brustkrebs oder gynäkologischen Tumoren. Sekundäre Ziele umfassten die explorative Analyse von Faktoren, die mit dem Risiko von Nebenwirkungen oder Therapieanpassungen der zielgerichteten Therapie assoziiert waren.

Beschreibung der Studienteilnehmerinnen

Brustkrebspatientinnen und solche mit weiteren gynäkologischen Tumoren aller Tumorstadien, welche im Network Oncology (NO) Register von Januar 2012 bis Januar 2022 registriert waren und zielgerichtete Therapien erhielten, wurden in die Studie aufgenommen. Die Studie umfasste 242 Patientinnen, von denen 160 (66,1 %) nur zielgerichtete Therapie erhielten, während 82 (33,9 %) zusätzlich Helixor VA auf Patientinnenwunsch und nach Maßgabe des Arztes erhielten.

Datenquelle und Bewertung

Demografische Daten, Diagnose- und Behandlungsinformationen wurden aus dem NO-Register extrahiert. Unerwünschte Wirkungen (AEs) wurden gemäß den ICH-Richtlinien und den Common Terminology Criteria for Adverse Events (CTCAE) Version 5 bewertet.

Statistische Methoden

Die kontinuierlichen Variablen wurden als Median mit Interquartilsabstand (IQR) beschrieben, während die kategorialen Variablen als Häufigkeiten und Prozentsätze angegeben wurden. Adjustierte multivariate logistische Regressionsanalysen wurden durchgeführt, um Assoziationsfaktoren zu ermitteln. Alle statistischen Analysen wurden mit der freien R-Software (Version 4.2.2, R core team, Vienna, Austria) durchgeführt.

Ergebnisse

Insgesamt wurden 242 Patientinnen mit Brust- oder anderen gynäkologischen Tumoren in die Studie eingeschlossen, von denen 160 (66,1 %) zielgerichtete Therapie erhielten und 82 (33,9 %) zusätzlich Helixor VA. Die Gruppen waren bezüglich der Baseline Parameter ausbalanciert ohne signifikante Unterschiede und die häufigste Krebsart war Brustkrebs (87,6 %).

Zielgerichtete Therapie

Die Mehrheit der Patientinnen erhielt eine zielgerichtete Therapie mit monoklonalen Antikörpern (mAB) (79,8 %, vermutlich bezogen auf n = 242), gefolgt von CDK 4/6-Inhibitoren (10,7 %) und Immun-Checkpoint-Inhibitoren (5,4 %, Tab. 1).

Tab. 1: Aufteilung der zielgerichteten Therapie COMB *vs.* CTRL Gruppe

Zielgerichtete Therapie	**Kontrolle (n = 160)**	**Kombination (n = 82)**
Monoklonale Antikörper, n (%)	136 (85,0)	70 (85,4)
CDK4/6 Inhibitor, n (%)	17 (10,6)	9 (11,0)
Immune Checkpoint Inhibitor, n (%)	8 (5,0)	5 (6,1)
Tyrosinekinaseinhitibor, n (%)	4 (2,5)	2 (2,4)
PARP Inhibitor, n (%)	3 (1,9)	1 (1,2)

Die durchschnittliche Dauer der zielgerichteten Therapie betrug 295,5 Tage. In der COMB Gruppe wurden bei 68 % der Patientinnen Helixor A, bei 26 % Helixor M und bei 5 % der Patientinnen Helixor P angewendet (Tab. 2).

Tab. 2: Zusammensetzung der Helixor VA Präparate

Helixorpräparate	**Total n (%)**
Helixor, total	82 (100)
Helixor A	56 (68,3)
Helixor M	21 (25,6)
Helixor P	4 (4,9)
Helixor, not specified	1 (1,2)

Unerwünschte Ereignisse, Therapieanpassungen und Behandlungsunterbrechungen

Insgesamt traten 10 unerwünschte Ereignisse (AEs) bei 242 Patientinnen auf, entsprechend einer Gesamtfrequenz von 4,13 %, Die häufigsten waren Übelkeit und Erbrechen (Pertuzumab, Niraparib) und allgemeine Beschwerden sowie Hautreaktionen (Trastumzumab, Trastuzumab/Pertuzumab, Pazopanib) an der Applikationsstelle.

Es wurden keine AEs in der Gruppe mit zusätzlichem Helixor VA beobachtet (COMB), im Vergleich zu 6,25 % in der Gruppe ohne Helixor VA (CTRL), $\chi^2 = 0{,}107$, p-value = 0,99, (Abb. 1). Die Gruppe mit zusätzlichem Helixor VA zeigte keine Nebenwirkungen und tendenziell niedrigere Raten der Dosisreduktion und Therapieunterbrechungen im Vergleich zur Gruppe ohne Helixor VA. In der Kontrollgruppe wurden fünf Dosisreduktionen und fünf Therapieunterbrechungen aufgrund von AEs beobachtet, während in der Gruppe mit zusätzlichem Helixor VA eine Dosisunterbrechung und drei Dosisreduktionen auftraten.

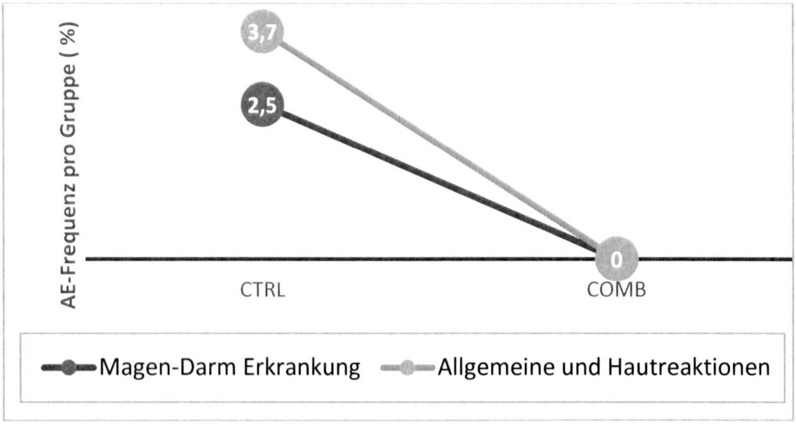

Abb. 1: Vergleich der AE-Rate COMB *vs.* CTRL Gruppe

Assoziationen und Risikofaktoren

Die adjustierte multivariate Analyse zeigte einen negativen Zusammenhang zwischen dem Auftreten von AEs oder Therapieanpassungen und der Helixor VA-Anwendung (Abb. 2).

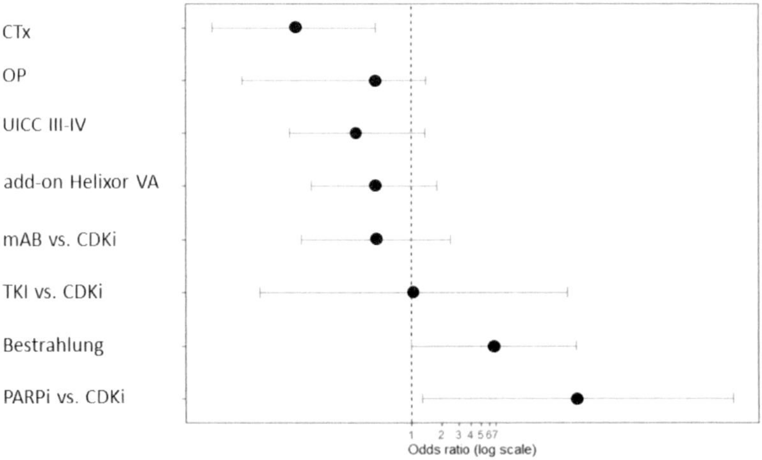

Abb. 2: Wahrscheinlichkeit von AEs, Dosisreduzierung oder Abbruch der zielgerichteten Therapie und damit verbundene Faktoren

Strahlentherapie und PARP-Inhibitoren erhöhten signifikant die Wahrscheinlichkeit von AEs oder Therapieanpassungen, während eine vorherige Chemotherapie mit einer signifikanten Reduktion von AEs und Therapieanpassungen assoziiert war. Die kombinierte Therapie von zielgerichteter Therapie und Helixor VA zeigte keine signifikanten Unterschiede in der AE-Frequenz im Vergleich zur alleinigen zielgerichteten Therapie.

Diskussion und Schlussfolgerung

Die vorliegende Studie liefert erste Erkenntnisse über die Sicherheitsaspekte der kombinierten Anwendung von zielgerichteter Therapie und Helixor VA bei Brust- und gynäkologischen s.o. Krebspatientinnen. Die Ergebnisse legen nahe, dass die zusätzliche Gabe von Helixor VA das Sicherheitsprofil der zielgerichteten Therapie positiv beeinflusst. Es wurde eine Tendenz zu niedrigeren AE-Raten und besserer Therapieadhärenz in der Gruppe mit Helixor VA beobachtet. Frühere Studien haben gezeigt, dass zusätzlich verabreichtes Helixor VA zur Chemotherapie die Nebenwirkungsraten reduziert und die Standard-Krebstherapie aufrechterhält (Piao *et al.* 2004). Unsere Ergebnisse stehen im Einklang mit drei anderen Beobachtungsstudien, die die Sicherheit der kombinierten Behandlung von VA-Extrakten mit monoklonalen Antikörpern, Immun-Checkpoint-Inhibitoren und zielgerichteten Therapien einschließlich mABs, ICIs und TKIs bei onkologischen Patienten beschreiben (Schad *et al.* 2016; Thronicke *et al.* 2017; 2018a; 2018b). Weitere klinische Studien mit größeren Kohorten sind erforderlich, um die Ergebnisse zu bestätigen und die Anwendbarkeit auf verschiedene Krebsarten zu prüfen.

Interessenkonflikt

Die Autoren haben die folgenden Interessenkonflikte in Bezug auf die Forschung, die Autorenschaft und/oder Veröffentlichung dieses Artikels: FS berichtet über Zuschüsse von Astrazeneca (Reisekosten und Honorare für Vorträge), Helixor Heilmittel GmbH (Reisekosten und Honorare für

Vorträge), Zuschüsse von der Abnoba GmbH und Zuschüsse von der Iscador AG, außerhalb der eingereichten Arbeit. PG berichtet über Zuschüsse von Ipsen Pharma, Miltenyi (Honorare für Vorträge), Helixor Heilmittel GmbH (finanzielle Forschungsunterstützung). Die anderen Autoren haben erklärt, dass keine konkurrierenden Interessen bestehen. Es wurden keine Zahlungen für andere Aspekte der eingereichten Arbeit erhalten. Es gibt keine Patente, Produkte in der Entwicklung oder vermarktete Produkte, die zu deklarieren sind. Es bestehen keine anderen Beziehungen/Bedingungen/Umstände, die einen potenziellen Interessenkonflikt darstellen.

Literatur

Bar-Sela G, Wollner M, Hammer L et al: Mistletoe as complementary treatment in patients with advanced non-small-cell lung cancer treated with carboplatin-based combinations: A randomised phase II study. Eur J Cancer. 2013; 49: 1058–1064.

Bock PR, Friedel WE, Hanisch J et al.: Efficacy and safety of long-term complementary treatment with standardized European mistletoe extract (Viscum album L.) in addition to the conventional adjuvant oncologic therapy in patients with primary non-metastasized mammary carcinoma. Results of a multi-center, comparative, epidemiological cohort study in Germany and Switzerland. Arzneimittelforschung. 2004; 54: 456–466.

Braal CL, Jongbloed EM, Wilting SM et al.: Inhibiting CDK4/6 in Breast Cancer with Palbociclib, Ribociclib, and Abemaciclib: Similarities and Differences. Drugs. 2021; 81: 317–331.

Büssing A: Immune Modulation Using Mistletoe (Viscum album L.) Extracts Iscador. Arzneimittelforschung. 2006; 56: 508–515.

Chan CY, Tan KV, Cornelissen B: PARP Inhibitors in Cancer Diagnosis and Therapy. Clin Cancer Res. 2021; 27: 1585–1594

National Cancer Institute. Targeted Therapy to Treat Cancer. https://www.cancer.gov/about-cancer/treatment/types/targeted-therapies (accessed November 11, 2022).

Piao BK, Wang YX, Xie GR et al.: Impact of complementary mistletoe extract treatment on quality of life in breast, ovarian and non-small cell lung cancer patients. A prospective randomized controlled clinical trial. Anticancer Res. 2004; 24: 303–310

Schad F, Axtner J, Kröz M et al.: Safety of Combined Treatment with Monoclonal Antibodies and Viscum album L. Preparations. Integr Cancer Ther. 2016; 17: 41–51.

Thronicke A, Steele ML, Grah C et al.: Clinical safety of combined therapy of immune checkpoint inhibitors and Viscum album L. therapy in patients with advanced or metastatic cancer. BMC Complement Altern Med. 2017; 17: 534.

Thronicke A, Oei SL, Grah C et al.: Nivolumab-induced toxicity profile in patients with advanced or metastasized lung cancer treated with Viscum album L. extracts. Abstract. In Proceedings of the German Cancer Congress, Berlin, Germany, 21–24 February 2018.

Thronicke A, Oei SL, Merkle A et al.: Clinical Safety of Combined Targeted and Viscum album L. Therapy in Oncological Patients. Medicines. 2018; 5: 100.

Dr. Anja Thronicke[1], Dr. Shiao Li Oei[1], PD Dr. Patricia Grabowski[2], PD Dr. Friedemann Schad[1, 2]

[1] Forschungsinstitut Havelhöhe, Berlin, Deutschland

[2] Interdisziplinäre Onkologie und Palliativmedizin, Gemeinschaftskrankenhaus Havelhöhe Berlin Deutschland

Korrespondenzadresse:

fschad@havelhoehe.de

Prospektive Beobachtungsstudie zur Kombinationstherapie von Immun-Checkpoint-Inhibitoren und *Viscum album* L. beim fortgeschrittenen Lungenkarzinom (PHOENIX-III)

Prospective Observational Study of Advanced Lung Cancer Patients Treated With a Combination of Immune Checkpoint Inhibitors and *Viscum album* L. Extract (PHOENIX-III)

Shiao Li Oei, Klaudia Kunc, Marcus Reif, Ulrike Weissenstein, Timo Weiß, Hannah Wüstefeld, Harald Matthes, Christian Grah

Zusammenfassung

Hintergrund: Erste klinische Erfahrungen mit der Zusatzbehandlung mit *Viscum album* L. Extrakt (VA) deuten auf eine positive Wirkung bei Patienten mit fortgeschrittenem oder metastasiertem nichtkleinzelligem Lungenkrebs (NSCLC) hin. Das primäre Ziel dieser Studie ist es, Machbarkeit und das Sicherheitsprofil der Kombinationstherapie aus Immun-Checkpoint-Inhibitoren (ICI) und VA bei NSCLC Patienten zu evaluieren.

Methoden: Klinischer Verlauf, Tumoransprechraten, unerwünschte Ereignisse und Lebensqualität werden nach drei und sechs Monaten evaluiert. Für alle Parameter werden deskriptive Statistiken erstellt.

Ergebnisse: Insgesamt wurden 104 Patienten mit fortgeschrittenem oder metastasiertem NSCLC zwischen 7/2016 und 1/2022 in die Studie aufgenommen. Die klinischen Verläufe für unterschiedliche Therapieschemata (Pembrolizumab als Monotherapie oder in Kombination mit Chemotherapie; Zweitlinientherapie mit Nivolumab) wurden beobachtet, dokumentiert und ausgewertet. Eine Immun-Checkpoint-Inhibitor-Therapie in Kombination mit einer Misteltherapie wurde von 87 (86 %) NSCLC Patienten durchgeführt.

Schlussfolgerungen: Die Machbarkeitsanalyse ergab, dass 86 % der gesamten Studienkohorte mit einer Kombinationstherapie aus Checkpoint-Immuninhibitoren und Misteltherapie behandelt werden konnten.

Es ergaben sich keine Hinweise auf ein vermehrtes Auftreten von therapiebedingten unerwünschten Ereignissen.
Schlüsselwörter: Immun-Checkpoint-Inhibitoren, nichtkleinzelliger Lungenkrebs, *Viscum album* L.

Summary

Background: Initial clinical experience with the addition of *Viscum album* L. extract (VA) suggests a positive effect in patients with advanced or metastatic non-small cell lung cancer (NSCLC). The primary objective of this study was to evaluate the safety profile and efficacy of immune checkpoint inhibitors (ICIs) in combination with VA in NSCLC patients.
Methods: Clinical progression, tumor response rates, adverse events, and quality of life will be evaluated at three and six months. Descriptive statistics will be generated for all parameters.
Results: A total of 104 patients with advanced or metastatic NSCLC were enrolled between 7/2016 and 1/2022. Clinical outcomes for different treatment regimens (pembrolizumab as monotherapy or in combination with chemotherapy; second-line nivolumab) were observed, documented and analyzed. Immune checkpoint inhibitor therapy in combination with mistletoe therapy was initiated in 87 (86 %) NSCLC patients.
Conclusions: The feasibility analysis revealed that 86 % of the entire study cohort could be treated with a combination therapy of immune checkpoint inhibitors and mistletoe therapy. There were no indications of an increased incidence of treatment-related adverse events.
Keywords: Immune checkpoint Inhibitors, non-small cell lung cancer, *Viscum album* L.

Einführung

Lungenkrebs ist weltweit die häufigste krebsbedingte Todesursache (Siegel *et al.* 2022), wobei das nichtkleinzellige Lungenkarzinom (NSCLC) 85 % aller Lungenkrebsfälle ausmacht. Immuntherapien mit PD-1/PD-L1-Inhibitoren, so genannten Immun-Checkpoint-Inhibitoren (ICI), haben sich inzwischen als Standardtherapie etabliert und können ein dauerhaftes Ansprechen auf die Krebstherapie bewirken (Lee and Kim 2023). Unterschiedliche ICI-Therapieschemata in Abhängigkeit von verschiedenen tumorhistologischen Parametern, Immuntherapie allein als Mono-

oder in Kombination mit Chemotherapie als Erstlinientherapie haben sich etabliert (Saxena *et al.* 2020) und Eingang in onkologische Leitlinien gefunden. Obwohl die Nebenwirkungen und die Beeinträchtigung der Lebensqualität nicht so schwerwiegend sind wie bei einer Chemotherapie, kann die Immun-Checkpoint-Blockade zu leichten, schweren und sogar tödlichen unerwünschten Ereignissen führen. Die Behandlung mit I-CIs, die mit einer Aktivierung von T-Zellen einhergeht, kann zu einem einzigartigen Spektrum von Toxizitäten führen, die als immunbedingte unerwünschte Ereignisse (immune-related adverse events – irAE) bezeichnet werden und alle Organsysteme betreffen können (Chennamadhavuni *et al.* 2022; Ramos-Casals *et al.* 2020). Daher ist ein sorgfältiges Management von irAEs bei der Behandlung mit ICIs wichtig (Poto *et al.* 2022; Trinh *et al.* 2019). Andererseits konnte auch gezeigt werden, dass das Auftreten hochgradiger irAEs mit einem besseren Ansprechen und einem längeren Gesamtüberleben korreliert (Guezour *et al.* 2022).

Viscum album L. (VA) ist in Deutschland zur subkutanen adjuvanten und palliativen Behandlung von malignen Tumorerkrankungen zugelassen und für die Verbesserung der gesundheitsbezogenen Lebensqualität zeigen systematische Reviews und Metaanalysen einen signifikanten Effekt mittlerer Größe (Loef, Walach 2020). Zu den Wirkmechanismen der Mistel in der Krebstherapie gehören die Hemmung der Zellproliferation, die Entzündungshemmung und die Immunmodulation (Oei *et al.* 2019; Szurpnicka *et al.* 2020). Erste klinische Erfahrungen mit der additiven Misteltherapie zu Immun-Checkpoint-Inhibitoren liegen bei Patienten mit fortgeschrittenem Krebs vor und es wurde keine Zunahme unerwünschter Ereignisse beobachtet (Thronicke *et al.* 2017).

Am Lungenkrebszentrum des Gemeinschaftskrankenhauses Havelhöhe (GKH) wurden im Rahmen einer prospektiven PHOENIX-III-Studie Patienten mit fortgeschrittenen oder metastasierten NSCLC, die eine Kombinationstherapie aus ICIs und VA-Extrakten erhielten, in Bezug auf klinischen Verlauf, Therapiesicherheit, Therapieverträglichkeit und Überleben evaluiert. Primärziel dieser Studie ist, die Machbarkeit und das Sicherheitsprofil der Kombinationstherapie aus ICIs und VA bei NSCLC Patienten zu beschreiben.

Methoden

Bei der vorliegenden Studie handelt es sich um eine Anwendungsbeobachtung, bei der die Auswahl der eingeschlossenen Patienten nach ärztlicher Beurteilung und Empfehlung durch die Tumorkonferenz erfolgte. In diese Studie wurden NSCLC Patienten im UICC Stadium IIIB-IV beiderlei Geschlechts eingeschlossen, für die eine Kombinationstherapie von ICIs und VA in der Erst- oder Folgelinie geplant wurde. Die demographischen und klinischen Daten der Studienteilnehmer wurden erhoben und im Verlauf der Studie nach drei und nach sechs Monaten ausgewertet. Bewertet wurden der klinische Gesamtverlauf, die Therapietreue, die Tumoransprechrate (TRR), unerwünschte Ereignisse und Arzneimittelwirkungen, der Trial Outcome Index (TOI) des FACT-L Lebensqualitätsfragebogens und das Gesamtüberleben. Deskriptive Statistiken werden für alle Parameter erstellt.

Die Planung, Durchführung und Auswertung dieser Studie folgt neben den gesetzlichen Vorgaben des AMG den Empfehlungen des BfArM/PEI und der GCP-Leitlinie und wurde von der Ethikkommission der Charité Berlin positiv bewertet (Antragsnummer: EA1/231/16).

Ergebnisse und Diskussion

Im Zeitraum von Juli 2016 bis Januar 2022 wurden im von der Deutschen Krebsgesellschaft zertifizierten Lungenkrebszentrum des GKH insgesamt 1.200 Lungenkrebspatienten behandelt, davon ca. 800 Patienten mit fortgeschrittenem oder metastasiertem NSCLC. Etwa 400 Patienten erhielten vom Tumorboard eine Therapieempfehlung für eine Behandlung mit PD-1/PD-L1-Inhibitoren gemäß den jeweiligen aktuellen onkologischen Leitlinien. Es wurden insgesamt 110 NSCLC Patienten für diese Studie rekrutiert. 104 Patienten hatten eine gesicherte Histologie eines fortgeschrittenen oder metastasierten NSCLC, der mit einem PD-1/PD-L1-Inhibitor-Schema behandelt werden konnte, und gaben ihr schriftliches Einverständnis zum Studieneinschluss (Abb. 1).

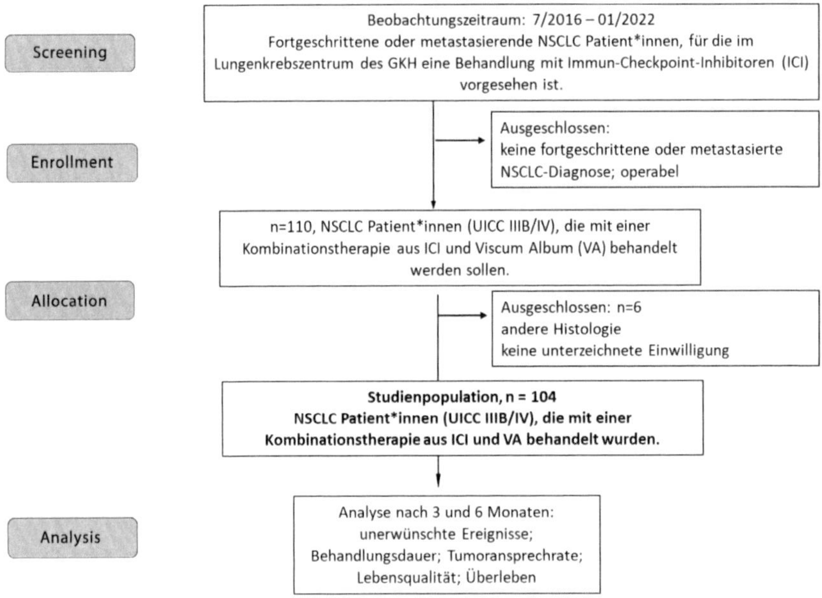

Abb. 1: Flussdiagramm der Studienpopulation. ICI: Immun-Checkpoint-Inhibitor.

Die Hauptmerkmale der gesamten PHOENIX-III-Kohorte sind in Tabelle 1 dargestellt.

Die 104 Patienten wurden entsprechend aktuellen onkologischen Leitlinien und dem Studienprotokoll untersucht und wurden über ihre individuellen anstehenden onkologischen Therapieoptionen wie radiologische Bestrahlung, Chemotherapie und weitere zielgerichtete Therapien aufgeklärt. Allerdings widerriefen drei Patienten kurz nach Studienbeginn ihre Einwilligung, so dass lediglich 101 Patienten die studienspezifischen Fragebögen zur Lebensqualität beantworteten. Die gesamte onkologische Behandlung erfolgte gemäß den Leitlinien und der individuellen, partizipativen Entscheidung durch die Patienten und ihre Onkologen. Dies wurde im Studienregister dokumentiert.

Tab. 1: Patienteneigenschaften

n = 104	**n (%)**
Anzahl der Patienten, n (%)	104 (100 %)
Alter, Jahre, median (ICS)	67 (60–74)
Geschlecht (männlich), n (%)	56 (54)
Rauchstatus	
• ehemals/aktuell	92 (88)
• nie	8 (8)
• nd	4 (4)
ECOG, n (%)	
• 0	32 (31)
• 1	54 (52)
• 2	13 (12)
• 3	2 (2)
• nd	3 (3)
UICC Stadium, n (%)	
• III	14 (13)
• IV	84 (81)
• nicht anwendbar (Rezidiv)	6 (6)
Histologie	
• Adenokarzinom	75 (72)
• Plattenepithelkarzinom	20 (19)
• Sarkomatiodes NSCLC	3 (3)
• Adenoid-zystisches Karzinom	1 (1)
• NSCLC nicht näher bezeichnet	5 (5)
PD-L1 Expressionsstatus	
• positiv	1 (1)
• ≥ 50 %	59 (57)
• < 50 %	41 (39)
• nd	3 (3)

n = Anzahl; nd = nicht bekannt; % = in Prozent der Gesamtpatientenzahl; ECOG = Performance-Status der Eastern Cooperative Oncology Group; UICC = Union for International Cancer Care

Für alle 104 Patienten der Studienkohorte war gemäß Tumorboard-Empfehlung eine kombinierte ICI-VA-Behandlung geplant, die jedoch in einigen Fällen aus verschiedenen Gründen (Komorbiditäten, Verschlechterung des Krankheitsverlaufs, Wunsch der Patienten) nicht begonnen oder geändert wurde. Letztlich hatten 87 (86 %) der Studienkohorte tatsächlich mit einer ICI/VA-Kombinationstherapie begonnen. Die onkologischen Therapien, die für die Patienten im Verlauf vom jeweiligen Studieneinschluss bis maximal 6 Monate danach dokumentiert wurden, sind in Tabelle 2 aufgelistet.

Tab. 2: Charakteristika der onkologischen Therapien

n = 101	**n (%)**
Radiologische Bestrahlung, n (%)	38 (38)
Erstlinie ICI Therapie	83 (82)
Pembrolizumab, n (%)	86 (85)
Nivolumab, n (%)	8 (8)
Azetolizumab, n (%)	1 (1)
Keine ICI Therapie begonnen	6 (6)
Viscum album – Art der Anwendung, n (%)	
• subkutan	64 (63)
• intravenös	1 (1)
• subkutan und intravenös	22 (22)
Keine *Viscum album* Therapie begonnen	14 (14)
Kombinationstherapie ICI und VA	87 (86)

n = Anzahl; % = in Prozent der Gesamtpatientenzahl

Pembrolizumab als Monotherapie oder in Kombination mit Chemotherapie gehört inzwischen zur Standardtherapie bei NSCLC, und 85 % der Patienten der dokumentierten Studienkohorte begannen eine Pembrolizumab-Immuntherapie (Tab. 2). Vor 2016 lag noch keine Zulassung für eine Erstlinientherapie mit Pembrolizumab vor, was dazu führte, dass acht Patienten mit einer Therapie in der Zweitlinie mit Nivolumab in Kombination mit VA behandelt wurden.

Für 49 Patienten, bei denen eine PD-L1 Expression ≥ 50 % detektiert wurde, war eine Erstlinien Pembrolizumab-Monotherapie kombiniert mit VA vorgesehen. In vier Fällen wurde aus individuellen Gründen (Akute Erkrankung, Verschlechterung des Krankheitsverlaufs, kurzfristige Therapieumstellung, Wunsch der Patienten) mit dieser Therapie nicht wie geplant begonnen. Letztlich erhielten 45 Patienten eine Erstlinien-Kombinationstherapie mit Mono-Pembrolizumab und subkutanen VA-Applikationen und diese 45-er Subkohorte ist vergleichbar mit der Keynote 24-Kohorte (Reck *et al.* 2016). Für diese Subkohorte wurde mit der Durchführung von Sicherheitsanalysen und der Beschreibung der aufgetretenen therapiebedingten unerwünschten Ereignisse, insbesondere der irAEs, begonnen. Es ist bekannt, dass eine hohe Tumoransprechrate auch mit einer erhöhten Inzidenz von auftretenden irAEs korreliert (Guezour *et al.* 2022), von besonderer Brisanz ist hier das Auftreten von Pneumonitis. So werden für Pembrolizumab Real-World-Pneumonitis-Inzidenzen von 19 % bis 22 % berichtet (Yin *et al.* 2022). Die Auswertung dieser Subgruppe wird zeigen, ob die Inzidenz von irAEs in dieser 45er-Subkohorte niedriger ist als in vergleichbaren publizierten Pembrolizumab-Studien ohne VA.

Für eine weitere Subkohorte mit PD-L1 Expression < 50 % wurde Pembrolizumab in Kombination mit Chemotherapie und VA als Erstlinientherapie festgelegt. Diese Subkohorte wird hinsichtlich Therapieadhärenz, Sicherheit und Wirksamkeit analysiert werden. In einer dritten Subkohorte fassen wir alle Patienten zusammen, die in der zweiten, oder dritten Behandlungslinie die Kombination eines PD-1/PD-L1 Inhibitors und eines VA-Präparates erhielten. Auch diese Subkohorte wird hinsichtlich Therapieadhärenz, Sicherheit und Wirksamkeit analysiert werden.

Bekannt ist, dass eine ICI-Therapie die Überlebensraten von NSCLC-Patienten nachweislich erheblich verbessern kann (Reck *et al.* 2022; Suresh *et al.* 2018). Real-World-Daten hatten ergeben, dass die Kombinationstherapie aus Chemotherapie und VA-Therapie positiv mit einem verbesserten Gesamtüberleben von fortgeschrittenen oder metastasierten NSCLC-Patienten assoziiert ist (Schad *et al.* 2018). Kürzlich konnte nun-mehr auch gezeigt werden, dass bei fortgeschrittenen oder metastasierten NSCLC-Patienten unabhängig von Alter, Geschlecht, Tumorstadium oder onkologischer Behandlung die Kombinationstherapie mit ICIs und VA mit einem signifikant verbessertem Überleben verbunden ist (Schad *et al.* 2024). Die prospektiven Ergebnisse der Subgruppenanalyse unserer Behandlungsgruppe von unerwünschten Wirkungen, insbesondere irARs sind vor diesem Hintergrund von besonderer Bedeutung.

Schlussfolgerungen

Die Misteltherapie kann etablierte Standardkrebstherapien sinnvoll ergänzen. Erste Analysen zur Machbarkeit und Sicherheit einer Kombinationstherapie mit Immun-Checkpoint-Inhibitoren sind vielversprechend, 86 % der gesamten Studienkohorte begannen mit einer ICI/VA Kombinationstherapie. Hinweise auf ein vermehrtes Auftreten von therapiebedingten unerwünschten Ereignissen gibt es bisher nicht. Die laufenden Evaluationen dieser Kombinationstherapie kann möglicherweise die Entwicklung von immunbezogenen unerwünschten Ereignissen verhindern oder ihr entgegenwirken, ohne das Tumoransprechen zu beeinträchtigen. Darüber hinaus könnte die Zahl der Therapieabbrüche reduziert und ein besseres Ansprechen des Tumors sowie ein längeres Überleben erreicht werden. Da es sich um eine Beobachtungsstudie und nicht um eine randomisierte Studie handelt, sind prospektive randomisierte Studien erforderlich.

Interessenkonflikte

CG berichtet über Zuschüsse von AstraZeneca, Takeda, Novartis, Chiesi, Iscador, außerhalb der eingereichten Arbeit. MR ist Mitarbeiter der Firma Iscador AG. Es bestehen keine weiteren relevanten Beschäftigungs- oder Beratungsbeziehungen.

Literatur

Chennamadhavuni A, Abushahin L, Jin N, Presley CJ, Manne A: Risk Factors and Biomarkers for Immune-Related Adverse Events: A Practical Guide to Identifying High-Risk Patients and Rechallenging Immune Checkpoint Inhibitors Front Immunol. 2022; 13:779691. doi:10.3389/fimmu.2022.779691.

Lee J, Kim EH: Mechanisms underlying response and resistance to immune checkpoint blockade in cancer immunotherapy Frontiers in oncology. 2023; 13:1233376. doi:10.3389/fonc.2023.1233376

Loef M, Walach H: Quality of life in cancer patients treated with mistletoe: a systematic review and meta-analysis BMC complementary medicine and therapies. 2020; 20:227. doi:10.1186/s12906-020-03013-3.

Oei SL, Thronicke A, Schad F: Mistletoe and Immunomodulation: Insights and Implications for Anticancer Therapies Evidence-based complementary and alternative medicine: eCAM 2019:5893017. doi:10.1155/2019/5893017.

Poto R, Troiani T, Criscuolo G et al.: Holistic Approach to Immune Checkpoint Inhibitor-Related Adverse Events. Front Immunol. 2022; 13:804597. doi:10.3389/fimmu.2022.804597.

Ramos-Casals M et al.: Immune-related adverse events of checkpoint inhibitors Nature Reviews Disease Primers. 2020; 6:38. doi:10.1038/s41572-020-0160-6.

Reck M, Remon J, Hellmann MD: First-Line Immunotherapy for Non-Small-Cell Lung Cancer Journal of clinical oncology : official journal of the American Society of Clinical Oncology. 2022; 40: 586–597. doi:10.1200/jco.21.01497.

Reck M et al.: Pembrolizumab versus Chemotherapy for PD-L1-Positive Non-Small-Cell Lung Cancer The New England journal of medicine. 2016; 375:1823-1833. doi:10.1056/NEJMoa1606774.

Schad F, Thronicke A, Hofheinz R-D, Matthes H, Grah C: Patients with Advanced or Metastasised Non-Small-Cell Lung Cancer with Viscum album L. Therapy in Addition to PD-1/PD-L1 Blockade: A Real-World Data Study Cancers (Basel). 2024; 16: 1609.

Schad F, Thronicke A, Steele ML, Merkle A, Matthes B, Grah C, Matthes H: Overall survival of stage IV non-small cell lung cancer patients treated with Viscum album L. in addition to chemotherapy, a real-world observational multicenter analysis PloS one. 2018; 13:e0203058. doi:10.1371/journal.pone.0203058.

Siegel RL, Miller KD, Fuchs HE, Jemal A: Cancer statistics, 2022 CA: a cancer journal for clinicians. 2022; 72: 7–33 doi:10.3322/caac.21708

Sugisaka J et al.: Relationship between Programmed Cell Death Protein Ligand 1 Expression and Immune-related Adverse Events in Non-small-cell Lung Cancer Patients Treated with Pembrolizumab JMA journal 2020; 3: 58–66. doi:10.31662/jmaj.2019-0005.

Suresh K, Naidoo J, Lin CT, Danoff S: Immune Checkpoint Immunotherapy for Non-Small Cell Lung Cancer: Benefits and Pulmonary Toxicities Chest. 2019; 154: 1416–1423. doi:10.1016/j.chest.2018.08.1048.

Szurpnicka A, Kowalczuk A, Szterk A: Biological activity of mistletoe: in vitro and in vivo studies and mechanisms of action Arch Pharm Res. 2020; 43:593–629. doi:10.1007/s12272-020-01247-w.

Thronicke A, Steele ML, Grah C, Matthes B, Schad F: Clinical safety of combined therapy of immune checkpoint inhibitors and Viscum album L. therapy in patients with advanced or metastatic cancer BMC complementary and alternative medicine. 2017; 17:534. doi:10.1186/s12906-017-2045-0.

Trinh S, Le A, Gowani S, La-Beck NM: Management of Immune-Related Adverse Events Associated with Immune Checkpoint Inhibitor Therapy: a Minireview of Current Clinical Guidelines Asia-Pacific journal of oncology nursing. 2019; 6:154–160. doi:10.4103/apjon.apjon_3_19.

Dr. Christian Grah[1, 2], Dr. Hannah Wüstefeld[1, 2], Dr. Shiao Li Oei[2], Klaudia Kunc[2], Timo Weiß[2], Dr. Marcus Reif[3], Prof. Dr. Harald Matthes[4, 5]

[1] Pneumologie, Gemeinschaftskrankenhaus Havelhöhe, Berlin; Deutschland

[2] Forschungsinstitut Havelhöhe, Berlin; Deutschland

[3] Gesellschaft für Klinische Forschung e. V., Berlin; Deutschland

[4] Gemeinschaftskrankenhaus Havelhöhe
[5] Institut für Sozialmedizin, Epidemiologie und Gesundheitsökonomie; Charité – Universitätsmedizin Berlin; Deutschland

Korrespondenzadresse:
christian.grah@havelhoehe.de

Sicherheit, Verträglichkeit, therapeutische Wirksamkeit und Lebensqualität (LQ) von Patienten mit malignen urogenitalen Tumorerkrankungen unter der Behandlung mit Iscucin® Populi – Ergebnisse einer nichtinterventionellen Studie (NIS)

Safety, Tolerability, Therapeutic Efficacy and Quality of Life (QoL) Assessment of Patients With Malignant Urogenital Tumors Upon Treatment With Iscucin® Populi – Results of a Non-interventional Study (NIS)

Jennifer E. Felenda, Claudia Turek, Florian C. Stintzing

Zusammenfassung

In der komplementärmedizinischen Tumortherapie werden häufig Mistelpräparate angewendet. Iscucin® Populi (WALA Heilmittel GmbH, Bad Boll, Deutschland) ist eine Zubereitung der Pappelmistel, die in der anthroposophischen Medizin dem Stoffwechsel-Gliedmaßen-System zugeordnet wird. Auf dieser Basis werden diese Präparate oft in der Behandlung von urogenitalen Tumorerkrankungen, wie Blasen- und Prostatakarzinomen, eingesetzt. Im Zuge einer nichtinterventionellen Studie wurden in acht onkologischen Praxen in Deutschland Daten zur Verträglichkeit und Anwendung von Iscucin® Populi sowie zum Therapieverlauf inklusive Lebensqualität von 72 Patientinnen und Patienten mit malignen urogenitalen Tumorerkrankungen erfasst. Die Intention-to-treat-Analyse umfasste 69 Patientinnen und Patienten, davon waren 96 % männlich und das mittlere Alter betrug 71,1 Jahre. 87 % litten an einem Prostatakarzinom und 15 % an einem Harnblasentumor. Iscucin® Populi wurde in individuellen Dosierungen bei allen Schweregraden kurativ, adjuvant oder palliativ meist zusätzlich zur konventionellen Therapie gemäß Leitlinien verordnet. Die globale Verträglichkeit und Wirksamkeit wurden mit gut bis sehr gut beurteilt.

Auftretende Nebenwirkungen waren vor allem Fieber und Lokalreaktionen, welche ohne Maßnahmen und Folgeschäden ausheilten. Während der Studie nahm die Zahl der Patientinnen und Patienten mit Progression ab, während mehr in Remission gingen. Zu Studienbeginn kam es bei 29 Patientinnen und Patienten bereits zu einem Vorkommnis bezüglich eines Rezidivs, eines Zweitmalignoms oder/und Metastasen. Während der Behandlung kam es bei zehn Personen zu mindestens einem o. g. Ereignis oder zum Tod (n = 7). Die Ärzte und Ärztinnen beobachteten eine Stabilisierung des Tumorstatus, Teilremission, Tumormarkerrückgang, Verbesserung bzw. Stabilisierung des Allgemeinzustandes, allgemeine Kräftigung und Steigerung der Leistungsfähigkeit, psychische Stabilisierung und Stimmungsaufhellung, Rückgang der Kälteempfindlichkeit sowie Schmerzreduktion. Die Einschätzungen der Ärzte und Ärztinnen korrelierten mit den Patient-Reported Outcomes (PROs). Parameter wie emotionale und kognitive Funktionen, Schlafstörungen, Atemnot, Durchfall und Harnsymptome verbesserten sich signifikant. Die Iscucin® Populi-Therapie stieß bei den Personen auf eine hohe Akzeptanz. Über 90 % der behandelten Patientinnen und Patienten waren sehr zufrieden oder zufrieden mit der Therapie und würden sich wieder für diese entscheiden.

Iscucin® Populi eignet sich zur begleitenden komplementärmedizinischen Behandlung von malignen urogenitalen Tumorerkrankungen in Ergänzung zur konventionellen Therapie durch die positiven therapeutischen Wirkungen auf Tumorstatus, Allgemeinbefinden und Lebensqualität der Patientinnen und Patienten bei guter Verträglichkeit.

Schlüsselwörter: *Viscum album*, Mistel, Tumorstatus, Allgemeinbefinden

Summary

Mistletoe preparations are frequently applied in complementary medicine tumour therapy. Iscucin® Populi (WALA Heilmittel GmbH, Bad Boll, Germany) is a preparation made of mistletoe from poplar trees. In anthroposophical medicine, its potential is assigned to the metabolic-limb system. On this basis, the preparation is often used in treatment of urogenital tumor disease, for example bladder and prostate cancers.

Within a non-interventional study, data on the tolerability and use of Iscucin® Populi, as well as the course of therapy including quality of life, were collected from 72 patients with malignant urogenital tumors from eight oncology physicians in Germany.

In the intention-to-treat analysis, 69 patients (96 % males, mean age 71 years) suffered from prostate (87 %) and/or bladder (15 %) carcinoma. Iscucin® Populi was prescribed in individual dosages for all degrees of severity in a curative, adjuvant or palliative setting. This was usually in addition to conventional therapy according to medical guidelines. Global tolerability and effectiveness were assessed to be very good to good. The side effects that occurred were primarily fever and local reactions, which healed without any interference or subsequent damage. During the study, the number of patients with progression decreased, while more patients went in remission. At baseline, 29 patients already had an event regarding recurrence, second malignancy or/and metastases. During treatment, ten patients developed at least one event or died (n = 7). The physicians observed a stabilization of the tumor status, partial remission, decline in tumor markers, improvement or stabilization of the general condition, general strengthening and increase in performance, psychological stabilization and improvement in mood, reduction in sensitivity to cold and reduction in pain. Physicians' assessments correlated with patient-reported outcomes (PROs). Parameters such as emotional and cognitive functions, sleep disorders, shortness of breath, diarrhea and urinary symptoms improved significantly. The Iscucin® Populi therapy was met with a high level of acceptance among patients. Over 90 % of the patients treated were very satisfied or satisfied with the therapy and would choose it again.
Iscucin® Populi is a suitable concomitant complementary medical treatment for malignant urogenital tumor diseases in addition to conventional treatment due to the positive therapeutic effects on the tumor status, general health and quality of life of the patients, as well as good tolerability.
Keywords: *Viscum album*, mistletoe, tumor status, general health

Einleitung

In der komplementärmedizinischen Tumortherapie werden im deutschsprachigen Raum am häufigsten Mistelpräparate angewendet, meist ergänzend zur konventionellen Behandlung (Kienle und Kiene 2005). Die Gewissheit, an einer Tumorerkrankung erkrankt zu sein sowie die daraufhin eingesetzten Therapien belasten die Patientinnen und Patienten physisch und psychisch in der Regel sehr. Daraus resultieren erhebliche Einschränkungen der Lebensqualität. Studien zur Wirksamkeit einer

Misteltherapie bei verschiedenen Tumorerkrankungen zeigten eine Verbesserung der Lebensqualität der Patienten, auch bedingt durch eine Reduktion der durch die Chemotherapie induzierten Nebenwirkungen, eine positive Beeinflussung des Schmerzempfindens und des Krankheitsverlaufs (u. a. Tumorremission) sowie tendenziell längere Überlebenszeiten (Kienle, Kiene 2005; Klein 2005; Lange-Lindberg *et al.* 2006).

Die Mistel besitzt immunstimulierende Eigenschaften und eine antitumorale Wirkung (Kienle, Kiene 2005; Klein 2005; 2009). Neben der unspezifischen Immunstimulation konnten antimutagene, DNA-stabilisierende Eigenschaften an peripheren mononukleären Zellen sowie zytotoxische und Apoptose-induzierende Effekte an malignen Zellen gezeigt werden (König, Mathers 2008). Mistelpräparate bewirken eine vermehrte Freisetzung von β-Endorphin, das eine stark analgetische und stimmungsaufhellende Wirkung hat. Dies kann zu einer Steigerung des Wohlbefindens und einer Abnahme der tumorbedingten Schmerzen und somit zu einer Verbesserung der Lebensqualität führen (Lange-Lindberg *et al.* 2006).

Die wirksamen Hauptbestandteile der Mistel sind Mistellektine (Glykoproteine) und Viscotoxine (Polypeptide), daneben enthält die Mistel auch Flavonoide, Phenylpropane, Alkaloide und Polysaccharide (Urech, Baumgarter 2015; Zuzak *et al.* 2004). Die Gehalte an Lektin und Viscotoxin sind abhängig vom Erntezeitpunkt, Erntejahr, Bodenbeschaffenheit und vom Wirtsbaum. Die Pappelmistel zählt zu den lektinreichen Mistelarten (Felenda *et al.* 2019). Mistelpräparate des Wirtsbaums Pappel werden in der anthroposophischen Medizin dem Stoffwechsel-Gliedmaßen-System zugeordnet wird. Daraus abgeleitet findet das Arzneimittel oft bei der Behandlung von Blasen- und Prostatakarzinomen Anwendung (Wilkens 2006).

Material und Methoden

Mit Hilfe dieser offenen, einarmigen, prospektiven und multizentrischen nichtinterventionellen Studie (NIS) wurden unter praxisnahen und routinemäßigen Bedingungen des klinischen Alltags Erkenntnisse über die Verträglichkeit und die Anwendung von Iscucin® Populi sowie über den

Therapieverlauf inklusive der Lebensqualität mit malignen, urogenitalen Tumorerkrankungen gewonnen. Zusätzlich wurde die Akzeptanz der Behandlung untersucht. Dabei wurde Anwendung und Dosierung von Iscucin® Populi Stärke A bis H (WALA Heilmittel GmbH, Bad Boll/Eckwälden, Deutschland) vom/ von der behandelnden Arzt/Ärztin individuell in Kenntnis des Erkrankungszustandes des Patienten und der Fachinformation/Gebrauchsinformation festgelegt. Im Rahmen dieser NIS wurden von Mai 2012 bis Januar 2020 Daten von 75 erwachsenen Patientinnen und Patienten mit malignen urogenitalen Tumorerkrankungen, denen Iscucin® Populi als therapeutische Maßnahme verordnet worden war, in acht onkologischen Praxen in Deutschland erfasst. Die Personen wurden dazu ca. 1 Jahr lang im vierteljährlichen Abstand (Beobachtungszeitpunkte: 0 (Baseline), 1, 2, 3 und 4) beobachtet. Die Entscheidung über die Therapie wurde unabhängig von der NIS im Vorfeld getroffen. Hinsichtlich weiterer Erkrankungen und Therapien bestanden keine Aufnahmebeschränkungen. Für die Lebensqualitätsabfragen wurden validierte Fragebögen (EORTC-QLQ-C30 und EORTC-QLQ-PR25 (prostatakarzinom-spezifisch)) der European Organisation for Research and Treatment of Cancer (EORTC) eingesetzt.

Ergebnisse

Es wurden 75 Patientinnen und Patienten in die NIS eingeschlossen, aber nur 72 Personen beobachtet, da von drei Personen keine gültige Einwilligungserklärung vorlag. Für weitere drei Personen lagen keine dokumentierten Verlaufsvisiten vor, so dass 69 Patientinnen und Patienten in die Intention-to-Treat- (ITT-) Population aufgenommen werden konnten, davon waren 96 % männlich und das mittlere Alter betrug 71,1 Jahre. 87 % litten an einem Prostatakarzinom und 15 % an einem Harnblasentumor. Die Tumorerkrankungen bestanden im Mittel schon seit 42,2 Monate vor Beginn der NIS. Bei 29 % der Patientinnen und Patienten lag die Erstdiagnose länger als 5 Jahre zurück. 14 Patientinnen und Patienten wiesen bei Beobachtungsbeginn Metastasen auf, die am häufigsten in den Knochen lokalisiert waren. 13 Patientinnen und Patienten (19 %) hatten bei

Beobachtungsbeginn ein Rezidiv und zwei Personen ein Zweitmalignom. Der Remissionsstatus der Patientinnen und Patienten zu Beginn der NIS war ausgeglichen mit jeweils um die 20 % auf alle Stadien verteilt, außer für „minimal response". Hier waren es nur 10 %.

57 % der Patientinnen und Patienten waren von Begleiterkrankungen, wie Gefäßerkrankungen, Herzerkrankungen sowie Stoffwechsel- und Ernährungsstörungen, betroffen. Fast alle Begleiterkrankungen wurden medikamentös behandelt.

Die neben der subkutanen Behandlung mit Iscucin® Populi eingesetzten Therapien bezüglich der malignen, urogenitalen Tumorerkrankung orientierten sich an den vorgeschlagenen Behandlungsoptionen in den entsprechenden Leitlinien (Andreesen *et al.* 2006; c/o Deutsche Krebsgesellschaft e.V. 2016; 2019). Eine operative Entfernung des Tumors (21) oder des betroffenen Organs (10) wird häufig als Erstbehandlung durchgeführt. Nach der Operation waren 73 % der operierten Patientinnen und Patienten Primärtumor-frei. Nur sechs Personen erhielten vor Beobachtungsbeginn eine Chemotherapie, davon handelte es sich bei drei Personen um eine Blaseninstillation mit Mitomycin. Acht Patientinnen und Patienten hatten schon im Vorfeld Iscucin® Populi verordnet bekommen, davon lag eine Verordnung allerdings schon mehrere Jahre zurück.

Anwendung von Iscucin® Populi

77 % der Patientinnen und Patienten erhielten Iscucin® Populi auf Veranlassung des Arztes/ der Ärztin und 70 % erhielten die Medikation auf eigenen Wunsch. Iscucin® Populi wurde meist als Ergänzung zur aktuellen Therapie (36 %), aber auch wegen unzureichender Wirkung anderer Präparate (24 %) verordnet. Bei 44 % der Patientinnen und Patienten war die Intention von kurativer, bei 34 % von adjuvanter und bei 21 % von palliativer Natur. Die Behandlungsschemata wurden individuell für jede Person vom Arzt/ von der Ärztin bestimmt. Teilweise wurden drei Ampullen der Stärke H auf einmal gegeben. Mit Ausnahme eines Patienten wurde Iscucin® Populi gemäß Fachinformation subkutan meist in Tu-

mornähe am Bauch injiziert. Diesem wurde Iscucin® Populi subkutan, intravenös und paraurethal verabreicht. Der behandelnde Arzt dokumentierte hier als „herausragende Veränderung" eine gute Toleranz dieser Applikationsart von Iscucin® Populi. Bei fast allen Patientinnen und Patienten (94 %) konnte im Verlauf der NIS eine wirksame Dosis von Iscucin® Populi anhand der Indizparameter gemäß Fachinformation ermittelt werden. Abzugrenzen von unerwünschten Ereignissen sind hierbei leichte lokale Reaktionen an der Injektionsstelle (< 5 cm) und leichte Temperaturerhöhungen (< 38°C) (Paepke 2018). Bei 58,9 % trat eine lokale Entzündungsreaktion, bei 85,7 % der Patientinnen und Patienten verbesserte sich das Allgemeinbefinden. Ebenfalls zeigten sich leichte Erhöhungen der Körpertemperatur. Bei über der Hälfte der Patientinnen und Patienten lag die wirksame Dosis bei Stärke H (entspricht 5 % Mistelextrakt), gefolgt von Stärke G (entspricht 0,25 % Mistelextrakt). Neun Personen beendeten die Therapie mit Iscucin® Populi vorzeitig, entweder auf eigenen Wunsch, Verordnung des Arztes / der Ärztin oder waren „Lost to Follow up".

Sicherheit und Verträglichkeit

Die globale Verträglichkeit und Wirksamkeit wurden als sehr gut (81 %) bis gut (15 %) beurteilt. Bei fünf Personen (7 %) traten insgesamt zehn nichtschwerwiegende unerwünschte Arzneimittelwirkungen (UAW) während der Therapie mit Iscucin® Populi auf. Auftretende Nebenwirkungen waren vor allem Fieber und Lokalreaktionen, welche ohne Maßnahmen und Folgeschäden ausheilten. Schwerwiegende UAWs traten nicht auf.

Therapieverlauf (therapeutische Wirksamkeit)

Bei 46 % der Patienteninnen und Patienten wurde die globale Wirksamkeit als sehr gut und bei 39 % der Patienteninnen und Patienten als gut eingeschätzt. Die häufigsten Gründe für eine sehr gute oder gute globale therapeutische Wirksamkeit waren Verbesserung/Stabilisierung des Allgemeinzustandes, stabiler Tumorstatus und Verbesserung der Lebensqualität. Bei sechs Personen (9 %) wurde die globale therapeutische Wirksamkeit als mäßig eingestuft, da ein Patient operiert werden musste und es bei fünf Personen zu einer Progression kam, wobei sich jedoch initial der Allgemeinzustand bei drei Personen verbesserte.

Klinischer Tumorverlauf

Bei Aufnahme der Patientinnen und Patienten befanden sich 24 % der Patientinnen und Patienten in einem progressiven Krankheitsstadium und 21 % in Vollremission. Am Ende der NIS war der Anteil der Patientinnen und Patienten mit einem progressiven Status gesunken (10 %). Der Anteil der Patientinnen und Patienten in Teilremission nahm im Verlauf ab, dafür stieg der Anteil an Patientinnen und Patienten mit Status „minimal response" um 17 % an.

Zu Beginn der Untersuchung hatten bereits 29 von 69 Patientinnen und Patienten ein Ereignis bezüglich Rezidive (19 %), Zweitmalignome (3 %) und Metastasen (21 %). Insgesamt trat im Studienverlauf bei zehn Personen mindestens ein Ereignis auf, davon waren drei Personen zu Beginn der Beobachtung ereignisfrei gewesen. Während der Studie wurden sieben Todesfälle dokumentiert. Vier davon wurden als tumorbedingt eingestuft, zwei Todesursachen waren unbekannt und ein Todesgrund war eine Bronchopneumonie, die nicht mit Iscucin® Populi in Zusammenhang stand. Weitere sieben Personen konnten nicht weiterverfolgt werden, so dass unklar war, ob ein Ereignis eintrat oder nicht (zensiert). Ereignisfrei waren somit insgesamt 30 Patientinnen und Patienten (Abb. 1).

Im Durchschnitt betrug die PSA-Konzentration zu Beginn der NIS 11,8 ng/ml. Im Beobachtungsverlauf sank der Mittelwert des PSA und die von den Ärzten/Ärztinnen als „klinisch signifikant" bewerteten Konzentrationen nahmen kontinuierlich ab. Weitere Tumormarker wurden nicht erfasst.

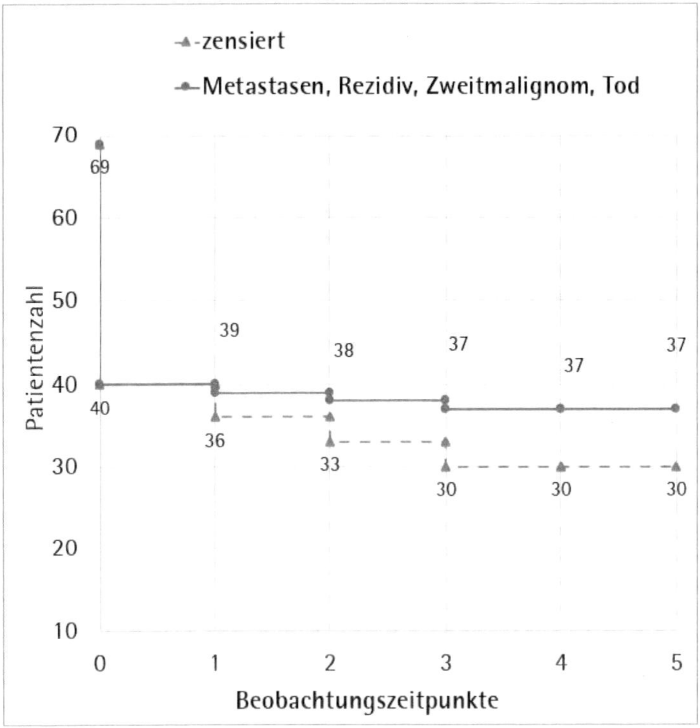

Abb.1: Kaplan-Meier-Kurve der ereignisfreien Zeit (Metastasen, Rezidiv, Zweitmalignom, Tod)

Gesundheits-/Leistungsstatus

Im Verlauf wurde ein leichter Rückgang des durchschnittlichen Karnofsky-Index von 98 auf 81 beobachtet.

Der Anteil der nicht kälteempfindlichen Patientinnen und Patienten stieg von 46 % auf 75 % an. Zu Beobachtungsbeginn waren zehn Patientinnen und Patienten (15 %) stark kälteempfindlich, im weiteren Verlauf keine Patientin/ kein Patient.

Herausragende Veränderungen wurden von den Ärzten/Ärztinnen bei 55 % der Patientinnen und Patienten dokumentiert. Am häufigsten wurde Verbesserung der Lebensqualität (37 %), gefolgt von Schmerzreduktion, Kräftigung/ Steigerung der Vitalität/ Leistungssteigerung und psychische Stabilisierung/ Stimmungsaufhellung genannt.

Lebensqualität (Tab. 1)

Zur Ermittlung der Lebensqualität wurde der Fragebogen EORTC-QLQ-C30 von den Patientinnen und Patienten zu allen Beobachtungszeitpunkten beantwortet. Es zeigten sich signifikant, verbesserte Werte bei „emotionaler Funktion", „kognitiver Funktion", „Atemnot", „Schlafstörungen" und „Durchfall". Besonders herauszuheben sind die Parameter „emotionale Funktion" (Median: 8,33) und „Müdigkeit" (Median: -8,20), da diese ebenfalls im Median eine Verbesserung zeigten.

Tab. 1: Ergebnisse der PROs

EORTC-QLQ-C30 Funktion-Skalen		**EORTC-QLQ-C30 Symptom-Skalen**		**EORTC-QLQ-PR25**	
emotionale Funktion	↑ *	Atemnot	↑ *	Harnsymptome	↑ *
kognitive Funktion	↑ *	Schlafstörungen	↑ *	Inkontinenzhilfe	↑
Rollenfunktion	↑	Durchfall	↑ *	behandlungs-bedingte Symptome	↑
physische Funktion	↑	Müdigkeit	↑	Darmsymptome	↑
soziale Funktion	↑	Verstopfung	↑	sexuelle Funktion	↑
globaler Gesundheitsstatus	↑	Schmerzen	↑	sexuelle Aktivität	↓
		Übelkeit und Erbrechen	↑		
		Appetitmangel	↔		
		finanzielle Probleme	↓		

↑ Verbesserung; ↓ Verschlechterung; ↔ keine Änderung;
* signifikante Ergebnisse

Im prostatakarzinomspezifische Fragebogen EORTC-QLQ-P25 zeigte sich eine Verbesserung bei den Parametern „Harnsymptome“, „Inkontinenzhilfe“ und „sexuelle Funktion“, wobei der Wert für „Harnsymptome“ im Vorher-Nachher-Vergleich signifikant war. Der Parameter „Harnsymptome“ zeigte ebenfalls im Median (-13,89) eine Verbesserung.

Akzeptanz

91 % der Patientinnen und Patienten waren sehr zufrieden oder zufrieden mit der Behandlung und 91 % würden wieder eine Misteltherapie mit Iscucin® Populi machen. Etwas mehr als die Hälfte der gab an, dass die Therapie mit Iscucin® Populi eine herausragende Veränderung mit sich gebracht hat. Am häufigsten berichteten die Patientinnen und Patienten über Kräftigung und Steigerung der Vitalität/ Leistungssteigerung sowie über eine verbesserte Lebensqualität und eine Verbesserung des Allgemeinzustandes.

Diskussion

Ursprünglich war geplant 180 Patientinnen und Patienten einzuschließen, jedoch wurde aufgrund schleppender Rekrutierung die NIS vorzeitig abgebrochen. Es war nicht möglich, weitere Ärzte/Ärztinnen mit genügend Kenntnis über Iscucin® Populi, die an der NIS hätten teilnehmen können, zu rekrutieren, so dass nur acht Praxen/Kliniken 75 Patientinnen und Patienten in die NIS aufgenommen werden konnten.

Die Charakteristika der Patientenpopulation in dieser NIS war der gewählten Indikation von malignen, urogenitalen Tumorerkrankungen geschuldet und fiel erwartungsgemäß aus. Ebenso der hohe Anteil an Prostatakarzinomen (87 %) mit schon länger zurückliegender Erstdiagnose, da diese die am häufigsten vorkommende Tumorerkrankung des Mannes ausmacht und die relativen 5- und 10-Jahres-Überlebensraten bei malignen, urogenitalen Tumorerkrankungen im Vergleich zu anderen Tumorarten hoch sind (RKI 2019; Tumorzentrum München 2008). Übergewicht, Rauchen, regelmäßiger Alkoholkonsum und Schadstoffbelastungen zählen zu den Risikofaktoren für die Entstehung von malignen, urogenitalen Tumoren (Tumorzentrum München 2008). In der NIS war über die Hälfte der Patientinnen und Patienten übergewichtig (46 %) oder adipös (12 %), was der Normalbevölkerung in Deutschland laut Gesundheitsberichtserstattung des Bundes (gbe-bund) entspricht (Gesundheitsberichterstattung des Bundes 2021). 29 % der Patienten waren ehemalige Raucher. Eine Schadstoffbelastung mit aromatischen Aminen, Azofarbstoffen, Trichlorethan, TCDD, Arsen oder Asbest und ein regelmäßiger Alkoholkonsum spielten in dieser NIS als Risikofaktor eine untergeordnete Rolle. Entsprechend dem Alter der Patientinnen und Patienten und ihrer Vorbelastungen waren 57 % von Begleiterkrankungen betroffen. Iscucin® Populi wurde in der Anwendung gemäß Fachinformation und in individuellen Dosierungen als kurativer, adjuvanter oder palliativer Therapieansatz, meist als Ergänzung zur aktuellen Therapie, aber auch wegen unzureichender Wirkung anderer Präparate oder auf Wunsch des Patienten/ der Patientin verordnet. Dies spiegelt die Behandlungspraxis und die Anwendung von komplementärmedizinisch angewendeten Mistelpräparaten wider. Abzugrenzen von den Indizparametern einer wirksamen Dosis sind UAWs von Mistelpräparaten. Zu den geläufigsten UAWs von Mistelpräparaten gehören überschießende lokale Reaktionen an der Injektionsstelle und grippeartige Symptome wie Fieber, Schüttelfrost, leichte gastrointestinale Beschwerden und Kopfschmerzen (Huber *et al.* 2011; Paepke 2018). In der aktuellen NIS waren alle aufgetretenen UAWs ohne zusätzliche Maßnahmen abgeklungen, alle Personen waren wiederhergestellt und es blieben keine Folgen zurück. Die Sicherheit von Iscucin® Populi wurde auch bereits von Huber *et al.* (2011) in einer Placebo-kontrollierten Studie an Probandinnen und Probanden dargelegt (Huber *et al.* 2018). Die globale Verträglichkeit von Iscucin® Populi wurde damit übereinstimmend in der vorliegenden NIS von den Ärzten/ Ärztinnen sehr oft (81 %) als sehr gut eingestuft.

Die globale Wirksamkeit wurde von den Ärzten/ Ärztinnen bei 86 % der Patientinnen und Patienten als sehr gut und gut eingeschätzt. Dies zeichnete sich auch im klinischen Tumorverlauf inklusive Stabilisation des Tumorstatus sowie der Verbesserung der Lebensqualität ab. Die Ärztinnen und Ärzte berichteten über Verbesserung/ Stabilisierung des Allgemeinzustandes, Kräftigung/ Steigerung der Vitalität/ Leistungssteigerung, Schmerzreduktion und psychische Stabilisierung/ Stimmungsaufhellung. Mistelpräparate bewirken eine vermehrte Freisetzung von β-Endorphin, das eine stark analgetische und stimmungsaufhellende Wirkung hat. Dies kann zu einer Steigerung des Wohlbefindens und einer Abnahme der tumorbedingten Schmerzen und somit zu einer Verbesserung der Lebensqualität führen (Lange-Lindberg *et al.* 2006). Ebenso berichteten Patientinnen und Patienten selbst über Kräftigung/Steigerung der Vitalität/Leistungssteigerung, verbesserte Lebensqualität und Verbesserung des Allgemeinzustandes und würden diese Therapie wieder machen.

Der Anteil der Patientinnen und Patienten mit einem progressiven Status sank während der Beobachtung ab, während sich prozentual gesehen mehr Patientinnen und Patienten in Vollremission befanden. Mehrere Patientinnen und Patienten kamen in den Status der „minimal response" während der Anwendung von Iscucin® Populi. Des Weiteren konnte ein Rückgang der Ereignisse bezüglich Rezidive, Zweitmalignom, Metastasen und/oder Tod verzeichnet werden. Da auch Patientinnen und Patienten mit weit fortgeschrittenen Tumorerkrankungen in die NIS aufgenommen wurden, welche im palliativen Stadium Iscucin® Populi bekamen, war das Auftreten tumorbedingter Todesfälle innerhalb der NIS bis zu einem gewissen Grad abzusehen. Von den Ärztinnen und Ärzten wurde berichtet, dass meist bis zum Tod das Allgemeinbefinden und die Lebensqualität der Patientinnen/Patienten sehr gut waren. Auch das prostataspezifische Antigen (PSA), welches ein Tumormarker für Prostatakarzinome darstellt und in der Früherkennung genutzt wird, sank im Laufe der NIS (c/o Deutsche Krebsgesellschaft e.V. 2019; Jungmayr 2017; RKI 2010, 2019). Patientinnen und Patienten sowie Ärztinnen und Ärzte sahen eine allgemeine Kräftigung und Steigerung der Vitalität sowie Leistungssteigerung durch die Therapie mit Iscucin® Populi, obwohl sich dies nicht in einem Anstieg des Karnofsky-Index zeigte. Jedoch die Stabilisierung der Thermoregulation konnte durch die Abnahme der Kälteempfindlichkeit der Patientinnen/Patienten bestätigt werden. Kienle und Kiene (2017) sowie Schad (2020) nannten als Wirkung der Mistelpräparaten die Normalisierung des Wärmeempfindens und die Verbesserung der „Durchwärmung“, v. a. bei Personen, die leicht frieren (Kienle, Kiene 2017; Schad 2020). Mehrere Studien zur Behandlung tumoröser Erkrankungen mit Mistelpräparaten zeigten eine Verbesserung der Lebensqualität (Kienle, Kiene 2017; Loef, Walach 2020; Paepke 2018; Schad 2020). Nach der Einteilung und Interpretation der Differenzlevel von King (1996) und Osoba *et al.* (1998) zeigte sich im Vorher-Nachher-Vergleich bei den Parametern „emotionale Funktion“, „kognitive Funktion“, „Atemnot“ und „Schlafstörungen“ eine moderate Verbesserung (King 1996; Osoba *et al.* 1998). Leichte Verbesserungen waren bei „physischen Funktion“, „Rollenfunktion“, „globaler Gesundheitsstatus“, „Müdigkeit“ und „Durchfall“ zu sehen. Auch Kienle, Kiene (2017), Paepke (2018) sowie Schad (2020) konnten in Reviews und Metaanalysen zu Studien mit Mistelpräparaten feststellen, dass sich Emotionalität, Konzentrationsfähigkeit, Schlaf sowie Fatigue und Diarrhoe verbesserten (Kienle, Kiene 2017; Paepke 2018; Schad 2020). Im Gegensatz zur Studienanalyse von Kienle und Kiene (2017) sowie Schad (2020) zeigte sich in der NIS keine Appetitsteigerung (Kienle, Kiene 2017; Schad 2020). Leichte Verbesserungen traten bei „Darmsymptome“, „behandlungsbedingte Symptome“ und der „sexuellen Aktivität“ auf. Moderate Verbesserungen gab es bei den Parametern „Harnsymptome“, „Inkontinenzhilfe“ und „sexuelle Funktion“.

Zusammenfassung/Ausblick

Iscucin® Populi wird in der Anwendung gemäß Fachinformation und individuellen Dosierungen nach Anweisung des Arztes/ der Ärztin in der Alltagspraxis verordnet. Durch eine Behandlung mit Iscucin® Populi kann sich der Tumorstatus stabilisieren und die Lebensqualität in vielen Parametern verbessert werden. Durch die hohe therapeutische Akzeptanz von Iscucin® Populi seitens der Patientinnen und Patienten und die gute Verträglichkeit, ist eine Behandlung mit Iscucin® Populi bei allen Schweregraden von malignen, urogenitalen Tumorerkrankungen als kurativer, adjuvanter oder palliativer Therapieansatz in Erwägung zu ziehen.

Danksagung

Die Autoren danken allen Patientinnen und Patienten für die Teilnahme an dieser nichtinterventionellen Studie sowie allen teilnehmenden Praxen und Kliniken für die Beobachtung und Dokumentation der Personen. Der Anfomed GmbH wird für die umfassende Auswertung der Daten gedankt.

Interessenkonflikt

Ein Interessenkonflikt besteht nicht. Die Autorinnen und Autoren waren zum Zeitpunkt der Datenerhebung und -auswertung Mitarbeitende der WALA Heilmittel GmbH.

Literatur

Andreesen R, Böhle A, Bokemeyer C et al.: F4 Harnblasenkarzinom. In: Garbe C, Albers P, Beckmann MW et al. (Hrsg.): Kurzgefasste interdisziplinäre Leitlinien 2006 (Deutsche Krebsgesellschaft e.V.) München: Zuckschwerdt; 2006: 259–265.

Deutsche Krebsgesellschaft e.V.: Interdisziplinäre Leitlinie der Qualität S3 zur Früherkennung, Diagnose und Therapie der verschiedenen Stadien des Prostatakarzinoms, 2019. https://www.leitlinienprogramm-onkologie.de/leitlinien/prostatakarzinom (Stand: 05.03.2021).

Deutsche Krebsgesellschaft e.V.: S3-Leitlinie Früherkennung, Diagnose, Therapie und Nachsorge des Harnblasenkarzinoms, 2016. https://www.leitlinienprogramm-onkologie.de/leitlinien/harnblasenkarzinom (Stand: 05.03.2021).

Felenda J, Turek C, Stintzing FC: Antiproliferative potential from aqueous Viscum album L. preparations and their main constituents in comparison with ricin and purothionin on human cancer cells. J Ethnopharmacol. 2019; 236: 100–107.

Gesundheitsberichterstattung des Bundes: Adipositas. https://www.gbe-bund.de/gbe (Stand: 14.07.2021).

Huber R, Lüdtke H, Wieber J et al.: Safety and effects of two mistletoe preparations on production of Interleukin-6 and other immune parameters – a placebo controlled clinical trial in healthy subjects. MC Complement Altern Med. 2011, 11: 116–128.

Jungmayr P: Chamäleon zwischen Organ- und Tumormarker. DAZ. 2017; 157: 1756–1759.

Kienle GS, Kiene H: Klinische Studien zur Misteltherapie der Krebserkrankung – Eine Übersicht. Der Merkurstab. 2017; 70: 176–186.

Kienle GS, Kiene H: Kontrollierte Studien zur Misteltherapie der Krebserkrankungen. Eine systematische Übersicht. In: Scheer R, Bauer R, Becker H et al. (Hrsg.): Fortschritte in der Misteltherapie. Essen: KVC; 2005: 405–421.

King MT: The interpretation of scores from the EORTC quality of life questionnaire QLQ-C30. QoL Res. 1996; 5: 555–567.

Klein R: Effekte von Mistelextrakten auf immunkompetente Zellen in vitro und in vivo und ihre mögliche Bedeutung für die Therapie von Tumorerkrankungen und andere klinische Entitäten. In: Scheer R, Bauer R, Becker H et al. (Hrsg.): Fortschritte in der Misteltherapie. Essen: KVC; 2005: 207–221.

Klein R: Effekte von Mistelextrakten auf immunkompetente Zellen in vitro und in vivo. In: Scheer R, Alban S, Becker H et al. (Hrsg.): Die Misteltherapie in der Tumortherapie 2. Essen: KVC; 2009: 185–193.

König M, Mathers MJ: Misteltherapie in der urologischen Onkologie. Blickpunkt Der Mann. 2008; 6: 28–32.

Lange-Lindberg AM, Velasco-Garrido M, Busse R: Misteltherapie als begleitende Behandlung der Toxizität der Chemotherapie maligner Erkrankungen. DAHTA-Bericht 4, 2006, DIMDI.

Osoba D, Rodrigues G, Myles J et al.: Interpreting the significance of changes in health-related quality-of-life scores. J Clin Oncol. 1998; 16: 139–144.

Paepke D: Die Misteltherapie in der Onkologie. Im Focus Onkologie. 2018; 21: 64–68.

Robert Koch-Institut (RKI): Krebs in Deutschland 2005/2006 – Häufigkeiten und Trends. Berlin: GEKID, 2010.

Robert Koch-Institut (RKI): Krebs in Deutschland 2015/2016 – Häufigkeiten und Trends. Berlin: GEKID, 2019.

Schad F: Misteltherapie in der Onkologie – Update der aktuellen Forschungsergebnisse. Erfahrungsheilkunde 2020; 69: 252–259.

Tumorzentrum München (Hrsg.). Urogenitale Tumoren – Empfehlungen zur Diagnostik, The preparation of mistletoe. Chemical constituents of Viscum album L.: Implications for the pharmaceutical preparation of mistletoe. Trans Res Biomed. 2015; 4: 11–23.

Wilkens J: Misteltherapie. Differenzierte Anwendung der Mistel nach Wirtsbäumen. Stuttgart: Sonntag; 2006: 79–84.

Zuzak T, Rist L, Viviani A et al.: Das Mistelpräparat Iscucin® – Herstellung, Analytik, Wirkung in vitro. Der Merkurstab. 2004; 54: 467–473.

Dipl. agrar-biol. Jennifer E. Felenda, Dr. Claudia Turek,
Prof. Dr. Florian C. Stintzing
WALA Heilmittel GmbH, Präklinische und klinische Forschung,
Bad Boll/ Eckwälden, Germany

Korrespondenzadresse:
florian.stintzing@wala.de

Viscum album as Potential Adjuvant Role in Standard Care of Resected Pancreatic Cancer

Chang Moo Kang

Summary

Background: Pancreatic cancer is among the most lethal malignancies of the gastrointestinal tract. Despite margin-negative pancreatectomy being the most effective monotherapy, only less than 20 % of patients have resectable disease. Even after resection, systemic metastasis is common, necessitating postoperative adjuvant chemotherapy. abnobaVISCUM® F, derived from *Viscum album*, has demonstrated potential in normalizing immune responses and inhibiting cancer cell proliferation. This study retrospectively investigates the oncologic impact of abnobaVISCUM® F on patients with resected pancreatic cancer.

Materials and Methods: A total of 604 patients who underwent radical resection for pancreatic cancer between January 2005 and December 2019 at Severance Hospital in Seoul, Korea, were reviewed. Patients were categorized into two groups based on the administration of abnobaVISCUM® F (*Viscum* group) or not (control group) during the postoperative period. Clinicopathologic characteristics, disease-free survival (DFS), and overall survival (OS) were compared using propensity score matching (PSM) to ensure balanced baseline characteristics between the groups.

Results: Out of 604 patients, 113 received postoperative abnobaVISCUM® F therapy. Initial comparisons revealed significant differences between the groups in terms of the timing of treatment initiation (post-2014), ASA scores, hospital stay duration, and preoperative CA19-9 levels. After PSM, no significant differences were observed in baseline characteristics between two groups. In the PSM cohort, the *Viscum* group showed a superior 1-year DFS (66.4 % vs. 55.2 %, $p = 0.015$) and a non-significant trend towards improved 1-year OS (93.2 % vs. 89.6 %, $p = 0.292$). Subgroup analyses indicated that the *Viscum* group had better DFS in patients with node-negative (pN0) status, R0 resection, and those not receiving adjuvant chemotherapy. Univariate and multivariate analyses identified *Viscum* therapy, positive lymph nodes, and lymphovascular invasion as significant factors affecting DFS. For OS, significant factors included adjuvant therapy and positive lymph nodes.

Conclusion: Postoperative administration of abnobaVISCUM® F significantly improves disease-free survival in patients with resected pancreatic cancer, particularly in those with node-negative, R0 resection, and without adjuvant chemotherapy. *Viscum* therapy, lymph node status, and lymphovascular invasion are critical factors influencing DFS, while adjuvant chemotherapy and lymph node status impact overall survival. These findings warrant further investigation through well-designed randomized controlled trials to confirm the therapeutic benefits of abnobaVISCUM® F in resected pancreatic cancer patients.
Keywords: Pancreatic cancer, pancreatectomy, adjuvant chemotherapy, *Viscum album*

A publication in a scientific journal is in preparation.

Conflict of interest

This study was supported by Abnoba Korea research grant (4-2021-0077): „Oncologic impact of postoperative abnobaVISCUM injection in resected pancreatic cancer".

Chang Moo Kang, M.D., Ph.D.[1,2]
[1] Division of HBP Surgery, Department of Surgery, Yonsei University College of Medicine, Seoul, South Korea
[2] Pancreatobiliary Cancer Center, Yonsei Cancer Center, Severance Hospital, Seoul, South Korea

Corresponding author:
cmkang@yuhs.ac

Pharmakokinetik von Mistellektinen nach intravenöser Applikation von Helixor® P bei gesunden Probanden

Pharmacokinetics of Mistletoe Lectins after Intravenous Administration of Helixor® P in Healthy Volunteers

Ann-Kathrin Lederer, Michael Schink, Sabine Rieger, Roman Huber

Zusammenfassung

Mistelpräparate haben zytotoxische und immunmodulierende Eigenschaften und werden nicht nur subkutan, sondern auch intravenös eingesetzt. Bisher gab es wenige pharmakokinetische Daten zur intravenösen Verabreichung, weswegen es Ziel der Studie war, die Pharmakokinetik und Sicherheit von Mistellektinen nach intravenöser Verabreichung eines Mistelpräparats zu untersuchen. Hierfür erhielten insgesamt 8 gesunde männliche Freiwillige eine einmalige Infusion von 2.000 mg Helixor® P. Es war möglich, bei allen Probanden Mistellektine nach der Infusion nachzuweisen. Die mittlere Halbwertszeit der Mistellektine im Serum betrug 7,02 ± 2,01 Stunden. Da es zu einem deutlichen Anstieg der Leberenzyme der Probanden kam, mussten wir die Studie vorzeitig beenden. Die Teilnehmer litten unter keinen leberspezifischen Symptomen und die Leberenzyme erholten sich im Verlauf vollständig. Der Schweregrad der arzneimittelinduzierten Leberschädigung wurde als leicht eingestuft. Wir konnten mit unserer Arbeit zeigen, dass die Pharmakokinetik von natürlichem Mistellektin deutlich länger ist als die von rekombinantem Mistellektin. Allerdings verursacht die Dosis von 2.000 mg Helixor P® bei Gesunden eine vorübergehende Hepatopathie. Bei Patienten und Patientinnen, die eine intravenöse Behandlung mit Helixor P® erhalten, sollten daher die Leberenzyme überwacht werden.

Schlüsselwörter: Klinische Phase I-Studie, *Viscum album*, Mistellektine, Pharmakokinetik, reversible Hepatopathie

Summary

Mistletoe lectins have cytotoxic and immunomodulating properties and are used not only subcutaneously but also intravenously. To date, there have been few pharmacokinetic data on intravenous administration, which is why the aim of the study was to investigate the pharmacokinetics and safety of intravenously administered mistletoe lectins. For this purpose, a total of 8 healthy male volunteers received a single infusion of 2,000 mg Helixor® P. It was possible to detect mistletoe lectins in all subjects after the infusion. The mean half-life of mistletoe lectins in serum was 7.02 ± 2.01 hours. As there was a significant increase in the subjects' liver enzymes, we had to terminate the study prematurely. The participants did not suffer from any liver-specific symptoms and the liver enzymes recovered completely after the study. The severity of the drug-induced liver damage was classified as mild. We were able to show that the pharmacokinetics of natural mistletoe is significantly longer than that of recombinant mistletoe. However, the dose of 2,000 mg Helixor P® causes transient hepatopathy in healthy individuals. Patients receiving intravenous treatment with Helixor P® should therefore have their liver enzymes monitored.

Keywords: Phase I clinical trial, *Viscum album*, mistletoe lectins, pharmacokinetics, reversible liver injury

Einleitung

Mistelpräparate werden außerhalb der eigentlichen Zulassung im Sinne eines Off-Label-Use beispielsweise zur Fieberinduktion auch intravenös verabreicht (Schläppi *et al.* 2017). In einer früheren Dosisfindungsstudie fanden wir eine gute Verträglichkeit von bis zu 2.000 mg Helixor® P, das einmal wöchentlich intravenös verabreicht wurde (Huber *et al.* 2017). Über die Pharmakokinetik von intravenös verabreichtem Helixor® P war bisher nur sehr wenig bekannt. Ziel der Studie war es daher, Informationen über die Pharmakokinetik und Sicherheit dieses intravenös verabreichten Mistelpräparates zu sammeln.

Material und Methoden

Die vorliegende monozentrische, offene, nicht kontrollierte Studie wurde zwischen Juni und Juli 2022 am Uni-Zentrum Naturheilkunde der Uniklinik Freiburg durchgeführt. Die Studie sollte die Pharmakokinetik von natürlichen Mistellektinen (enthalten in Helixor® P, einem standardisierten wässrigen Frischpflanzenextrakt aus *Viscum album* L. *austriacum* (Kiefernmistel)) innerhalb von 72 Stunden nach einer einmaligen Infusion von 2.000 mg des Mistelpräparats untersuchen. Hierfür wurden nur gesunde Nichtraucher im Alter von 18 bis 45 Jahren mit einem Body-Mass-Index (BMI) zwischen 18,5 und 28 kg/m² eingeschlossen. Interessenten mit Vorerkrankungen, regelmäßiger Medikamenteneinnahme, Infektionskrankheiten, klinisch relevanten Allergien oder Alkohol- oder Drogenmissbrauch konnten nicht eingeschlossen werden.

Als Sicherheitsparameter wurden diverse laborchemische Parameter gewählt, die u. a. den Elektrolythaushalt, die Funktion von Leber und Niere sowie die Zellzahlen im peripheren Blut abbilden.

Eine Übersicht aller Untersuchungszeitpunkte ist in Tabelle 1 dargestellt. Die klinische Studie mit der EudraCT-Nr. 2021-000601 wurde nach den Regeln der Guten Klinischen Praxis (GCP) geplant, durchgeführt und ausgewertet. Die Genehmigung der Studie durch das BfArM erfolgte am 19.01.2022. Die Ethikkommission des Uniklinik Freiburg erteilte am 20.04.2022 ein positives Votum (Nummer 21-1693). Außerdem wurde die Studie beim Deutschen Register für Klinische Studien registriert (DRKS-S00027485). Alle Studienteilnehmer haben nach detaillierter mündlicher Aufklärung eine schriftliche Einverständniserklärung zur Teilnahme abgegeben.

Tab. 1: Übersicht aller Untersuchungszeitpunkte (UZP) im Rahmen der Studie. (ML = Mistellektine, E-/A-Kriterien = Ein- und Ausschlusskriterien, UE = Unerwünschtes Ereignis, SUE = Schweres unerwünschtes Ereignis, SUSAR = Suspected Unexpected Serious Adverse Reaction)

Untersuchungszeitpunkt (UZP)[1] **Untersuchung/ Maßnahme**	Screening	UZP 0 vor/mit Beginn i.v.	UZP 1 0h	UZP 2 0,25h	UZP 3 0,5h	UZP 4 0,75h	UZP 5 1h	UZP 6 1,5h	UZP 7 2h	UZP 8 3h	UZP 9 4h	UZP 10 6h	UZP 11 8h	UZP 12 10h	UZP 13 12h	UZP 14 18h	UZP 15 24h	UZP 16 36h	UZP 17 48h	UZP 18 72h	UZP 19 Follow-up (Tag 14±3)	Studien-abschluss
Probandeninfo/Einverständniserklärung	X																					
E-/A-Kriterien incl. Alkohol-/Drogenabusus	X																					
Demograph. Daten/Größe	X																					
Gewicht/ Blutdruck/ Puls/ EKG	X																			X	X	
Körperliche Untersuchung	X																			X	X	
Körpertemperatur	X	X							X		X	X	X	X	X	X	←	[2]	→	X	X	
Blutentnahme Safety-Parameter	X																X		X	X	X	
Blutentnahme Ermittlung ML-Konz		X[3]	X	X	X	X	X	X	X	X	X	X	X	X	X	X	X	X	X	X	X	
Verabreichung des Prüfpräparats		X																				
UE/SUE/SUSAR-Erfassung		X	X	X	X	X	X	X	X	X	X	X	X	X	X	X	X	X	X	X	X	
Compliance		X	X	X	X	X	X	X	X	X	X	X	X	X	X	X	X	X	X	X	X	
Studienabschluss																						X

[1] Angabe der Zeiträume bezogen auf Ende der intravenösen Infusion (Infusionsdauer ca. 2.5 Stunden)

[2] Temperaturmessung 24 – 48 Stunden nach Verabreichung der Prüfmedikation: nach 24 Stunden alle 2 Stunden bis 40 Stunden nach Verabreichung, danach wieder nach 48 Stunden

[3] Blutabnahme zwingend vor Verabreichung der Prüfmedikation

Ergebnisse

Insgesamt wurden 8 Probanden (durchschnittliches Alter 29,6 ± 5,7 Jahre mit einem durchschnittlichen BMI von 24 ± 1,5 kg/m²) eingeschlossen. In allen Probanden konnten nach der Infusion Mistellektine im Serum nachgewiesen werden. Die Mistellektine waren bei einem Probanden bis nach 10 Stunden, bei fünf Probanden bis nach 12 Stunden, sowie bei jeweils einem Probanden bis nach 18 Stunden bzw. bis nach 24 Stunden noch nachweisbar. Die Halbwertszeit der Mistellektine im Serum lag bei 7,02 ± 2,0 Stunden.

Eine Übersicht über den Konzentrationsverlauf der Mistellektine im Serum zeigt Abbildung 1. Alle errechneten pharmakokinetischen Parameter werden in Tabelle 2 dargestellt.

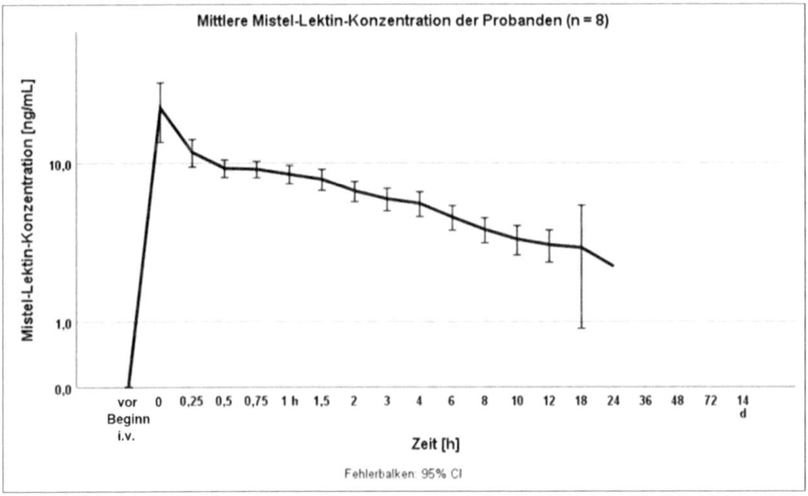

Abb. 1: Konzentration der Mistellektine im Serum während der Beobachtungsphase

Tab. 2: Errechnete pharmakokinetische Parameter

Parameter	N		Mittel-				Perzentile		
	Gültig	Fehl.	wert	Std	Min.	Max.	25	Median	75
λ [/h] (= Eliminationskonstante der gesamten Phase 0 – 24 h)									
Gesamt (n = 8)	8	0	0,107	0,033	0,067	0,166	0,085	0,097	0,128
$t_{1/2}$ [h] (= Halbwertszeit der gesamten Phase 0 – 24 h)									
Gesamt (n = 8)	8	0	7,023	2,011	4,179	10,376	5,458	7,169	8,187
k_e [/h] (= reine Geschwindigkeitskonstante der Elimination aus zentralem ins periphere Kompartiment)									
Gesamt (n = 8)	8	0	0,065	0,030	0,018	0,097	0,040	0,075	0,089
C_{max} [ng/mL] (= maximale Konzentration im Serum)									
Gesamt (n = 8)	8	0	18,99	7,403	10,00	30,90	14,40	16,75	24,35
Fläche unter der Kurve $_{(0-24\,h)}$ [ng * h/mL]									
Gesamt (n = 8)	8	0	68,35	50,12	33,11	176,12	36,88	45,38	86,54

Initial war der Einschluss von 12 Probanden für die Studie geplant. Nach Einschluss der ersten 8 Probanden fiel bei allen Probanden eine deutliche Erhöhung der Leberenzyme auf, so dass die Studie aufgrund des möglichen Risikos einer entsprechenden Leberschädigung für weitere Probanden vorzeitig beendet wurde. Die Alanin-Aminotransferase (ALT, auch GPT) stieg 72 Stunden nach Infusion von 23 ± 6 auf maximal 445 ±2 60 U/l, das absolute Maximum lag bei 892 U/I. Die Aspartat-Aminotransferase (AST, auch GOT) stieg 72 Stunden nach Infusion von 24 ± 3 auf maximal 318 ± 33 U/l, das absolute Maximum lag bei 474 U/I. Die Laktatdehydrogenase (LDH) stieg ebenfalls erheblich an, und zwar von 178 ± 18 auf ein Maximum von 334 ± 84 nach 72 Stunden. Die übrigen Werte, insbesondere auch die Leberfunktionsindikatoren wie die Gerinnung und der Bilirubinwert, blieben im Normbereich. Bei allen Probanden zeigt sich im Rahmen der Nachuntersuchung zwei Wochen nach Abschluss der Studie eine Normalisierung der Leberwerte.

Der Schweregrad der hier offenbar vorliegenden arzneimittelinduzierten Leberschädigung wurde nach den Common Terminology Criteria for Adverse Events (CTCAE,Version 5.0) für Kriterien für hepatobiliäre Störungen als gering (Grad 1) eingestuft („asymptomatisch oder leichte Symptome; nur klinische oder diagnostische Beobachtungen; Intervention nicht angezeigt") (U.S. Department of Health and Human Services 2017).

Insgesamt wurden 78 unerwünschte Ereignisse berichtet, davon 40 mit Kausalzusammenhang zum Prüfpräparat (hiervon in 24 Fällen möglicher und in 16 Fällen ein wahrscheinlicher Zusammenhang). Neben den bereits beschriebenen Abweichungen der Leberwerte, kam es weiterhin zu Veränderungen anderer Laborparameter wie der Anzahl der Leukozyten und der Lymphozyten sowie bei 3 Probanden zu Grippe-ähnliche Symptome und bei je einem Probanden zu einer Rötung bzw. Venenreizung des Infusionsarmes.

Diskussion

Wir berichten über die erste Studie, die die Pharmakokinetik der natürlichen Mistellektine nach intravenöser Infusion eines Mistelpräparats untersucht hat. Obwohl die Studie wegen unerwarteter Erhöhungen der Leberenzyme vorzeitig beendet werden musste, konnten wir anhand der Ergebnisse von 8 Probanden verschiedene Parameter der Pharmakokinetik berechnen. Unsere Studie konnte zeigen, dass die Halbwertszeit von natürlichem Mistellektinen länger ist als die Halbwertzeit von rekombinantem Mistellektinen (7 Stunden vs. 13 Minuten) (Schöffski *et al.* 2004). In einer früheren Phase-I-Studie mit Krebspatienten wurden 2.000 mg Helixor® P gut vertragen (Huber *et al.* 2017). Einer von 9 Patienten, die mit dieser Dosis behandelt wurden, hatte eine leichte bis mäßige Erhöhung der Leberenzyme, die sich aber trotz Verabreichung weiterer Infusionen spontan wieder normalisierte. Bei niedrigeren Konzentrationen hatte keiner der 21 in die Studie einbezogenen Patienten erhöhte Leberenzyme entwickelt. Der starke Anstieg der Leberenzyme bei allen Probanden unserer Studie war daher unerwartet. Im Gegensatz zur vorherigen Studie untersuchten wir junge, gesunde, körperlich aktive Männer. Ihr Leber- und Immunsystem scheint demnach viel empfindlicher auf Mistellektine zu reagieren als das von älteren Krebspatienten und -patientinnen. Alle Symptome klangen vollständig ab. Die erhöhten Leberenzyme normalisierten sich 6–8 Wochen nach der Infusion. Dennoch scheint die in dieser Studie verwendete Dosis von 2.000 mg aufgrund ihrer potenziell hepatotoxischen Wirkung nicht für die Erstbehandlung von Patienten und Patientinnen geeignet zu sein. Klinisch werden bei

Krebspatienten und -patientinnen meist niedrigere Dosierungen als 2.000 mg Helixor® P eingesetzt (Steele *et al.* 2014; Schläppi *et al.* 2017). Da die Leberenzyme in diesen Studien nicht untersucht wurden und die Datenbasis derzeit zu klein ist, um eindeutige Aussagen darüber zu treffen, welche intravenös verabreichten Dosen eine Erhöhung der Leberenzyme verursachen können, schlagen wir vor, dass die Leberenzyme bei Patienten und Patientinnen, die eine intravenöse Behandlung mit Helixor® P erhalten, überwacht werden sollten.

Schlussfolgerung

Die Pharmakokinetik der natürlichen Mistellektine ist deutlich länger als die des rekombinanten Mistellektins. Die Dosis von 2.000 mg Helixor® P scheint bei Gesunden eine vorübergehende Hepatopathie zu bewirken. Bei Patienten und Patientinnen, die eine intravenöse Behandlung mit Helixor® P erhalten, sollten daher die Leberenzyme überwacht werden.

Interessenkonflikte

Dr. Schink und Frau Rieger sind bei der Helixor Heilmittel GmbH beschäftigt. Prof. Dr. Huber erhielt von der Helixor Heilmittel GmbH finanzielle Unterstützung für die Durchführung der Studie.

Literatur

Huber R, Schlodder D, Effertz C, Rieger S, Tröger W: Safety of intravenously applied mistletoe extract – results from a phase I dose escalation study in patients with advanced cancer. BMC Complement Altern Med. 2017; 17 (1): 465. doi: 10.1186/s12906-017-1971-1

Schläppi M, Ewald C, Kuehn JJ, Weinert T, Huber R: Fever Therapy with Intravenously Applied Mistletoe Extracts for Cancer Patients: A Retrospective Study. Integr Cancer Ther. 2017; 16 (4): 479–484. doi: 0.1177/1534735416658121

Schöffski P, Riggert S, Fumoleau P et al.: Phase I trial of intravenous aviscumine (rViscumin) in patients with solid tumors: a study of the European Organization for Research and Treatment of Cancer New Drug Development Group. Ann Oncol. 2004; 15 (12): 1816–1824. doi: 10.1093/annonc/mdh469

Steele ML, Axtner J, Happe A, Kröz M, Matthes H, Schad F: Safety of Intravenous Application of Mistletoe (Viscum album L.) Preparations in Oncology: An Observational Study. Evidence-Based Complement Altern Med. 2014: 1–10. doi: 10.1155/2014/236310

U.S. Department of Health and Human Services. Common Terminology Criteria for Adverse Events (CTCAE). Version 5.0. 2017. https://ctep.cancer.gov/protocoldevelopment/electronic_applications/docs/ctcae_v5_quick_reference_5x7.pdf (accessed Feb 12, 2023).

Dr. Ann-Kathrin Lederer[1, 2], Dr. Michael Schink[3], Sabine Rieger[3], Prof. Dr. Roman Huber[1]

[1] Uni-Zentrum Naturheilkunde, Sir-Hans-A-Krebs Straße 55, Universitätsklinikum Freiburg, Deutschland

[2] Klinik für Allgemein-, Viszeral- und Transplantationschirurgie, Langenbeckstraße 1, Unimedizin Mainz, Deutschland

[3] Helixor Heilmittel GmbH, Fischermühle 1, Rosenfeld, Deutschland

Korrespondenzadresse:
roman.huber@uniklinik-freiburg.de

Mistletoe Therapy in Context of a Multimodal Treatment in a Patient With Severe Cancer-Survivorship-Fatigue-Syndrome With Comorbid Sleep Disorder: A Case Report

Misteltherapie im Rahmen einer multimodalen Behandlung bei einer Patientin mit schwergradigem Cancer-Survivorship-Fatigue-Syndrom und komorbider Schlafstörung: Ein Fallbericht

Timotheus Haeck, Ana-Paula Simões-Wüst, Sibylle Creutz v. Essen, Florian Strasser, Matthias Kröz

Summary

Background: Cancer-related fatigue (CRF) is a frequent and burdensome syndrome in cancer patients related to disturbed sleep. We report the case of a female patient suffering from severe chronic CRF triggered by a *carcinoma in situ* of the vocal cords and the consecutive surgical and radiological therapies. The CRF accompanied by cognitive fatigue and hypersomnia was aggravated by a post-traumatic-stress-disorder, anxiety and depression.

Treatment and Results: The patient was treated with a multimodal therapy (MT) over five years to tackle the complex dysregulation. The MT consisted of three mainstays: 1) subcutaneous (sc.) and intravenous (iv.) mistletoe applications; 2) cancer fatigue rehabilitative interventions (aerobic-, strength-training, relaxation-, mindfulness-, nutrition and psychotherapy); and 3) sleep-therapy. The sleep therapy was based on Cognitive Behavioral Therapy for Insomnia (CBTI), consisting of sleep hygiene, restriction and stimulus control. Additionally, *Zincum valerianicum* D3 and Bryophyllum 50 % chewable tablets were used to treat symptoms frequently associated with a Restless Legs Syndrome (RLS) and the associated periodic leg movements as well as an elevated supine sleeping position in order to reduce sleep apnea.

The mistletoe therapy starting in August 2018 largely consisted of sc.-injections with Iscador P (1.1 mg/week–20 mg/week), infusions of Helixor P (50 mg/week–550 mg/week) and abnobaVISCUM Fraxini D30 and endothermic infusions with Iscador M (12 mg–24 mg/infusion). Rehabilitative intervention and sleep therapy were started in June 2020 and in February 2022, respectively. With the mistletoe therapy and the rehabilitative therapy, the CRF was gradually reduced. Upon inducing a fever up to 39.5°C, the patient reported short-term reduction of the severe fatigue up to 2–3 days. Beginning with sleep therapy and lavender oil applications on the legs prior to sleep in February 22, RLS-symptoms in the patient were reduced. Additionally, improvements in daytime sleepiness, hypersomnia (from 12.5 h to 8–10h) and sleep quality were seen. Fatigue was measured using the Cancer Fatigue Scale (CFS-D), a decrease from 44/60 to 30.5/60 in the timeframe of February 22 to January 23 was observed. However, only a slight improvement was seen regarding neuropsychological dysfunction in the same time frame.

Conclusion: In this case, mistletoe therapy may have contributed to CRF treatment. Sustainable improvements in CRF were observed following the integration of rehabilitative and sleep therapy to the mistletoe therapy. This leads to the conclusion that further research on multimodal approaches to treat severe CRF is highly warranted.

Keywords: CRF, mistletoe therapy, cancer-fatigue rehabilitative interventions, sleep therapy, multimodal therapy

Zusammenfassung

Hintergrund: Tumorassoziierte Fatigue („cancer-related fatigue", CRF) ist ein häufiges und belastendes Syndrom in Krebspatienten welches mit gestörtem Schlaf verbunden ist. Wir stellen eine Patientin vor, die an schwerer chronischer CRF leidet, ausgelöst durch ein *carcinoma in situ* der Stimmbänder – Erstdiagnose 2017 – sowie den folgenden chirurgischen Eingriffen und der Strahlentherapie. Die CRF war begleitet von kognitiver Fatigue und Hypersomnie und wurde durch eine posttraumatische Belastungsstörung, eine Angststörung und Depression aggraviert.

Behandlung und Ergebnisse: Um die komplexe Dysregulation zu verbessern, wurde die Patientin über fünf Jahre mit einer multimodalen Therapie (MT) behandelt. Die MT bestand hauptsächlich aus drei Säulen: 1) subkutanen (sc.) und intravenösen (iv.) Mistelapplikationen, 2) CRF-Rehabilitationsinterventionen (Ausdauer- und Krafttraining, Entspannungs-, Achtsamkeits-, Ernährungs- und Psychotherapie) sowie 3) Schlaftherapie.

Die Schlaftherapie bestand aus Schlafhygiene und -restriktion, Stimuluskontrolle (CBTI), *Zincum valerianicum* D3 und Bryophyllum 50 % Kautabletten um das Restless-Legs-Syndrom (RLS)/Periodische Beinbewegungsstörung zu behandeln sowie einer Erhöhung des Rückenteils zur Reduktion von Schlafapnoe in Rückenlage.
Die Misteltherapie beginnend im August 2018 bestand hauptsächlich aus subkutanen Injektionen mit Iscador P (1.1 mg/Woche–20 mg/Woche), Infusionen mit Helixor P (50 mg/Woche–550 mg/Woche), abnobaVISCUM Fraxini D30 und endothermen Infusionen mit Iscador M (12 mg-24 mg/Infusion). Die Rehabilitationsintervention startete im Juni 2020, die Schlaftherapie im Februar 2022. Unter der Misteltherapie und der Rehabilitationstherapie verbesserte sich die CRF langsam. Unter Mistelfiebertherapie mit Fieber bis zu 39.5°C, berichtete die Patientin über eine kurzzeitige Verbesserung der schweren Fatigue für bis zu 2–3 Tage. Beginnend mit der Schlaftherapie und zusätzlichen Lavendelöl-Einreibungen der Beine vor dem zu Bett gehen im Februar 22, reduzierten sich bei der Patientin die RLS-Symptome, die Tagesschläfrigkeit und Hypersomie (von 12.5h auf 8–10h). Die Schlafqualität verbesserte sich klinisch signifikant. Die Fatigue reduzierte sich auf der Cancer Fatigue Skala (CFS-D) von 44/60 zu 30.5/60 im Zeitraum von Februar 22 zu Januar 23. Die moderate, neuropsychologische Funktionsstörung verbessert sich hingegen nur leicht im gleichen Zeitraum.
Schlussfolgerung: Die Misteltherapie dürfte zur Behandlung der CRF beigetragen habe. Jedoch verbesserte sich die Fatigue nachhaltig unter Integration von Rehabilitationsinterventionen und Schlaftherapie. Weitere Forschung zu multimodalen Ansätzen zur Behandlung schwerer Fatigue ist daher sehr gerechtfertigt.
Schlüsselwörter: CRF, Misteltherapie, CRF-Rehabilitationsinterventionen, Schlaftherapie, multimodale Therapie

Introduction

Fatigue is – with an overall pooled prevalence of 52 % according to a recent metanalysis – the most frequent problem in cancer patients (Fabi *et al.* 2020; Ma *et al.* 2020). It is defined by the National Comprehensive Cancer Network as a distressing, persistent and subjective sense of physical, emotional and/or cognitive tiredness or exhaustion related to cancer or cancer treatment that is not proportional to recent activity and interferes with usual functioning (Berger *et al.* 2015). According to Berger (Berger *et al.* 2015), CRF is perceived by patients as the most distressing symptom associated with cancer and its treatment.

Current recommendations to treat CRF are physical exercise, psychoeduation and Cognitive Behavioral Therapy (CBT) and mindfulness-oriented therapies. Furthermore, giving information and counselling to help understanding CRF and to educate about ways to either prevent fatigue, avoid it becoming a chronic condition or to manage it (Fabi *et al.* 2020).

Many cancer survivors find fatigue as a significant problem which is not adequately addressed by healthcare providers (Thong *et. al.* 2020). To tackle that complementary and integrative approaches have started to be explored. One complementary approach is treatment with mistletoe extracts. Treatment with mistletoe extract has shown a moderate effect on fatigue in cancer patients according to a meta-analysis, it is to note that impact on cognitive fatigue was not assessed (Pelzer *et al.* 2022). Furthermore, a recent trial has shown promising results using a multimodal approach of both standard and complementary therapies (Kröz *et. al.* 2023).

We report of a patient suffering from CRF and a sleep disorder aggravated by Restless Legs Syndrome (RLS). The patient was treated with a multimodal therapy consisting of mistletoe injections, aerobic training, relaxation techniques, mindfulness and Cognitive Behavioral Therapy for Insomnia (CBTI) which was adapted for CRF and RLS. These therapies were combined with the mainstay therapy consisting of Bryophyllum 50 % chewable tablets (CT) and *Zincum valerianicum* D3/D30.

Material and methods

Patient information

The 48-year-old female patient was first diagnosed with *carcinoma in situ* on the left vocal cord in August 05 and underwent a resection via microlaryngoscopy. Papillomatose recurrences in 2006 and 2015 were also removed using microlaryngoscopy. In 2017, a further recurrence of a *carcinoma in situ* was treated with radiation therapy.

The CRF was present in different episodes post-operationally and was exacerbated by the radiation therapy that followed in the years 2017–2018. The CRF symptomatology was amplified by a wide variety of factors including a chronified pain syndrome in the neck, moderate to severe anxiety and depression, post-traumatic stress disorder (PTSD), chronic stress through the restricted ability to speak and disturbed sleep Additionally, the patient presented with a controlled bronchial asthma. Following a surgical repair of diastasis recti in July 2021, the patient developed a new onset sleeping disorder symptomatology related to RLS.

Clinical findings and diagnostic assessment

The CRF was formally diagnosed using the diagnostic interview for cancer related fatigue syndrome at the initial visit to the Cancer Fatigue Clinic (CFC) in June 20. In this context blood analysis was done and repeated in the course of treatment to exclude/treat other somatic causes of fatigue. The severity of the fatigue was quantified throughout the therapy using the brief fatigue inventory (BFI) as a mainstay assessment. To assess depression the BDI-II was used. In the sleep clinic, the German version of the Cancer Fatigue Scale (CFS-D) and the Fatigue Numerical Scale (FNS) were used to assess the CRF. For the RLS, the diagnostic criteria of the International Restless Legs Syndrome Study Group were used. The patient reported FNS was used regularly to assess the fatigue before, during and after fever therapy and reported to the treating physicians. Additionally, sleep diaries were used for the assessment of patient sleep using a rating of 0 being the worst sleep quality to 10 being the best sleep quality, as well as the sleep time (in hours) and the sleep efficiency (sleep time/time in bed in percentages). The sleep was documented over the course of two weeks.

Therapeutic interventions

In the oncology department of Klinik Arlesheim the patient was treated with various mistletoe preparations as follows; treatment at the walk-in clinic was mainly performed with Helixor P (50–550 mg) as *i.v.* mistletoe preparations, supported by abnobaVISCUM Fraxini D30 – excluding a trial with additional Helixor A (50 mg) in August 2019. At home, the patient mainly used s.c. injections with Iscador P (1.073–15 mg per week). Furthermore, the patient received endothermic injections during her inpatient stays that were primarily done with Iscador M (12–24 mg/infusion).

In the CFC the patient continued a cancer-fatigue specific rehabilitation program, which was started in stationary setting (July and August 20). It consisted of aerobic, strength and balance exercise regimen. Additionally, educating the patient on a regimen of mind and body interventions (e.g. breathing) as well as various relaxation techniques. In CBT the patient was able to train coping skills and learn various approaches on how to better manage her energy resources and sleep problems. Furthermore, the patient was set up on dietary intervention with a Mediterranean diet and restricted intake of non-animal proteins, which were allowed only two days a week except for eggs. Psychotherapy (CBT and psychoeducation) was also done to improve her posttraumatic stress disorder, anxiety and depression. For anxiety, mirtazapine had been prescribed by a third party physician starting from September 19 with a dose of 15 mg. It was increased to 30 mg in February 20 and reduced to 15 mg starting from October 22.

In the sleep clinic, the patient was started on a therapy of Bryophyllum 50 % CT and *Zincum valerianicum* D3. Furthermore, a RLS and CRF adapted CBTI were performed upon physician visits. The most recent medication regimen (01/23) was Bryophyllum 50 % CT (0-0-0-2 if needed) and *Zincum valerianicum* D3 (0-0-0-20° – autonomously increased up to 0-0-0-25°).

In October 2022, the patient took the initiative of starting an intermittent hypo/hyperoxic training and began to change her diet to a ketogenic one. For an overview over the different treatments in relation to the fatigue see Figure 1.

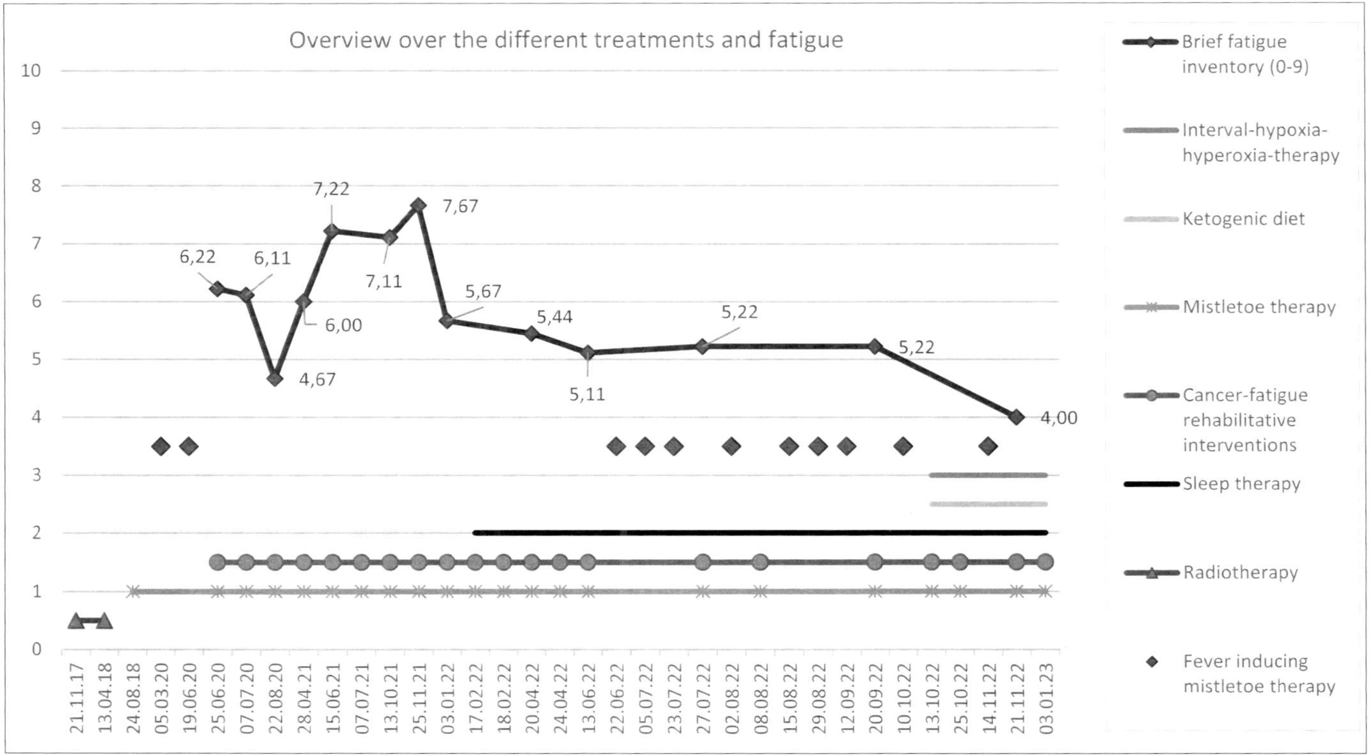

Fig. 1: Overview over the different treatments and fatigue

Results

The mistletoe therapy and cancer fatigue rehabilitative interventions lead to a decrease in CRF. This can be seen on the BFI scale with a decrease from 6.22/10 points in the first visits to CFC clinic to 5.67/10 in the last visit before sleep therapy started in 01/22. Additionally, mistletoe therapy with fever induction up to 39.5°C resulted in a short-term reduction of the severe fatigue (Fatigue-Numerical Scale (FNS) values reduced from 6/10 (morning) and 9/10 (afternoon) to 3/10 (morning) and 5–6/10 (afternoon) up to 2–3 days).

The BDI-II showed with 20/63 points a moderate depression in April 21. The score reduced to a minimal/light depression (12-14/63) beginning with June 22. In the sleep medicine office, the CFS-D was used to assess the CRF, a decrease from 44/60 points in August 22 to 30.5/60 in January 23 was observed. Over the course of the treatment, hypersomnia decreased from a maximum of 12.5h in February 22 to 8–10h in August 22 and the patient did not experience any more daytime sleepiness. Parallel, sleep efficiency increased from 66.8 % to 80.3 % – according to the sleep diary. The sleep quality first increased from 7.1/10 in 02.22 to 8.1/10 in 08.22 but decreased back to 6.9/10 in 11/22.

Once the multimodal treatment comprised all therapies, a further reduction in CRF is seen on the BFI scale from 5.67/10 in January 22 to 4.00/10 in the last visit to the CFC November 22. An overview with selected graphical data representing the results can be seen in Figure 2.

Discussion

In a patient suffering from severe CRF after *carcinoma in situ* of the vocal cords we see a sustainable improvement in fatigue following multimodal therapy. Furthermore, temporary improvements in CRF lasting 2–3 days are reported by the patient following fever inducing mistletoe therapy.

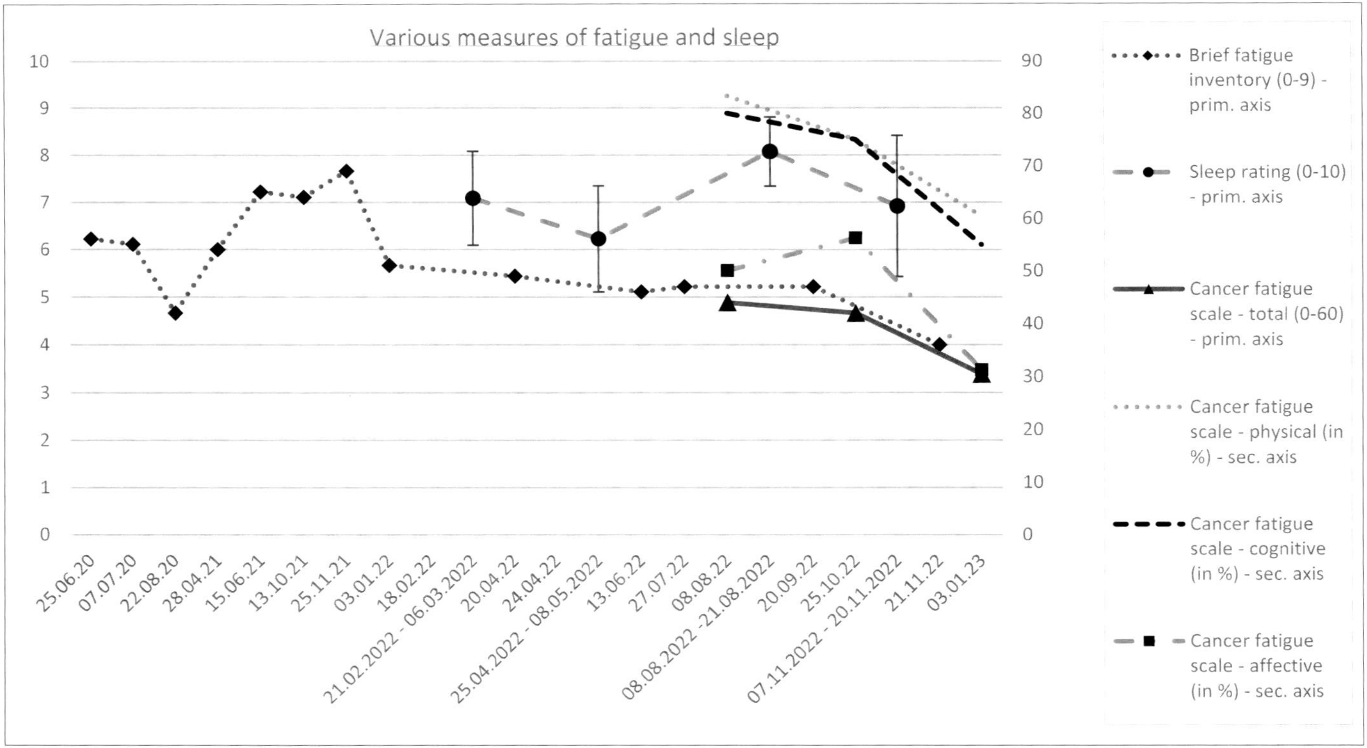

Fig. 2: Various measures of fatigue and sleep

Besides that, the patient also presented with sleep disturbances. These are known to be closely linked in terms of prevalence – although being distinct conditions – often occurring as part of a multi-symptom cluster, where a targeted treatment of either symptom may positively affect the other (Roscoe *et al.* 2007). This might explain the further reduction in CRF after hypersomnia and sleep efficiency improved. Although we must state that the sleep quality improvement was only temporary.

We don't expect that Mirtazepine had influenced the CRF-improvements clinically relevant. The anxiety level barely changed over the course of the treatment. The depression score dropped already in June 22 to 12/63 – before the sustainable improvements in the CRF-scores happened.

We describe here a complex case of severe CRF with different aggravations and sustainable improvements with multimodal treatment. Therefore, it is difficult to say which treatment had what kind of influence on the CRF – especially since the CRF and comorbidities seem to be interconnected and many treatments tackle more than one condition. A review analyzing the effect of mistletoe treatment in CRF e.g., showed a reduction of CRF in 60 % of the analyzed trials, but an even more frequent improvement of sleep disturbances was found in 66.6 % of those trials. (Kröz *et al.* 2016) What can be stated after all, is that the three treatment elements seemed to have add-on effects rather than cancelling each other out.

Further research could focus on prospective studies with a combined therapy of mistletoe injections, cancer-fatigue rehabilitative interventions and sleep therapy.

Conclusion

In this case, mistletoe therapy may have contributed to CRF treatment. Sustainable improvements in CRF were observed following the integration of rehabilitative and sleep therapy to the mistletoe therapy. This leads to the conclusion that further research on multimodal approaches to treat severe CRF is highly warranted.

Authors affiliations/conflict of interest

TH, APSW, SCvE and MK are employees of Klinik Arlesheim. Weleda AG supported research at Klinik Arlesheim.

References

Berger AM, Mooney K, Alvarez-Perez A et al.: Cancer-Related Fatigue, Version 2.2015. J Natl Compr Canc Netw. 2015; 13 (8): 1012–1039.

Fabi A, Bhargava R, Fatigoni S, et al.: Cancer-related fatigue: ESMO Clinical Practice Guidelines for diagnosis and treatment. Ann Oncol. 2020; 31 (6) : 713–723.

Kröz, M., Quittel, F., Reif, M. et al.: Four-year follow-up on fatigue and sleep quality of a three-armed partly randomized controlled study in breast cancer survivors with cancer-related fatigue. Sci Rep 2023; 13: 2705.

Kröz M, Büssing A, Reif M, et al.: Besteht eine Indikation für die Misteltherapie in der Behandlung von Cancer-related Fatigue und Insomnie bei Krebspatienten? – Ein Review. In: Scheer R, Alban S, Becker H, et al. (Hrsg.): Die Mistel in der Tumortherapie 4. Essen: KVC; 2016: 287–298.

Ma Y, He B, Jiang M, et al.: Prevalence and risk factors of cancer-related fatigue: A systematic review and meta-analysis. Int J Nurs Stud. 2020; 111: 103707.

Pelzer F, Loef M, Martin DD, et al.: Cancer-related fatigue in patients treated with mistletoe extracts: a systematic review and meta-analysis. Support Care Cancer. 2022; 30 (8): 6405–6418.

Roscoe JA, Kaufman ME, Matteson-Rusby SE, et al.: Cancer-related fatigue and sleep disorders. Oncologist. 2007; 12 Suppl 1: 35–42.

Thong MSY, van Noorden CJF, Steindorf K, et al.: Cancer-Related Fatigue: Causes and Current Treatment Options. Curr Treat Options Oncol. 2020; 21(2): 17.

Timotheus Haeck[1], Prof. Dr. phil. II Ana Paula Simões-Wüst[1, 2], Sibylle Creutz v. Essen[1, 3] , PD Dr. med. Florian Strasser[4], PD Dr. med. Matthias Kröz[1, 5, 6, 7]

[1] Department of Research, Klinik Arlesheim, Arlesheim, Switzerland
[2] Department of Obstetrics, University Hospital Zurich, Zurich, Switzerland
[3] Department of Oncology, Klinik Arlesheim, Arlesheim, Switzerland
[4] Cancer Fatigue Clinic, Schaffhausen, Switzerland
[5] Sleep medicine, Klinik Arlesheim, Arlesheim, Switzerland
[6] Institute for Integrative Medicine, University Witten/Herdecke, Witten, Germany
[7] Research Institute Havelhöhe, Berlin, Germany

Corresponding author:
timotheus.haeck@klinik-arlesheim.ch

Clinical Regression of Chondrosarcoma Applying High Doses of *Viscum album* Extracts (VAE) by Intratumoral Injection: A Case Report

Joon Beom (John) Park, Inmyung Oh, Sunjoo Chung, Taek Joon Yoon, JongBae Kim

Summary

Mistletoe lectins (ML/VAL) are known to induce apoptotic cell death. Intratumoral applications of *Viscum album* extract (VAE) have induced local tumor response in various cancer entities for variant carcinomas. A 46-year-old male patient suffering from chondrosarcoma had two large-sized masses (40 cm x 25 cm x 17 cm) and a satellite tumor (8 cm x 14 cm x 3 cm). The patient was treated with by 24 times abnobaVISCUM F (fraxini) 20 mg intratumoral injections and concomitant administration of 19 times Helixor A (abietis) 100 mg IV infusions weekly. 32 weeks after treatment the tumoral parenchyma showed a significant regression (> 70 % of the tumor size). These treatments aimed to improve survival and QoL by reducing tumor burden and symptoms, such as shortness of breath, coughing, hemoptysis, and cachexia. Retrospectively, on average, the lectin amount in one ampoule of abnobaVISCUM F 20 mg was 205.2 ng/ml. As eight ampoules of abnobaVISCUM F 20 mg (total 160 mg) were injected into the patient a day by intratumoral application, up to 1,642 ng/ml of mistletoe lectin (ML) was injected as the extending maximum high-dose in safety. The concentration of VAL was determined by ELISA. Reference mistletoe lectin was isolated using an immunoaffinity column with lectin-specific monoclonal antibodies.

Keywords: Mistletoe, chondrosarcoma, intratumoral mistletoe injection, *Viscum album*, lectin.

Introduction

Chondrosarcomas are malignant tumors, comprise an estimated 20 % of primary malignant bone tumors, second only to osteosarcoma. Chondrosarcoma is a type of bone cancer that starts in cartilage cells. Cartilage is the smooth connective tissue that protects the ends of bones and lines most joints. Chondrosarcoma mainly affects the cartilage cells of the thighbone (femur), shoulder, or pelvis. Less often, it starts in the knee, ribs, skull, and trachea. Björnsson and colleagues (1998) found a 5-year survival rate of 89 % for grade 1 chondrosarcoma and 57 % for the combined group of patients with Grade 2 and Grade 3 tumors. Chondrosarcomas frequently grow slowly, and can be present for several years before a patient consults a doctor. Pain in the absence of a pathologic fracture can be important in helping to differentiate an enchondroma from a low-grade chondrosarcoma (Inwards *et al.* 2021).

Intralesional curettage with adjuvant local therapy (i.e., intralesional cryotherapy, phenol, liquid nitrogen, or argon-beam laser) has emerged as an effective treatment for tumors of the long bones classified as Grade 1 chondrosarcomas or atypical/borderline tumors, provided the tumors show no radiologic evidence of aggression (*i.e.*, cortical permeation or soft tissue extension) (Meftah *et al.* 2013; Dierselhuis *et al.* 2016). In patients with higher grade chondrosarcomas of the extremities or chondrosarcoma of any grade involving the axial skeleton the tumors are usually resected. (Gelderblom *et al.* 2008). Chondrosarcomas do not respond to standard chemotherapy, and local recurrence rates vary from 15 % to 28 %, depending on the type of surgical procedure. Occasionally, recurrent tumors are of a higher histologic grade (Schwab *et al.* 2007).

We here studied whether *Viscum album* would show tumoral cell death and necrosis effects when injected into tumors of connective tissue cancer such as chondrosarcoma, and what would be the highest dose of lectin that could safely be used in a patient.

Material and methods

A 46-year-old male patient was diagnosed with chondrosarcoma with pleural and lung metastasis in the lower and posterior parts of the 7th and 8th ribs in the left chest in September 2016. In October 2016, the chest wall resection of the 7th and 8th ribs was performed. Histological findings were 7.4 x 7.0 x 6.6 cm sized mass, grade 2, resection margin < 0.1 cm involvement, parietal pleural invasion positive, necrosis and lymphovascular invasion were negative. Postoperative radiation therapy for the left chest wall was performed 30 times at 45 GY/25 fx.

After 14 months, exploratory thoracotomy and mass excision were performed again due to recurrence at the previous operative site. After the second operation, chemotherapy with ifosfamide and doxorubicin for six cycles was applied, and some adverse effects of chemotherapy were seen. Surgery and subsequent chemotherapy was effective and tumor growth was retarded as demonstrated by CT.

However, in the following 11 months, the tumor mass grew, and the invasion of the left lung's pleural and metastatic infiltration in the pulmonary parenchyma further expanded significantly. As a result, the additional chemotherapy was performed again with VIP (etoposide + ifosfamide + cisplatin) twice, followed by palliative chemotherapy with adriamycin and dacarbazine four times and palliative radiation therapy to the large left chest wall and pleural mass in 52 Gy/13fx.

Patient pathway

In July 2020, the patient underwent his final chemotherapy. Following this, the patient was transferred to a hospice ward because of the advancement of tumor extension and correlated general symptoms in resisting the effect of conventional treatments. One week after the end of the conventional treatments, the patient came to the mistletoe clinic at New Breath Hospital. We conducted our intratumoral injection and simultaneous intravenous injection treatment using VAE.

Tumor characteristics

When the patient first came to New Breath Hospital, he had two tumor masses. Masses of the same nature were located somewhat close to each other. The very large external tumoral mass that had grown out of the chest wall occupied from just below the left shoulder joint to the 8th rib laterally, back neck and lateral and posterior chest walls were invaded by enlarged tumoral mass from the middle of posterior triangle with left trapezius muscle to the entire left scapula and surrounding soft tissues posteriorly. The anterior wall of the chest protruded into a diffuse lump from the left sub-clavicular point to 3rd to 6th intercostal level of left anterior chest wall. The large tumoral tissue connected between anterior, lateral, and posterior wall was 400 mm[A] x 250 mm[B] x170 mm[C] in size. The depth of mass from the chest wall was 150 mm. The smaller tumor was 180 mm[D] x 140mm[E] x 20mm(depth). Both masses were palpably hard in-depth and more little soft in the dermal and epidermal layers (Fig. 1). Inside the thoracic cavity, the tumor had extensively invaded the lung parenchyma of all three lobes (Fig. 2).

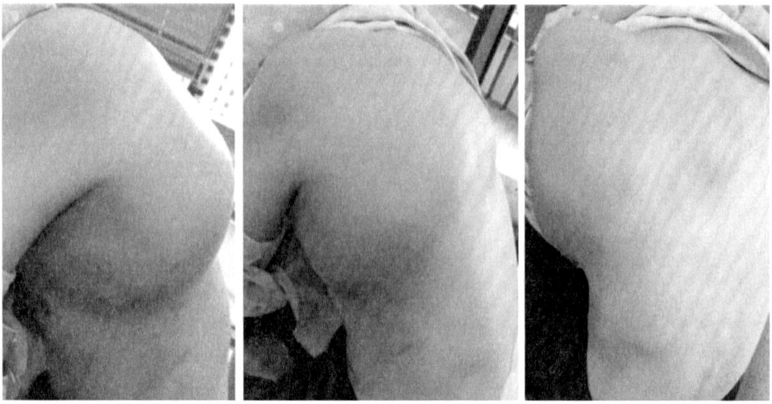

Fig. 1: External appearance of the patient's advanced large chondrosarcoma

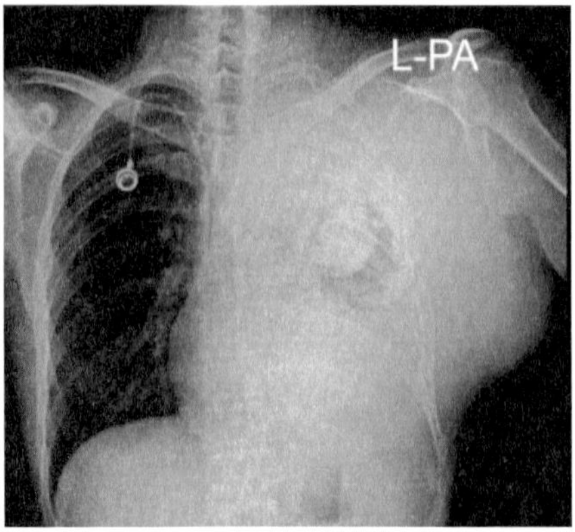

Fig. 2: Chest X-Ray showing chondrosarcoma invaded to left lung cavity

Viscum album intratumoral and intravenous injections

We initiated a set of continual treatments with intratumoral injection of abnobaVISCUM F 20 mg (Abnoba GmbH) preparation into the large tumor mass and intravenous administrations of Helixor A 100 mg (Helixor Heilmittel GmbH) mixed with saline solution.

First, to induce the patient's immune physiology and sensitize the mistletoe component, abnobaVISCUM F 0.02 mg, the smallest unit, was injected subcutaneously. At the same time, abnobaVISCUM F 0.2 mg was injected into the tumor mass. Three days after this first injection, another dose of abnobaVISCUM F 0.02 mg was applied subcutanously and an intratumoral injection of abnobaVISCUM F 2 mg was carried out (Table 1).

Strong immediate drug adverse effects were not observed in the patient, but there were three time pyrexia over 38.5 °C at the nights at home in the following weeks. We proceeded the intratumoral injections according to the following protocol: 1) one time 20 mg injection, followed by 5 times 40 mg, 3 times 60 mg, 6 times 80 mg 5 times 100 mg, and 5 times 120 mg a week mostly while this treatment protocol confronted actively to the tumor burden with vigorous intensity, and was continued two weeks interval when the tumor size was decreased significantly after three months later. Finally, the intratumoral injection dose reached 160 mg of abnobaVISCUM F (Table 2).

In parallel with intratumoral injection for resolution of a large tumor mass, intravenous Helixor therapy was administered to stop the aggravation of various cancerous complications at the terminal stage of the patient, maintain the equilibrium of cells and immune system, and raise QoL. Starting with Helixor A 100 mg, from the second injection, we infused Helixor A 200 mg mixed with 500 ml of normal saline solution once regularly at weekly intervals.

Table 1: Intratumoral and intravenous treatments with *Viscum album* preparation on the patient (1 to 17 week)

Week of treatment	abnobaVISCUM F® 20 mg intra-tumoral injection	abnobaVISCUM F® 20 mg subcutaneous	Helixor A® IV mixing with n/s 250 ml	Clinical remarks
1	0.2 mg (Tues) 2 mg (Fri)	0.02 mg	100 mg	Starting Tx under Off-Label agreement Existed hemoptysis
2	20 mg	0.2 mg		
3	40 mg	2 mg		decresed hemoptysis
4	—	—	200 mg	more soften on sarcoma mass
5	40 mg	2 mg	—	fever 37.3, chilling after one day
6	40 mg		—	No aggravated tumor extension
7	40 mg	2 mg	—	tolerable to increased VAE aount
8	40 mg (Fri)	2 mg	200 mg (Tue)	dark sanguneous mucid fluid aspirated. fever 37.7
9	120 mg (Mon)	—	200 mg (Tue)	starting decreased tumor mass locally
10	40 mg (Fri)	—	200 mg (Tue)	
11	60 mg (Fri)	—	200 mg (Tue)	significantly decreased external(lat & post) tumor contour
12	60 mg (Fri)	—	250 mg (Tue)	after one time injection on ant. upper chest, decreased tumor contour and size
13	80 mg (Fri)	—	250 mg (Tue)	decresed hemoptysis and pain on injected tumor site
14	80 mg (Fri)	—	250 mg (Tue)	more exercise and diet
15	120 mg (Fri)	—	—	tolerable to increased VAE aount
16	—	—	250 mg (Tue, Thur)	
17	—	—	250 mg (Tue)	

Table. 2: Intratumoral and intravenous treatments with *Viscum album* preparation on the patient (18 to 34 week)

Week of treatment	abnobaVISCUM F® 20 mg intratumoral injection	Helixor A® IV mixing with n/s 250 ml	abnobaVISCUM F® 20 mg IV with n/s250 ml	Clinical remarks
18	80 mg(Mon)	200 mg (Fri)	—	
19	120 mg(Thur)	200 mg (Tue)	—	
20	100 mg	250 mg (Tue)	—	
21	—	250 mg	—	
22	100 mg	250 mg	—	
23	120 mg (Tue), 40 mg(Fri)	250 mg	40 mg	
24	160 mg	—	—	tolerable to increased VAE aount
25	100 mg (Tue)	—	60 mg (Thur)	
26	120 mg (Mon)	—	60 mg (Thur)	
27	120 mg (Mon)	—	80 mg (Thur)	
28	120 mg (Tue)	—	80 mg (Thur)	
29	140 mg	—	80 mg (Thur)	
30	—	—	80 mg (Thur)	heatochezia d/t stercoral colitis on colonoscopy. No evidence of active bleeding on Abdo CT angio.
31	—	—	40 mg	
32	—	—	80 mg (Thur)	
33	160 mg	—	100 mg (Thur)	tolerable to increased VAE aount
34	-	—	100 mg (Thur)	
TOTAL	**29 times**	**18 times**	**11 times**	

One week after the second time injection of mistletoe, the mass of the tumor started to fluctuate without any added manipulation, and when the lesion formed was aspirated with 18 gauge needles, the aspirated content was bloody sanguineous color containing necrotic tissues which was of mucoid nature and the amount was about 140 to 200 ml weekly. For example, when 5 ml of abnobaVISCUM F 20 mg (corresponding to 100 mg) were injected, approximately 200 ml +/- 20 ml of tissue fluid was removed by syringe aspirations. When 8 ampoules were injected, approximately 300 ml of tissue fluid was aspirated (Fig. 3).

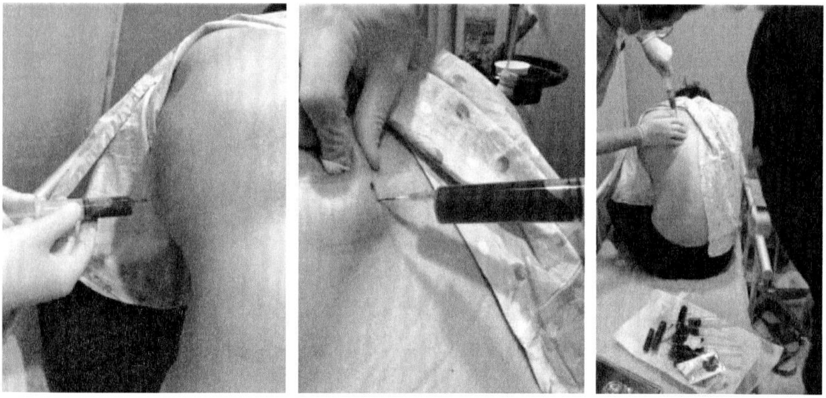

Fig. 3: Intratumoral injections with VAE and aspirating the necrotic tumor weekly

Measuring maximum dose and safety of VAE intratumoral injection

The lectin component found in *Viscum album* preparation has been shown to cause cancer cell necrosis (Majeed *et al.* 2021; Hajtó *et al.* 2005). The aim of our study was to determine the safe dosage of VAE that can be directly injected into tumors. The safety criteria used in this study for assessing the effects of VAE injection were as follows: 1. Absence of anaphylactic symptoms, i.e., diastolic BP less than 60mmHg or tachycardia exceeding 100/min. 2. No systemic allergic reactions. 3. No respiratory distress.

However, the cases of manageable pyrexia occurring within two days after injection were not considered part of the safety evaluation criteria.

To achieve this, we reviewed our clinical experience in this case to determine the maximum usable dose of VAE that we have safely administered through intratumoral injection into solid chondrosarcoma tumor. To find out the highest possible dose of VA lectin that can be administered intratumorally to the patient using abnobaVISCUM F 20 mg once, we measured the lectin content in abnobaVISCUM F 20 mg. For this purpose, we conducted a test on five ampoules (labeled N1 to N5) of abnobaVISCUM F 20 mg. We conducted a Sandwich ELISA analysis using a polyclonal antibody as a capture antibody and a monoclonal antibody (8b11-2C5) that responded well to the lectin antigen (Fig. 4).

The standard material used for this analysis was a previous lectin, and we determined the lectin antigen concentration in the samples. The amount of lectin in abnobaVISCUM F 20 mg and Helixor A 100 mg was measured using the Bradford (Majeed *et al* 2021) assay. We measured an average amount of 205.2 ng/ml of lectin from blind-tested five ampoules of abnobaVISCUM F 20 mg (Table 3).

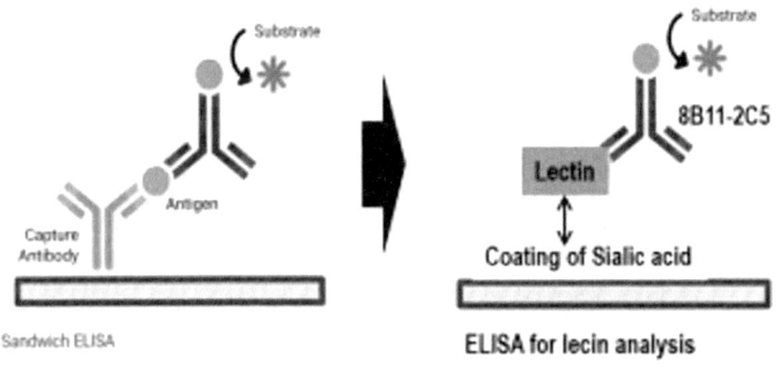

Fig. 4: ELISA Analysis Measuring Lectin of VAE, abnobaVISCUM F 20 mg

Table 3: The lectin concentration after 54-fold dilution of one sample of abnobaVISCUM F 20 mg (Two-Site Sandwich ELISA, Bradford Assay by Park & Yoon for this research)

abnobaVISCUM F® 20 mg Sample (blind labeled)	**N1**	**N2**	**N3**	**N4**	**N5**
M (ng/ml)	201.8	214.8	195.0	201.2	213.2
SD	+/-0.1	+/-6.7	+/-2.8	+/-1.3	+/-19.8

Based on this finding, we assumed that the maximum safe amount of lectin that can be administered to a patient on the day eight ampoules of abnobaVISCUM F 20 mg are injected for intratumoral injection is 1,642 ng/ml.

Results

We share the outcomes of our study that involved multiple intratumoral injections of *Viscum album* into a large chondrosarcoma mass. Our primary goals were to improve the patient's life expectancy, enhance their quality of life by decreasing tumor burden, and examine the direct antitumoral impact of *Viscum album* on connective tissue cancers, such as chondrosarcoma. We conducted our intratumoral injection and simultaneous intravenous injection treatments using VAE so that we could evaluate VAE therapies' effectiveness independently, excluding chemotherapy and other therapeutic factors.

We observed clinical effectiveness in the large tumor of advanced chondrosarcoma through treatments with intratumoral injections with VAE, reducing tumor mass by over 70 %. Certainly, there was a remarkable decrease in the externally grown tumor mass where we performed intratumoral injections, but not until internal increased tumor extension in the lung cavity.

The patient well tolerated a dose of up to 160 mg of abnobaVISCUM F 20 mg. This treatment increased the patient's life expectancy from less than a month to 11 months. It was demonstrated that intratumoral injection treatment with VAE for chondrosarcoma may be a viable option during the course of treatment from the beginning. To the best of our knowledge, this is the first report about treating chondrosarcoma and even large chest wall chondrosarcoma with VAE intratumoral injections experiencing partial regression.

Discussion

Lectin-inducing apoptosis of *Viscum album* is well known (Büssing, Schietzel 1999). Several case reports about intratumoral applications of VAE showed durable remission in different types of cancer (cutaneous squamous cell carcinoma, adenoid cystic carcinoma, breast cancer, Merkel-cell carcinoma, cutaneous B-cell lymphoma, and malignant melanoma (Werthmann *et al.* 2018). Many authors reported that the high cytotoxic, apoptotic, and immunologic properties of VAE may have been pivotal in inducing the remissions in intratumoral injections (Werthmann *et al.* 2013; 2014; Orange *et al.* 2010).

This case of chondrosarcoma tumor was reduced significantly by VAE intratumoral injections and aspirations weekly. We suppose that the entire amount of lectin and viscotoxin injected into a large tumor mass may contribute to destroying cancer cells and vessels in connective tissues and that the amount of those is not absorbed wholly into the bloodstream. Further research on the blood concentration of lectin and viscotoxin, while we do intratumoral injections to large malignant tumors, is needed to set a tolerated maximum dose of *Viscum album* intratumorally.

The declined tumor induced improving this patient's general symptoms, chronic inflammation, malignant cachexia, and breathing difficulty. Clearly, the patient's survival period was extended. The patient's cause of death was an acute respiratory failure at home due to acute respiratory and cardiac failure in the cardio-pulmonary system by extensive tumor invasion into the pericardiac space, mediastinum, and main bronchus of this aggressive chondrosarcoma.

Surgical resection is undoubtedly necessary as a first-line treatment for chondrosarcoma. However, it is essential to note that even in cases where there is chondrosarcoma, regardless of first diagnosis or recurrence and tumor size, intralesional VAE therapy is supposed to affect tumor mass necrosis and provide a higher potential of curing when used in conjunction with resection and chemotherapy and radiation.

Conclusion

We observed the tumor cell necrosis and death of chondrosarcoma by intratumoral injections high-dose VAE. It was demonstrated that intratumoral injection treatment with VAE for chondrosarcoma may be a viable option for treating this kind of tumor. Even chondrosarcoma, a very resistant to conventional therapies, was observed to cause significant tumor regression due to the dose-dependent effects of VAE with up to 1,642 ng/ml of lectin amount of VAE at once for intratumoral injection. The quantified lectin content of abnobaVISCUM F 20 mg is to contribute to setting the standard for maximum usage of intratumoral injection for achieving tumoral regression by apoptosis-induced cell death and clinical safety.

Acknowledgments

We remember and express our gratitude to this patient, who showed courage and love for living beautifully until the end of his life. We are deeply grateful to Nam Sang-Ok, Chairman of LB Bridge Co. Ltd., for his encouragement and cooperation in completing this study and presenting it at the 8th Mistletoe Symposium.

Conflict of interest

This study has no conflict of interest with the German manufacturers of the mistletoe products (Abnoba GmbH and Helixor Heilmittel GmbH), nor with the pharmaceutical companies in South Korea (LB Bridge and Dalim Biotech). The choice of abnobaVISCUM F and Helixor A as therapeutic drugs was made based on the doctor's clinical judgment.

References

Björnsson J, McLeod RA, Unni KK, Ilstrup DM, Pritchard DJ: Primary chondrosarcoma of long bones and limb girdles. Cancer. 1998; 83 (10): 2105–2119. doi:10.1002/(sici)1097 0142(19981115)83:10<2105::aid-cncr9>3.3.co;2-l.

Büssing A, Schietzel M: Apoptosis-inducing properties of Viscum album L. extracts from different host trees, correlate with their content of toxic mistletoe lectins. Anticancer Res. 1999; 19 (1A): 23–28.

Dierselhuis EF, Gerbers JG, Ploegmakers JJW et al.: Local treatment with adjuvant therapy for central atypical cartilaginous tumors in the long bones. Journal of Bone and Joint Surgery. 2016; 98 (4): 303–313. doi:10.2106/jbjs.o.00472.

Gelderblom H, Hogendoorn PCW, Dijkstra SD et al.: The clinical approach towards chondrosarcoma. The Oncologist. 2008; 13 (3): 320–329. doi:10.1634/theoncologist.2007-0237.

Hajtó T, Hostanska K, Berki T, Pálinkás L, Boldizsár F, Németh P: Oncopharmacological perspectives of a plant lectin (Viscum album agglutinin-I): Overview of recent results from in vitro experiments and in vivo animal models, and their possible relevance for clinical applications. Evid Based Complement Alternat Med. 2005; 2 (1): 59–67. doi:10.1093/ecam/neh058.

Inwards CJ, Carter JM, Oliveira AM: Tumors of the Osteoarticular System. In: Fletcher CDM: Diagnostic Histopathology of Tumors. Philadelphia: Elsevier; 2021: 2002–2066.

Majeed M, Hakeem KR, Rehman RU: Mistletoe lectins: From interconnecting proteins to potential tumour inhibiting agents. Phytomedicine Plus. 2021; 1 (3): 100039. doi:10.1016/j.phyplu.2021.100039

Mavrogenis AF, Angelini A, Drago G et al.: Survival analysis of patients with chondrosarcomas of the pelvis. J Surg Oncol. 2013; 108 (1): 19–27. doi:10.1002/jso.23351.

Meftah M, Schult P, Henshaw RM: Long-term results of intralesional curettage and cryosurgery for treatment of low-grade chondrosarcoma. J Bone Joint Surg Am. 2013; 95 (15): 1358–1364. doi:10.2106/jbjs.l.00442.

Orange M, Fonseca M, Lace A et al.: Durable tumour responses following primary high dose induction with mistletoe extracts: two case reports. Eur J Integr Med. 2010; 2: 63–69.

Schwab JH, Wenger D, Unni K et al.: Does local recurrence impact survival in low-grade chondrosarcoma of the long bones? Clin Orthop Relat Res. 2007; 462: 175–180. doi: 10.1097/BLO.0b013e3180caac2c.

Werthmann PG, Helling D, Heusser P et al.: Tumour response following high-dose intratumoural application of Viscum album on a patient with adenoid cystic carcinoma. BMJ Case Rep. 2014:bcr2013203180. doi: 10.1136/bcr-2013-203180.

Werthmann PG, Huber R, Kienle GS: Durable Clinical Remission of a Skull Metastasis under Intralesional Viscum album Extract Therapy: Case Report. Head Neck. 2018; 40 (7): E77–E81. doi: 10.1002/hed.25320.

Werthmann PG, Sträter G, Friesland H, Kienle GS: Durable response of cutaneous squamous cell carcinoma following high dose peri-lesional injections of Viscum album extracts – a case report. Phytomedicine. 2013; 20: 324–327.

Joon Beom (John) Park, MD, PhD[1]; Inmyung Oh, MD[2]; Sunjoo Chung, MD[2]; Taek Joon Yoon, PhD[3]; JongBae Kim, PhD[1]

[1] Mistletoe Research Center, New Breath Hospital, Seoul, South Korea

[2] Mistletoe Cancer Clinic, New Breath Hospital, Seoul, South Korea

[3] DoGenBio, Independent Researcher & Consultant, Seoul, South Korea.

Corresponding author:

gdjbpark1106@gmail.com

Mistletoe and Pharmacological Ascorbate: An Innovative Integrative Oncology Protocol for BCG-refractory High-grade Bladder Cancer

Devra Davis, Dugald Seely, Christopher Morash, Mikail Kogan, Nasha Winters, Jeffrey A. Jones

Summary

There is currently a global shortage of Bacillus Calmette-Guerin (BCG), the standard. Complete remission has been achieved for a 77-year-old female with high-grade NMIBC, refractory to BCG therapy, using pharmacologic ascorbate (PA) and mistletoe. Standard of care for patients that have failed BCG includes cystectomy and hysterectomy/prostatectomy with high rates of complications. Because the patient wished to avoid further surgery, an innovative integrative oncology protocol was adapted from a report (Rose *et al.* 2015) of successful treatment of bladder cancer with the instillation of mistletoe. This novel therapy included an 8-week induction phase of treatment for high-grade disease that entailed intravesical mistletoe into bladder with intravenous pharmacological ascorbate (PA) and *mali* and subcutaneous *pini* mistletoe, followed by a maintenance phase of intravenous, intravesical and subcutaneous treatments every 3 months for 3 consecutive weeks for 3 years, with twice yearly treatments thereafter. Transurethral Bladder Resection (TURB), cytology and MRI show no signs of recurrent disease at 90 months as assessed by cytology and MRI. Typical recurrence in such cases is 70 % within 5 years. Additional cases are being recruited internationally to evaluate the value of this therapy, with collaborations in Canada, Germany, China and the United States.

Keywords: NMIBC, BCG-refractory, pharmacologic ascorbate, mistletoe, integrative oncology, case series, integrative oncology

Introduction

The high recurrence and progression rates of non-muscle-invasive bladder cancer (NMIBC) pose significant treatment challenges, especially in cases refractory to standard of care with instillation into the bladder of Bacillus Calmette Guerin (BCG). Recurrence ranges up to 70 % in 5 years. While cases of low-grade disease can be managed and do not result in increased mortality, cases of high-grade disease that fail BCG can progress and typically result in cystectomy and hysterectomy or prostatectomy. Complete Remission (CR) for NMIBC high-grade disease was achieved in a 77-year-old female with combined therapies of intravenous and bladder instillation of *mali* mistletoe, subcutaneous *pini* mistletoe, and pharmacological ascorbate (PA) (Davis *et al.* 2023). This report briefly explains the underlying pharmacological foundations for this innovative treatment and provides the integrative oncology protocol that can be employed to recruit additional cases. In light of the global shortage of BCG and the relative ease and low cost of production and administration of mistletoe and pharmacological ascorbate, it will be important to evaluate this treatment further, including the relative merits of various sources of mistletoe and their types of extraction and impact on quality of life.

Several reports have noted significant benefit from including PA in oncology treatments in combination with immuno- or chemotherapies for several cancers. (Bazzan *et al.* 2018; Lykkesfeldt, Tveden-Nyborg 2019) Cantley, Yun 2020; Magri *et al.* 2020) Others indicate the positive role of nutriceuticals in enhancing immune function. Before treatment with PA can be carried out at the high doses involved in this case of up to 100 grams during initiation patients must be evaluated for G6PD deficiency (Rees *et al.* 1993), to avoid hemolysis.

Material and methods

Patient background

A 77-year-old nonsmoking female with a history of environmental carcinogen exposure and prior diagnosis of benign neoplasia, progressing to high-grade CIS of the bladder and refractory to standard of care with BCG was successfully treated with intravesical (Douglass, Schoenberg 2016). subcutaneous and intravenous mistletoe and PA. CR for 7.5 years confirmed by cytology, MRI, and TURB. Mistletoe was provided through

Uriel Pharmacy, which sources material through Helixor® Preparations are non-fermented, aqueous fresh plant extracts from two and a half years old mistletoe shoots (leaves, stems, flowers, berries) harvested to include all the seasonally different constituents. The mistletoe comes exclusively from regional wild collection. Mistletoe extracts from fir trees (Helixor® A), from apple trees (Helixor® M) and from pine trees (Helixor® P) are processed.

Table 1: Timeline of Relevant Environmental Exposures for Bladder Cancer in Nonsmoking Female Born 1946

Date	Incident	Chemical
1948	Killer-smog survivor from Donora, PA, USA; ultrafine particulates	Zinc refinery, coke and coal smoke
1950–1953	Handwashing	Gasoline-benzene, toluene, and other aromatic hydrocarbons; kerosene
1948–1956	Playground on slag dump	Cadmium, lead, other heavy metals
1950–1956	Swimming	Coal mine lake
1956–1960	Play with homemade rocket fuel; backyard chemistry experiments	Nitrogen oxides, phenol
1963–1966	Work as a laboratory technician	Phenols
1982–1983	Postdoctoral laboratory immunology	Chloroform, phenols, acrylamide

Table 2: Timeline of Diagnosis and Treatment interventions

Date	Diagnosis	Treatment
2012–2015	Benign neoplasia with low malignancy potential, confirmed by TURB	Routine cystoscopic surveillance, 2x/year
2016	High-grade carcinoma *in situ*, with no muscle involvement, confirmed by TURB	One postoperative treatment: Intravesical dose of 40 mg of mitomycin in 20 ml of sterile water
		Induction treatment: Six weeks of 81 mg of BCG, with maintenance at 3-month intervals, following Southwest Oncology Protocol
6-2016 9-2016	High-grade carcinoma *in situ*, with no muscle involvement TURB shows refractory	Southwest Oncology Group BCG Initiation Treatment
9-2016		Induction with integrative multimodal protocol (Table 3A) Integrative, multimodal protocol maintenance (Table 3B)
11-2016	No sign of tumor confirmed by TURB	
2017–2018		Maintenance protocol once monthly treatments (table 3B)
		Cystoscopic and cytologic monitoring every 3 months with no evidence of bladder disease, confirmed by TURB

Abbreviations: BCG = Bacillus Calmette-Guerin; TURB = transurethral bladder resection.

Integrative oncology treatment induction phase

For 8 weeks, the patient underwent an induction treatment combining intravenous pharmacologic ascorbate (Carr, Cook 2018) and mistletoe, detailed in Table 3A.

Table 3A: Combined Intravenous and Intravesical, Integrative Induction Protocol for Treatment of High-Grade *Carcinoma in Situ* of the Bladder.

Once weekly	Three times per week	Once weekly	Twice weekly
Escalating doses of Helixor® intravesical mistletoe *mali*, at 400 mg, 800 mg, 1200 mg, 1600 mg, and 2000 mg, retained for 2 hours	Alternating days: Subcutaneous doses of 50 mg of mistletoe and 50 mg of abietis	Intravenous mistletoe *mali*, escalating up to 1200 mg, in 100 ml increases	Intravenous vitamin C: 75 grams in 750 ml of sterile water increases to 100 grams in 1000 ml of sterile water with 4 ml (165 mg) Mg; 3 ml (117 mg) K, 50 mg each of Zn, Cr, Se; and one gram of B-12, infused over 1.5 hours and protected from light

Integrative oncology maintenance treatment protocol

Following induction, a maintenance protocol was implemented as outlined in Table 3B (Integrative Multimodal Maintenance Protocol, administered for 3 weeks every 3 months for 3 years). Subsequent maintenance was administered bi-annually for 3 weeks from years 5–7.

Table 3B: Integrative Multimodal Maintenance Protocol

November 2017 to November 2020— For 3 Weeks Every 3 Months			November 2019— Present Maintenance
Weekly	**Three times per week**	**Twice weekly**	**Monthly**
1200 mg of intravesical mistletoe *mali*	40 mg of subcutaneous mistletoe *pini*	Intravenous ascorbate at 25 grams in 250 ml sterile water, 2 ml (78 mg) K, 1 mg K	600 mg of intravenous mistletoe mali; 50 grams of intravenous ascorbate

Supplementary treatments

In addition to the primary treatment protocol of PA and mistletoe, the patient was prescribed a regimen of nutraceuticals aimed at supporting overall health and potentially enhancing treatment efficacy. The specifics of the nutraceutical regimen during the induction and maintenance phases are detailed in Table 4: Induction nutraceuticals which provides the daily dosages of various supplements, including curcuma longa, vitamin D (Bernardi *et al.* 2002), omega-3 fatty acids, ubiquinone (Co-Q 10), melatonin, and a blend of medicinal mushrooms, among others. These supplements were selected for their potential anti-inflammatory, antioxidant, and immune-supportive properties.

Table 4: Induction Nutraceuticals

Period			
Daily	1804 mg of *Curcuma longa* rhizome (Euro-Medica Green Bay, WI, USA)	5000 IU of Vitamin D (Pure) Sudbury, MA USA)	Omega-3 BID—borage seed, flax seed, and deep-sea fish oil; DHA, ALA,
			EPA, GLA; organics
	200 mg of ubiquinone Co-Q 10 (L Apothecary Suffield, Connecticut, USA)	20 mg of melatonin at night qd, started at 3 mg and slowly increased to qd 20 mg (Pure)	One gm BID inonotus (Chaga)
	Obliquus (Host Defense, Olympia WA , USA): • One gram BID Stamets 7 Royal • 214 mg of Sun Blazei (*Agaricus brasiliensis f. blazei*) mycelium • 214 mg of Cordyceps (*Cordyceps militaris*) mycelium • 214 mg of Reishi (*Ganoderma lucidum s.l.*) mycelium • 214 mg of Maitake (*Grifola frondosa*) mycelium • 214 mg of Lion's Mane (*Hericium erinaceus*) mycelium • 214 mg of Chaga (*Inonotus obliquus*) mycelium • 214 mg of Mesima (*Phellinus linteus*) mycelium		
During Induction	Probiotics: 50 billion, 12 different strains (Renew Life Extra Care, Durham, NC , USA)		
During Maintenance	• 20 billion CFU of live bacteria from 14 probiotic strains (Megafood Fort Lauderdale, FL, USA) • 10 mg *qd* of melatonin (Pure) • 4 grams of FiberSmart, made with flaxseed, probiotics and L-glutamine (Renew Life, Durham, NC , USA)		
Abbreviations: ALA = alpha lipoic acid; DHA = dehydroascorbate acid; EPA = eicosapentaenoic acid; GLA, gamma-linolenic acid			

Results

The integrative treatment protocol resulted in CR, with the patient remaining cancer-free for over 90 months. The treatment was well tolerated, with the anticipated increase in temperature and no other significant adverse effects.

Discussion

The successful use of PA and mistletoe in treating high-grade NMIBC refractory to therapy suggests a promising alternative or adjunctive treatment option. This case underscores the potential benefits of integrative approaches in oncology, warranting further investigation. Evidence is growing that mistletoe may well function in ways that stimulate immunological response to cancer (Schötterl *et al.* 2019), parallel to those believed to operate with BCG (Redelman-Sidi *et al.* 2014; Johnson, Winters 2022).

Conclusion

This case study demonstrates the potential efficacy of combining pharmacologic ascorbate and mistletoe in treating NMIBC refractory to BCG therapy, contributing to the growing body of evidence supporting integrative cancer care approaches. Typical recurrence in such cases is 70 % within 5 years. Additional cases are being recruited internationally to evaluate the value of this therapy, with collaboration in Canada, Germany, China and the United States. The relatively low cost and toxicity of this treatment are especially noteworthy in light of both the global shortage of BCG and the growing costs of oncology treatments overall.

Acknowledgements

The authors wish to thank the patient for her participation, the healthcare team for their dedication, Marion Debus for constructive comments on an earlier draft, and Candace Woodbury and Miles Zaud for editorial assistance.

Conflict of interest

The authors declare no conflict of interest.

References

Abnoba GmbH: Intravesical Mistletoe Extract in Superficial Bladder Cancer: A Phase III Efficacy Study. clinicaltrials.gov; 2022 (accessed January 19, 2023). https://clinicaltrials.gov/ct2/show/NCT02106572.

Bazzan AJ, Zabrecky G, Wintering N, Newberg AB, Monti DA: Retrospective Evaluation of Clinical Experience With Intravenous Ascorbic Acid in Patients With Cancer. Integrative Cancer Therapies 17. 2018; 912–920. doi: 10.1177/1534735418775809.

Bernardi RJ, Johnson CS, Modzelewski RA, Trump DL: Antiproliferative Effects of 1α,25-Dihydroxyvitamin D3 and Vitamin D Analogs on Tumor-Derived Endothelial Cells. Endocrinology. 2002; 143, 2508–2514. doi: 10.1210/endo.143.7.8887.

Cantley L, Yun J: Intravenous High-Dose Vitamin C in Cancer Therapy [WWW Document]. RAS Dialogue, NIH National Cancer Institute. 2020; URL https://www.cancer.gov/research/key-initiatives/ras/ras-central/blog/2020/yun-cantley-vitamin-c.

Carr AC, Cook J: Intravenous Vitamin C for Cancer Therapy – Identifying the Current Gaps in Our Knowledge. Front Physiol. 2018;9:1182.

Cumberbatch MGK, Cox A, Teare D, Catto JWF: Contemporary occupational carcinogen exposure and bladder cancer. JAMA Oncology. 201;5 1: 1282–1290. doi: 10.1001/jamaoncol.2015.3209.

Davis DL, Seely D, Morash C, Armstrong J, Meng M, Lowe P, Kogan M: Complete Remission of BCG-Refractory High-grade Bladder CIS and Pharmacologic Ascorbate and Mistletoe. Altern Ther Health Med. 2023; 29 (4): 6–17.

Douglass L, Schoenberg M: The Future of Intravesical Drug Delivery for Non-Muscle Invasive Bladder Cancer. Bladder Cancer. 2016; 2 (3): 285–292. doi: 10.1001/jamaoncol.2015.320910.3233/BLC-160056.

Flaig TW, Spiess PE, 2019. NCCN Clinical Practice Guidelines in Oncology (NCCN Guidelines®) Bladder Version 4.2019–July 10, 2019.

Johnson S, Winters N, Blanning A et al.: Mistletoe and the Emerging Future of Integrative Oncology. Spencertown: Steiner Books; 2023.

Klimant E, Wright H, Rubin D, Seely D, Markman M: Intravenous vitamin C in the supportive care of cancer patients: a review and rational approach. Curr Oncol. 2018; 25: 139–148. doi: 10.3747/co.25.3790.

Koutros S, Silverman DT, Baris D et al.: Hair dye use and risk of bladder cancer in the New England bladder cancer study. Int J Cancer. 2011; 129: 2894–2904. doi: 10.1002/ijc.26245.

Lykkesfeldt J, Tveden-Nyborg P: The Pharmacokinetics of Vitamin C. Nutrients. 2019; 11: 2412. https://doi.org/10.3390/nu11102412.

Magrì A, Germano G, Lorenzato A et al.: High-dose vitamin C enhances cancer immunotherapy. Sci Transl Med. 2020; 12 (532):eaay8707. doi: 10.1126/scitranslmed.aay8707.

Patel S, Goyal A: Recent developments in mushrooms as anti-cancer therapeutics: a review. 3 Biotech. 2012; 2 (1): 1–15. doi: 10.1007/s13205-011-0036-2.

Redelman-Sidi et al.:The mechanism of action of BCG therapy for bladder cancer – a current perspective. Nat Rev Urol. 2014; 11 (3): 153–162. doi: 10.1038/nrurol.2014.15.

Rees DC, Kelsey H, Richards JD: Acute haemolysis induced by high dose ascorbic acid in glucose-6-phosphate dehydrogenase deficiency. BMJ. 1993; 306 (6881): 841–842. doi: 10.1136/bmj.306.6881.841.

Rose A, El-Leithy T, vom Dorp F et al.: Mistletoe Plant Extract in Patients with Nonmuscle Invasive Bladder Cancer: Results of a Phase Ib/IIa Single Group Dose Escalation Study. J Urol. 2015; 194 (4): 939–943. doi: 10.1016/j.juro.2015.04.073

Schötterl S, Miemietz JT, Ilina EI, Wirsik NM et al.: Mistletoe-Based Drugs Work in Synergy with Radio-Chemotherapy in the Treatment of Glioma In Vitro and In Vivo in Glioblastoma Bearing Mice. Evid

Based Complement Alternat Med. 2019: 1376140. doi: 10.1155/2019/1376140.

Schötterl S, Mittelbronn M, Lentzen H, Naumann U: Effects of mistletoe lectins on the natural killer (NK) cell activity against glioma cells. In: Scheer R et al. (Eds.): Die Mistel in der Tumortherapie 4. Essen: KVC; 149–160.

Devra Davis, PhD, MPH[1], Dugald Seely, FABNO[2], Christopher Morash, MD, FACS[3], Mikail Kogan, MD[4], Nasha Winters, FABNO[5], Jeffrey A. Jones, MD[6]

[1] Environmental Health Trust, Teton Village, WY, USA

[2] Ottawa Center for Integrative Oncology, Canada

[3] University of Ottawa Hospital, Canada

[4] George Washington University School of Medicine & Health Sciences, Washington, DC, USA

[5] Metabolic Terrain Institute of Health, Tucson, Arizona, USA

[6] Baylor College of Medicine, Houston, Texas, USA

Corresponding Author:
ddavis@ehtrust.org

Anwendung eines lipophilen Extraktes aus *Viscum album* bei aktinischer Keratose, kutanem Plattenepithelkarzinom und Basalzellkarzinom

Viscum album Lipophilic Extract in Actinic Keratosis, Cutaneous Squamous Cell Carcinoma and Basal Cell Carcinoma

Karolina Königsberger, Wilfried Tröger, Marcus Reif, Dorothea Schläpfer, Konrad Urech, Marion Debus, Thomas Meisermann, Andrea Diehl, David D. Martin, Stephan Baumgartner

Zusammenfassung

In dieser retrospektiven Fallserie wird über Sicherheit und die Wirksamkeit einer Mistelharzcreme berichtet, die bei aktinischen Keratosen, kutanen Plattenepithelkarzinomen und Basalzellkarzinomen angewendet wurde.
Es wurden 55 Patienten mit 74 Läsionen dokumentiert.
Die klinischen Ansprechraten (vollständige und partielle Remissionen) für einzelne Läsionen lagen bei 78 % für Plattenepithelkarzinomen, 70 % für Basalzellkarzinomen und 71 % für aktinischen Keratosen.
Fünf Patienten hatten Nebenwirkungen, darunter Erytheme und Entzündungsreaktionen von meist mäßigem Schweregrad, die vollständig abklangen. In einem Fall wurde die Therapie vorübergehend pausiert, in vier Fällen wurde sie ohne Unterbrechung fortgesetzt.
Schlüsselwörter: Lipophiler Mistelextrakt, topische Anwendung, nichtmelanomatöser Hautkrebs, aktinische Keratose

Summary

This retrospective case series reports on the safety and efficacy of a mistletoe resin cream applied to actinic keratosis, cutaneous squamous cell carcinomas and basal cell carcinomas. 55 patients with 74 lesions were documented.

The clinical response rates (complete and partial remissions) for individual lesions were 78 % for squamous cell carcinoma, 70 % for basal cell carcinoma and 71 % for actinic keratosis.
Five patients had side effects, including erythema and inflammatory reactions of mostly moderate severity, which resolved completely. In one case, therapy was temporarily paused, in four cases it was continued without interruption.
Keywords: *Viscum album* lipophilic extract, topical treatment, non-melanoma skin cancer, actinic keratosis

Hintergrund und Fragestellung

Für das kutane Plattenepithelkarzinom und das Basalzellkarzinom ist die chirurgische Exzision die Standardtherapie (Fahradyan 2017). Mögliche Gründe für Ausnahmen können großflächige, multifokal verteilte, unklar begrenzte Läsionen an kritischen Lokalisationen aber auch Komorbiditäten, hohes Alter oder der Wille der Patienten sein (Linos *et al.* 2013; Micali *et al.* 2014; Collins *et al.* 2019). Es gibt nur wenige Möglichkeiten nichtinvasiver topischer Therapien (Deutsche Dermatologische Gesellschaft 2017/18; Leitlinienprogramm Onkologie – Deutsche Krebsgesellschaft 2020).

Die Aktinische Keratose ist eine Vorstufe des kutanen Plattenepithelkarzinoms und wird im Allgemeinen topisch behandelt (Leitlinienprogramm Onkologie – Deutsche Krebsgesellschaft 2020). Jedoch können auch hier unangenehme Nebenwirkungen gepaart mit geringer Wirksamkeit auftreten (Koch *et al.* 2021).

Diese Studie (Königsberger, 2022; Königsberger *et al.* 2024) berichtet über topische Behandlungen von aktinischen Keratosen (AK), kutanen Plattenepithelkarzinomen (cSCC) und Basalzellkarzinomen (BCC) mit einer Creme aus lipophilem Mistelextrakt.

Patienten und Methodik

Viscum album Lipophiler Extract (VALE) wird aus der europäischen Kiefernmistel durch überkritische CO_2-Extraktion gewonnen. Der Extrakt wird als Creme in 10 %iger Konzentration mit raffiniertem Sesamöl als Hauptbestandteil und geringen Konzentrationen von gereinigtem Wasser, Wollfett, Bienenwachs, Ethanol und Emulgatoren hergestellt. VALE ist derzeit als „*Viscum album Herba Extractum resinosum* 10 %, Crème" (Iscador AG, Schweiz) für die topische Anwendung erhältlich. In der Regel wird VALE ein bis zwei Mal täglich topisch auf die betreffenden Läsionen aufgetragen, vorzugsweise okklusiv in der Nacht.

Es wurde eine retrospektive Fallserienstudie durchgeführt, um die Sicherheit und Wirksamkeit einer topischen Anwendung von 10 % VALE zu bewerten. Die Planung und Durchführung der Studie orientierte sich an den GCP- und GEP-Leitlinien (Deutsche Gesellschaft Für Epidemiologie, 2021; Committee for Human Medicinal Products 2002). Die Berichterstattung orientierte sich an den PROCESS-Leitlinien für Fallserien (Agha *et al.* 2018).

Primäre Studienziele waren die Art und Häufigkeit von unerwünschten Arzneimittelwirkungen (UAW) gemäß den Common Terminology Criteria for Adverse Events, Version 5.0 (CTCAE) (National Cancer Institute 2017) und das klinische Ansprechen auf die Behandlung mit VALE, das gemäß der Klassifikation der Response Evaluation Criteria in Solid Tumors (RECIST) (Schwartz *et al.* 2016) dokumentiert wurde. Sekundäre Ziele waren unter anderem die Zeit vom Beginn der Behandlung mit VALE bis zum besten klinischen Ansprechen.

Die Studie wurde von der Ethikkommission der Universität Witten/Herdecke genehmigt (Nr. 146/2020) und im Deutschen Register für Klinische Studien unter der ID: DRKS00023229 registriert. Vor Studienbeginn haben die Patienten schriftlich eingewilligt an der Studie teilzunehmen und auch der Verwendung von Fotodokumentationen zugestimmt.

Es wurden Falldokumentationsbögen an Ärzte gegeben, die in ihren Zentren VALE in der Zeit von November 2013 bis Juni 2020 zur Behandlung von kutanen Plattenepithelkarzinomen, Basalzellkarzinom und aktinischen Keratosen eingesetzt hatten. Zusätzlich zu den Zielparametern wurden auch Risikofaktoren, Begleittherapien, Begleiterkrankungen sowie weitere diagnostische und therapeutische Informationen dokumentiert.

Die pseudonymisierten Daten der Falldokumentationsbögen wurden in ein Tabellenkalkulationsprogramm (MS EXCEL) übertragen mit dem die absoluten und relativen Häufigkeiten sowohl bezüglich der Patienten als auch bezüglich der einzelnen Läsionen berechnet wurden.

Es wurden Risikofaktoren, Begleittherapien und Begleiterkrankungen sowie weitere diagnostische und therapeutische Informationen dokumentiert, die Einflussgrößen sein könnten. Die hierfür nötigen statistischen Tests wurden mit dem Programm WinPepi (Abramson 2011) durchgeführt.

Ergebnisse

In dieser retrospektiven Datenerhebung an sechs Studienzentren in Deutschland, der Schweiz und Österreich konnten 55 Patienten (31♀, 24♂, mittleres Alter: 72) dokumentiert werden, bei denen 74 Hautläsionen im Zeitraum zwischen dem 29.11.2013 und dem 25.06.2020 mit der Mistelharz-Creme behandelt worden waren.

Die Einzelfallanalyse mit Fotodokumentation ergab vielversprechende Behandlungsverläufe (Abb. 1–3).

Die klinischen Ansprechraten (vollständige + partielle Remissionen) für einzelne Läsionen lagen bei 78 % für cSCC, 70 % für BCC und 71 % für AK (Tab. 1). Die Komplettremissionsraten für einzelne Läsionen lagen bei 56 % für cSCC, 35 % für BCC und 15 % für AK. Bei cSCC und BCC wurden kürzere Zeiten bis zum besten klinischen Ansprechen beobachtet (Abb. 4). Bei fünf Patienten wurden unerwünschte Arzneimittelwirkungen gemeldet, darunter Erytheme und Entzündungsreaktionen von meist mäßigem Schweregrad, die vollständig abklangen. In einem Fall wurde die Therapie vorübergehend pausiert, in vier Fällen wurde sie ohne Unterbrechung fortgesetzt.

Das explorative statistische Testen auf die Einflussgrößen Geschlecht, Alter, Diagnose, Hauttyp, UV-Exposition, Fläche, Körperseite, Okklusion und Compliance ergab keinen signifikanten Zusammenhang mit der klinischen Response. Auffällig war der inverse Zusammenhang von Remissionen und Verhornungsgrad.

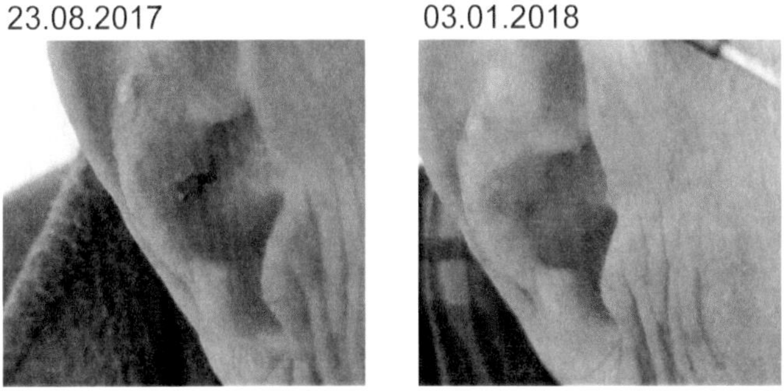

Abb. 1: 97 Jahre alter Patient mit partieller Remission einer aktinischen Keratose nach 27 Monaten

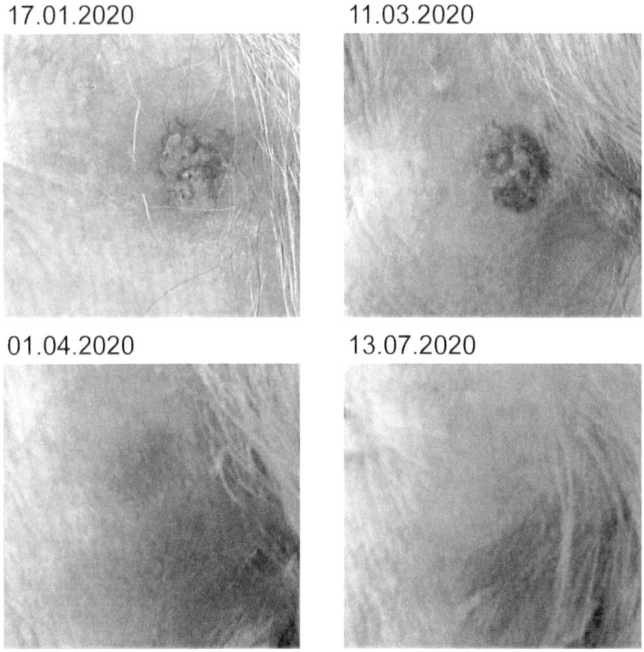

Abb. 2: 96 Jahre alte Patientin mit kompletter Remission eines Plattenepithelkarzinoms nach 6 Monaten

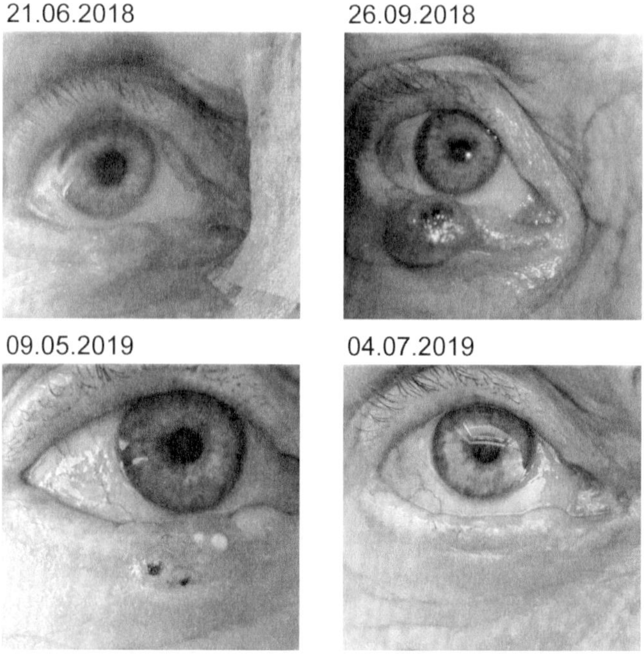

Abb. 3: 77 Jahre alter Patient mit kompletter Remission eines Basalzellkarzinoms nach 12 Monaten

Tab. 1: Klinischer Verlauf von AK, cSSC und BCC gemäß RECIST

	Aktinische Keratose	**Plattenepithel-karzinom**	**Basalzellkarzinom**
Total	48 (100 %)	9 (100 %)	17 (100 %)
Klinische Response Rate	34 (71 %)	7 (78 %)	12 (70 %)
RECIST-Kriterien			
partielle Remission	27 (56 %)	2 (22 %)	6 (35 %)
keine Änderung	14 (29 %)	1 (11 %)	4 (24 %)
Progression	0 (0 %)	1 (11 %)	1 (6 %)

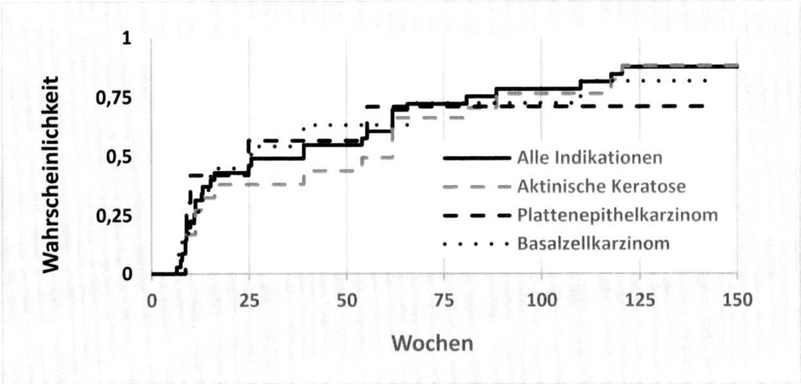

Abb. 4: Zeit bis zum besten klinischen Ansprechen

Schlussfolgerung

Diese retrospektive Fallserie zeigt, dass VALE eine sichere topische Anwendung bei AK, cSCC und BCC ist. Während der Anwendung wurden komplette und partielle Remissionen beobachtet.

Prospektive Studien könnten die Wirksamkeit von VALE nachweisen. Hierbei sollten stark verhornte Läsionen ausgeschlossen oder vor Therapie mit VALE abgetragen werden.

Interessenkonflikt

Die gemeinnützigen Organisationen Verein für Krebsforschung e.V. und Gesellschaft für klinische Forschung sind Mehrheitsaktionäre der Iscador AG, die VALE 10 % Creme in der Schweiz produziert. Karolina Königsberger war zum Zeitpunkt der Studie Mitarbeiterin des Vereins für Krebsforschung. Wilfried Tröger und Konrad Urech sind Mitarbeiter des Vereins für Krebsforschung. Marcus Reif ist Teilzeitmitarbeiter bei der Gesellschaft für Klinische Forschung und bei der Iscador AG. Stephan Baumgartner ist Teilzeitmitarbeiter des Vereins für Krebsforschung und der Iscador AG. David D. Martin erklärt, dass er keinen Interessenkonflikt hat.

Literatur

Abramson JH: WINPEPI updated: computer programs for epidemiologists, and their teaching potential. Epidemiologic Perspectives & Innovations. 2011; 8 (1): 1.

Agha RA, Borrelli MR, Farwana R et al.: The PROCESS 2018 statement: Updating Consensus Preferred Reporting of Case Series in Surgery (PROCESS) guidelines. Int J Surg. 2018; 60: 279–282.

Collins A, Savas J, Doerfler L: Nonsurgical Treatments for Nonmelanoma Skin Cancer. Dermatologic Clinics. 2019; 37 (4): 435–441.

Committee for Human Medicinal Products: Guidelines for Good Clinical Practice E6 (R2). 2016. https://www.ema.europa.eu/ en/documents/scientific-guideline/ich-e-6-r2-guideline-good-clinical-practice-step-5_en.pdf (accessed May 7, 2020).

Deutsche Dermatologische Gesellschaft, ADO, Deutsche Krebsgesellschaft, AWMF: S2k-Leitlinie Basalzellkarzinom der Haut. Aktualisierung 2017/18.

Deutsche Gesellschaft für Epidemiologie: Leitlinien und Empfehlungen zur Sicherung von Guter Epidemiologischer Praxis (GEP). September 2018. https://www.dgepi.de/assets/Leitlinien-und-Empfehlungen/Leitlinien_fuer_Gute_Epidemiologische_Praxis_GEP_vom_September_2018.pdf (accessed June 6, 2020).

Fahradyan A, Howell AC, Wolfswinkel EM et al.: Updates on the Management of Non-Melanoma Skin Cancer (NMSC). Healthcare (Basel). 2017; 5 (4).

Koch E, Wessely A, Steeb T et al.: Safety of topical interventions for the treatment of actinic keratosis. Expert Opin Drug Saf. 2021: 1–14.

Königsberger K: Anwendung eines Harz-Extraktes aus Viscum album bei aktinischer Keratose, kutanem Plattenepithelkarzinom und Basalzellkarzinom. Fakultät für Gesundheit. Dissertation: Universität Witten/Herdecke; 2022: 89.

Königsberger K, Urech K, Reif M et al.: Viscum album Lipophilic Extract in Actinic Keratosis, Cutaneous Squamous Cell Carcinoma and Basal Cell Carcinoma: A Retrospective Case Series. Complement Med Res. 2024; 31 (3): 241–252.

Leitlinienprogramm Onkologie – Deutsche Krebsgesellschaft, DK, AWMF: S3 Leitlinie Aktinische Keratose und Plattenepithelkarzinom der Haut, Langversion 1.1, 2020. https://www.leitlinienprogramm-onkologie.de/leitlinien/aktinische-keratose-und-plattenepithelkarzinom-der-haut (accessed January 4, 2020).

Linos E, Parvataneni R, Stuart SE et al.: Treatment of nonfatal conditions at the end of life: nonmelanoma skin cancer. JAMA Internal Medicine. 2013; 173 (11): 1006–1012.

Micali G, Lacarrubba F, Nasca MR et al.: Topical pharmacotherapy for skin cancer: part II. Clinical applications. Journal of the American Academy of Dermatology. 2014; 70 (6): 979 e1-12; quiz 9912.

National Cancer Institute: Common Terminology Criteria for Adverse Events (CTCAE) v5.0. https://ctep.cancer.gov/protocolDevelopment/electronic_applications/ctc.htm#ctc_50 (accessed April 2, 2021).

Schwartz LH, Litiere S, de Vries E et al.: RECIST 1.1-Update and clarification: From the RECIST committee. European Journal of Cancer. 2016; 62: 132–137.

Dr. Karolina Königsberger[1,2], Dr. Wilfried Tröger[2], Dr. Marcus Reif[3], Dr. Dorothea Schläpfer, Dr. Konrad Urech[2], Dr. Marion Debus[5], Dr. Thomas Meisermann[6], Andrea Diehl[7], Prof. Dr. David D. Martin[1], Prof. Dr. Stephan Baumgartner[1,2]

[1] Institut für Integrative Medizin, Universität Witten/Herdecke, Deutschland

[2] Society for Cancer Research, Arlesheim, Schweiz

[3] Society for Clinical Research, Berlin, Deutschland

[4] Dermatological Practice, Salzburg, Österreich

[5] Klinik Arlesheim, Schweiz

[6] Therapeutikum Merkur, Wien, Österreich

[7] Medicus Gesundheitszentrum, Querschied, Deutschland

Korrespondenzadresse:
w.troeger@vfk.ch

Classification and Minimum Clinically Important Difference of the German Version of the Cancer Fatigue Scale (CFS-D)

Klassifikation und minimale klinisch relevante Differenz der deutschen Version der Cancer Fatigue Scale (CFS-D)

Markus Reif, Roland Zerm, Christoph Gutenbrunner, Matthias Kröz

Summary

Cancer-related fatigue (CRF) is a major factor of quality of life in cancer patients. The Cancer Fatigue Scale (CFS-D) is a robust 15-item inventory covering physical, cognitive, and affective fatigue. We conducted a classification procedure for best separating no/minor from moderate/clinically relevant fatigue. Data of 285 patients came from 3 studies including a) 57 patients with different cancer diagnoses, below them 21 breast (BC) and 7 colorectal (CRC) cancer patients and 57 matched healthy controls; b) 41 BC- and 25 CRC-patients with chemotherapy; and c) 105 BC-patients studied in a longitudinal interventional trial. Four groups with increasing mean CFS-D could be distinguished who in cut-off analyses were categorized regarding their CFS-D values. We identified those CFS-D threshold values that resulted in maximum χ^2-value and therefore best possible separation. Further, we conducted anchor analyses using the Fatigue Numerical Scale (FNS) and EORTC QLQ-C30 Fatigue scales. Finally, we estimated Minimum Clinically Important Differences (MCID) of CFS-D-sub-/scales based on published FNS- and EORTC-Fatigue MCIDs and compared them with patient ratings of therapy satisfaction and with well-being 4 years later. Cut-off and anchor analyses of the CFS-D global scale revealed a threshold range of 22–23 which we suggest to interpret as discrimination between no/minor and moderate fatigue, while a second threshold for discriminating between moderate and severe fatigue varied between 31 and 38 in the different datasets and could therefore not definitely be determined. Finally, a MCID value of 6 was derived. Subscale analyses yielded ambiguous results. The CFS-D global and cognitive fatigue scales revealed the highest chemotherapy and mistletoe sensitivity.

The CFS-D therefore is a reliable inventory indicating moderate or clinically relevant CRF at least for ≥23 and a conservative MCID-estimation at 6 points (10 %), enabling to capture individual dimensions of clinically relevant fatigue including chemotherapy- and mistletoe sensitivity.
Keywords: Cancer-related fatigue, CRF, Cancer-Fatigue Scale, CFS-D, classification, thresholds, minimum clinically important difference, mistletoe therapy

Zusammenfassung

Krebsbedingte Fatigue (CRF) ist ein wichtiger Faktor für die Lebensqualität von Krebspatienten. Die Cancer Fatigue Scale (CFS-D) ist ein robustes 15-Item-Inventar, das körperliche, kognitive und affektive Fatigue erfasst. Wir führten ein Klassifizierungsverfahren durch, um keine/geringe von mittelschwerer/klinisch relevanter Fatigue zu unterscheiden. Die Daten von insgesamt 285 Patienten stammten aus drei Studien: a) 57 Patienten mit verschiedenen Krebsdiagnosen, darunter 21 Brust (BC)- und 7 Darmkrebs (CRC)-Patienten sowie 57 gesunde Kontrollpersonen; b) 41 BC- und 25 CRC-Patienten, die eine Chemotherapie erhielten; und c) 105 BC-Patientinnen, die im Rahmen einer Längsschnittstudie untersucht wurden. Es konnten vier Gruppen mit ansteigenden mittleren CFS-D-Werten unterschieden werden, die in Cut-off-Analysen anhand dieser Werte kategorisiert wurden. Wir identifizierten diejenigen CFS-D-Schwellenwerte, die zu einem maximalen χ^2-Wert und damit zur bestmöglichen Trennung führten. Des Weiteren führten wir Ankeranalysen anhand der Fatigue Numerical Scale (FNS) und der EORTC QLQ-C30 Fatigue-Skala durch. Zuletzt schätzten wir die minimalen klinisch relevanten Unterschiede (Minimum Clinically Important Differences, MCID) der CFS-D-Sub-/Skalen auf der Grundlage der publizierten FNS- und EORTC-Fatigue-MCIDs und verglichen sie mit den Patienteneinschätzungen zur Therapiezufriedenheit und zum Wohlbefinden 4 Jahre später. Cut-off- und Anker-Analysen der CFS-D-Global-Skala ergaben einen Schwellenwertbereich von 22–23, den wir als Unterscheidung zwischen keiner/geringer und mäßiger Fatigue zu interpretieren vorschlagen, während ein zweiter Schwellenwert für die Unterscheidung zwischen mäßiger und schwerer Fatigue in den verschiedenen Datensätzen zwischen 31 und 38 variierte und nicht eindeutig bestimmt werden konnte. Außerdem wurde ein MCID-Wert von 6 abgeleitet. Die Analysen der Subskalen ergaben uneinheitliche Ergebnisse. Die CFS-D-Skalen zur globalen und kognitiven Fatigue zeigten die höchste Chemotherapie- und Mistelsensitivität.

Die CFS-D ist somit ein zuverlässiges Inventar, das eine moderate oder klinisch relevante CRF zumindest für ≥23 und einen konservativen MCID-Wert von 6 Punkten (10 %) besitzt und es ermöglicht, einzelne Dimensionen der Fatigue klinisch relevant zu erfassen, einschließlich der Chemotherapie- und Mistelsensitivität.
Schlüsselwörter: Krebsbedingte Fatigue, CRF, Cancer-Fatigue Scale, CFS-D, Klassifizierung, Schwellenwerte, minimaler klinisch wichtiger Unterschied, Misteltherapie

Introduction

Cancer-related fatigue (CRF) is one of the most common yet at the same time most complex symptoms experienced by cancer patients. Several studies reported moderate to severe CRF in cancer patients while undergoing treatment with radio-, chemo-, hormone and/or biological therapies (Stone *et al.* 2000; Lawrence *et al.* 2004). Particularly, the most recent meta-analysis found CRF prevalence in breast cancer (BC) patients receiving antineoplastic therapy to range between 50 and 95 % (Kang *et al.* 2023). CRF may persist for months or even years after successful treatment completion (Bower *et al.* 2000; 2006; Young, White 2006; Alexander *et al.* 2009; Kröz *et al.* 2010; 2014; Kang *et al.* 2023).

Therapy with mistletoe extracts (*Viscum album* extracts, VAE) has repeatedly been shown to exert a beneficial effect on CRF. Kienle *et al.* (2010) in a systematic review of VAE treatment assessing different aspects of health-related quality of life (QoL) concluded that patients reported benefits of VAE related to fatigue, sleep and a state of exhaustion. Similarly, a literature review by Kröz *et al.* (2016) identified six out of ten randomized controlled trials (RCT) on VAE therapy assessing fatigue in cancer patients, tiredness, and six of nine trials on insomnia or sleep quality, either as single item or as scale, to demonstrate significant reductions in fatigue under VAE treatment. In the most recent review and meta-analysis, which evaluated 12 RCTs including 1494 participants and in parallel seven retrospective non-randomized studies of intervention (NRSIs) including 2668 participants, Pelzer *et al.* (2022) found moderate effects of

VAE on fatigue similar in size to physical activity, which was regarded as gold standard at the time of conducting of these studies.

Assessment of CRF is challenging as there is no commonly agreed on definition (Jacobsen 2004). One definition that captures several important characteristics of CRF describes fatigue as „a subjective state of overwhelming and sustained exhaustion and decreased capacity for physical and mental work that is not relieved by rest" (Cella *et al.* 1998); while according to the National Cancer Comprehensive Network CRF is „a distressing, persistent, subjective sense of physical, emotional, and/or cognitive tiredness or exhaustion related to cancer or cancer treatment that is not proportional to recent activity and interferes with usual functioning" (Berger *et al.* 2015).

Various instruments have been used to assess CRF, including uni- and multidimensional fatigue scales, sometimes developed specifically for cancer patients (for a review see Seyidova-Khoshknabi *et al.* 2010; Agasi-Idenburg *et al.* 2010). However, since CRF is usually only one of several secondary outcome measures in clinical studies, it has regularly been assessed by only one or few questions as part of a multidimensional health-related QoL questionnaire, *e.g.*, by three items of the 30-item questionnaire of the European Organization on Research and Treatment of Cancer (EORTC QLQ-C30; Pelzer *et al.* 2022). What is needed is an instrument that includes sufficient items to capture the different qualities of CRF yet short enough to be administered repeatedly in clinical trials without further burdening this already fatigued patient group.

The Cancer Fatigue Scale (CFS) is a highly reliable and valid three-dimensional inventory with 15 items consisting of five-point Likert scales, providing one global scale ranging from 0 (no fatigue) to 60 (maximum fatigue), or three separate subscales on physical, cognitive and affective fatigue, respectively. The CFS was originally developed at the National Cancer Research Institute of Japan (Okuyama *et al.* 2000b), the validation of its German version (CFS-D) was published by Kröz *et al.* (2008). CFS and CFS-D have already been used in clinical studies (Okuyama *et al.* 2000a; 2001; Kröz *et al.* 2013; 2017).

In clinical routine and diagnostics, a tool with clear thresholds for distinguishing between minor and clinically relevant CRF can be very helpful for a physician's immediate decision making. Therefore, we performed a classification procedure to best distinguish between no/mild and moderate/severe fatigue and estimated the minimal clinically important differences (MCID). Also, the sensitivity of the CFS-D on changes in fatigue due to chemotherapy or mistletoe therapy was evaluated. From both analyses, an estimation of the minimum clinically relevant difference was strived for. Parts of the analyses described below were already presented (published in Kröz *et al.* 2009; 2013). In order to provide a comprehensive picture, we have compiled all previous and current analyses on the classification of CFS-D into an overview.

Material and methods

Patients

Patient data came from three studies:

- Study 1) From January 2003 to February 2004, 114 study participants (57 with a histologically confirmed malignancy of various entities, from which we selected the 21 BC- and 7 colorectal (CRC) patients, and an equally sized age- and gender-matched healthy control (C) group were tested, below others, on the CFS-D and the Fatigue Numerical Scale (FNS; Piper *et al.* 2008) (see Kröz *et al.* 2008).
- Study 2) From April 2003 to March 2007, chemotherapy sensitivity was measured in an observational validation study in 25 CRC patients, and mistletoe therapy responsiveness in 41 BC patients with concomitant mistletoe therapy (various mistletoe extracts were used in different dosages) under ongoing adjuvant chemotherapy a) from the first, or b) from the third cycle, each of whom received adjuvant or initially curative chemotherapy. For this purpose, the CFS-D was used to survey patients 1–5 days before the start of chemotherapy (T0) or 1–5 days before the start of the third chemotherapy cycle (T1), during chemotherapy, i.e. 1–5 days after the third cycle (T2), and 4–8 weeks (T3) after chemotherapy. Both groups were comparable in terms of age, Karnofsky Performance Index, carcinoma stage, surgery and chemotherapy. In line with the breast cancer study arm,

chemotherapy sensitivity was measured in CRC patients before, during and after completion of chemotherapy (Kröz *et al.* 2013).

- Study 3) Between June 2011 and March 2013, 126 breast cancer patients with a significant chronic cancer-related fatigue were randomized or assigned by preference, of whom 105 began either aerobic training (n = 20), a multimodal therapy (n = 34), or a combination of both programs (n = 51), respectively. The patients were assessed using, below others, the CFS-D and the EORTC QLQ-C30 up to 4 times, i.e. at baseline, after 10 weeks of intervention, and six months and four years afterwards. In addition, patients completed a survey on patient satisfaction after 6 months and on their perceived change in general health status after four years (Kröz *et al.* 2017; 2023).

Statistical analyses

From studies 1) and 2), four groups of subjects with increasing mean CFS-D could be distinguished (N ♀ /♂): C 65/27, CRC with mistletoe 27/34, BC with mistletoe 110/0 (BC^+), BC without mistletoe 30/0 (BC^-); subjects were also dichotomized into healthy controls *vs.* cancer patients.

First, we did a resampling analysis to check for mistletoe or chemotherapy sensitivity. For this purpose, 1000 separate data sets were prepared from the original data set using a bootstrap procedure, i.e. random sampling with replacement. For mistletoe sensitivity, CFS-D data at T2 (i.e., during chemotherapy) of each data set were compared between BC^+ and BC^- groups by Mann-Whitney's U test for independent groups. For chemotherapy sensitivity, CFS-D data of CRC patients were compared between T0 and T2 (i.e., before and during chemotherapy) by Wilcoxon's signed rank test for paired data. The test results are presented as a percentage of comparisons of BC or CRC patients, respectively, showing a statistically significant difference of $p < 5$ % (one-sided). For an interpretation of these sensitivities, we repeated these analyses with the functional and symptom dimensions of the EORTC QLQ-C30 and two fatigue-associated dimensions of the Herdecke Life Quality questionnaire (Initiative, Power & Interest item and Physical Complaint item, Ostermann *et al.* 2005).

Second, in cut-off analyses we iteratively categorized the CFS-D global scale into 2x2- (minor / major fatigue), 3x4- (no / minor-moderate / strong fatigue) and 4x4- (no / mild / moderate / severe fatigue) tables using moving thresholds, each time calculating the respective χ^2-values for between-category differences with respect to the patient groups (healthy / patients; or C / CRC / BC^+ / BC^-, respectively). We selected those CFS-D thresholds that resulted in maximum χ^2-values. In addition, receiver operating characteristic (ROC)-curves for the combination of minor / major fatigue *vs.* healthy / cancer patients were calculated for concordance.

With data from all three studies, we conducted external anchor analyses of the FNS or the EORTC QLQ-C30 Fatigue scale on the CFS-D global and subscales, respectively. Published threshold values of the FNS (4 / 7, Piper *et al.* 2008) and the EORTC QLQ-FA12 (40 / 70, in analogy to the FNS and to Friedrich *et al.* 2018) for minor-moderate and strong fatigue were chosen as reference. We used orthogonal regression analysis to estimate the CFS-D values that best corresponded to the FNS or EORTC QLQ-C30 thresholds. We chose the orthogonal regression method, since the sums of squares are calculated for the perpendicular rather than for the vertical distances to the regression line as in ordinary least squares regression. Thereby, we accounted for the fact that data of all three questionnaires may have similar measurement errors.

Using the same method, in sample 3) we also estimated MCIDs of the changes in CFS-D global and subscales from baseline to 10 weeks, 6 months and 4 years later, respectively, referring to the MCID of the EORTC QLQ-C30 Fatigue scale of 8 points suggested by Musoro *et al.* (2023) as external anchor for improvements in fatigue.

Finally, we graphically compared the descriptive statistics of the CFS-D for each category of the patients' therapy satisfaction or general well-being surveys after 10 weeks or 4 years, respectively, including the estimated CFS-D MCID as reference.

Results

Mistletoe and chemotherapy sensitivity

In the following a summary of the results first presented in Kröz *et al.* (2009) and in more detail in Kröz *et al.* (2013) is given. The percentages of re-sample comparisons with statistically significant differences for CRC and BC patients is shown in Table 1. For comparisons of CRC patients between before and during chemotherapy, a high rate of significant comparisons can indeed be seen in fatigue-associated scales (CFS-D, EORTC Cognitive and Physical Functioning, EORTC Fatigue scale) yet also in known adverse reactions of the chemotherapy like nausea/vomiting, pain, appetite loss and diarrhea, which supports the external validity of these analyses. The comparison of BC patients with or without mistletoe therapy during chemotherapy, on the other hand, shows similar and sometimes even higher rates of significant comparisons in fatigue-related scales. In contrast, differences between chemotherapy-related events are smaller (due to the fact that all BC patients have already received three cycles of chemotherapy) yet symptoms known to affect BC patients in particular like role functioning and mood / affectivity (CFS-D Affectivity, HLQ Initiative, Power & Interest, EORTC Role Functioning) show larger differences between BC patients receiving or not receiving mistletoe therapy; again supporting the external validity of the observed significant differences. It is noteworthy that the highest rate of significant comparison in both patient groups was observed for the CFS-D subscale 'Cognitive Fatigue', a symptom thought to be particularly responsive to mistletoe therapy.

Table 1: Rate of statistical comparisons showing significant differences (percentage of 1000 re-samples created by bootstrapping) in scales of the German version of the Cancer Fatigue Scale (CFS-D), Herdecke Life Quality questionnaire (HLQ) or EORTC QLQ-C30 (EORTC) (adapted from Kröz *et al.* 2013)

Questionnaire	**Colon cancer patients before *vs.* during chemotherapy**	**Breast cancer patients during chemotherapy with *vs.* without mistletoe therapy**
CFS-D Global score	39.4	50.7
CFS-D Physical fatigue	22.2	14.1
CFS-D Cognitive fatigue	86.4	67.4
CFS-D Affective fatigue	20.0	33.3
HLQ Initiative Power & Interest	8.1	34.3
HLQ Physical Complaints	8.9	10.3
EORTC Physical Functioning	47.5	50.5
EORTC Role Functioning	5.3	44.3
EORTC Emotional Functioning	3.6	5.9
EORTC Cognitive Functioning	32.5	30.6
EORTC Social Functioning	7.9	5.8
EORTC Global Health/QoL	8.7	11.7
EORTC Fatigue	33.3	34.7
EORTC Nausea and Vomiting	46.8	26.0
EORTC Pain	24.7	10.9
EORTC Sleep Disturbance	5.9	11.6
EORTC Appetite Loss	61.8	11.6
EORTC Constipation	10.1	7.3
EORTC Diarrhea	67.1	23.3

Cut-off analyses of relevant CFS-D thresholds

The following threshold values were found in the cut-off analyses for categorizing the CFS-D global scale into 2x2-, 3x4- and 4x4-tables:

Table 2: Results of the cut-off analyses aiming to best possibly categorize the four identified study subject groups into classes of increasing fatigue according to the χ^2 value of the respective test of a 2x2-, 3x4 and 4x4 table. C: control group; CRC: colorectal cancer patients; BC^+: breast cancer patients with mistletoe therapy, BC^-: breast cancer patients without mistletoe therapy

Categorization	Subject categories	CFS-D categories (tentative suggestion)	Threshold ...at CFS-D value 1	2	3
2x2 table	controls / cancer patients	Noneminor / manifest	29	-	-
3x4 table	C / CRC / BC^+ / BC^-	None-minor / moderate / burdensome	23	30	-
4x4 table	C / CRC / BC^+ / BC^-	None-minor / moderate / burdensome / possibly severe	23	30	34

In contrast to the 2x2-table, the ROC analysis striving for the best possible separating between healthy controls and cancer patients resulted in a CFS-D threshold of 23, thereby reflecting the lower threshold of the cut off analyses of both 3x4- and 4x4-tables.

Threshold estimation by orthogonal regression

The orthogonal regression analyses against the external anchors FNS (data sets 1 and 2, thresholds 4 and 7 for minor-moderate or strong fatigue, respectively) and the EORTC QLQ-C30 Fatigue scale (data set 3, thresholds 40 and 70 for minor with moderate and moderate with strong fatigue, respectively) revealed a narrow range of 21–23 for thresholds between no and minor with moderated fatigue, yet an inconsistently large range of 31–38 between moderate and strong fatigue (Table 3). Subscale analyses yielded ambiguous results, yet first explorative hints might indicate 'none-minor', 'moderate' or 'severe' fatigue below/above physical fatigue: 10 / 15, cognitive fatigue: 6 / 12, and affective fatigue: 4 / 7.

Table 3: CFS-D global scale threshold values between none-minor and moderate or moderate/severe fatigue, respectively, resulting from orthogonal regression analysis with external anchor questionnaires FNS or EORTC QLQ-C30 Fatigue scale

Data set	Anchor (thresholds)	Timepoint	Threshold ... at CFS-D global scale between	
			none-minor / moderate	moderate / severe
1	FNS (4 / 7)	-	22.2	34.1
2	FNS (4 / 7)	-	23.8	38.3
3	EORTC Fatigue (40 / 70)	T0 (baseline)	23.5	33.8
		T1 (10 weeks)	22.2	31.9
		T2 (6 months)	21.3	31.4
		T3 (4 years)	21.0	31.0

Minimum clinically important difference

Finally, the same orthogonal regression method was applied for an estimation of the MCID of the changes of the CFS-D global scale from baseline to the three post-baseline time points after 10 weeks, 6 months, and 4 years, respectively. On average, an MCID of 6 points, i.e. a change of 10 % of the CFS-D range could be derived from the individual MCID estimates (Table 4).

Table 4: CFS-D global scale MCID estimate resulting from orthogonal regression analysis with the external anchor questionnaire EORTC QLQ-C30 Fatigue scale

Data set	Anchor (MCID)	Change from baseline to	MCID for the CFS-D global scale
3	EORTC Fatigue (8 points)	T1 (10 weeks)	5.4
		T2 (6 months)	6.1
		T3 (4 years)	6.3

In a subsequent reliability analysis regarding the proposed MCID value of 6 points, the changes from baseline in the CFS-D global scale were descriptively presented as mean, median, interquartile (IQ) and 1.5 x IQ range, and more extreme individual outliers between the different survey categories of patients' general satisfaction at T1 (after 10 weeks of therapy) and patients' perceived change in their state of health from baseline until four years later (Figure 1).

Mean and median CFS-D values of both questionnaires indicate a clear association between better satisfaction / general health perception and lower fatigue. Moreover, the distribution of data with reference to the MCID value indicates that patients on average need to be at least fairly satisfied, or perceive to be at least somewhat better regarding their health status, to show improvements in the CFS-D global scale of at least the MCID threshold of 6 units.

Discussion and conclusions

The CFS-D is a compact reliable inventory indicating moderate or clinically relevant cancer-related fatigue at least for ≥23 and with a conservative MCID-estimation of 6 (10 %), indicating CFS-D to be able to capture individual dimensions of clinically relevant fatigue including chemotherapy- and mistletoe sensitivity. Thresholds for strong fatigue and CFS-D-subscales need further evaluation.

In a systematic review Agasi-Idenburg *et al.* (2010) evaluated the quality and user-friendliness of questionnaires capturing CRF. The authors reported on eleven multidimensional questionnaires and evaluated them according to different psychometric criteria and validity. The ranking of the CFS was in third place of the multidimensional questionnaires just below the Functional Assessment of Chronic Illness Therapy – Fatigue (FACIT-F) and Multidimensional Fatigue Inventory (MFI) and was evaluated by the authors as satisfactory with some gaps in quality assessment such as interpretability, responsiveness and reliability of reproducibility (Agasi-Idenburg *et al.* 2010). With the analyses shown in this article we could contribute to improving the interpretability and responsiveness of the CFS-D. For the CFS-D a good test-retest reliability is confirmed (Kröz et al 2008).

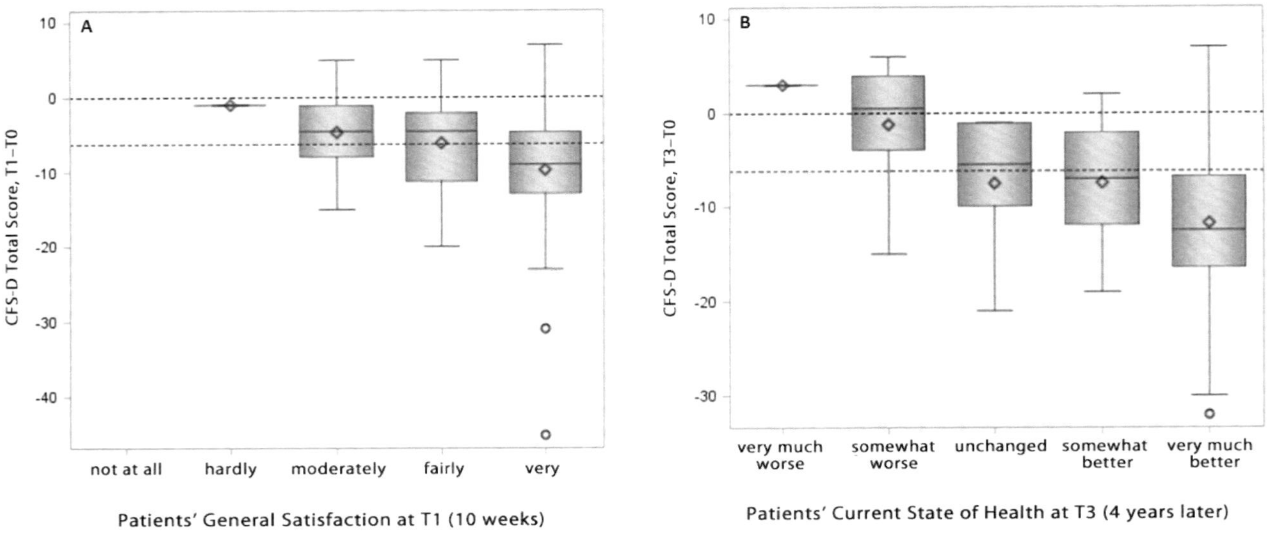

Fig. 1: Descriptive statistics of CFS-D values between the different categories of patients' survey; **A**: Patients' general satisfaction with therapies at T1; **B**: Patients' perceived change in their state of health from baseline until T3. Shown are mean, median, interquartile (IQ) and 1.5 x IQ range, and more extreme individual outliers. In addition, the proposed MCID of 6 points is indicated as reference line

In another systematic review Seyidova-Khoshknabi *et al.* 2011 judged the CFS as one of the five best validated scales besides, e.g., MFI, FACT-F, and Brief-Fatigue Inventory (BFI). Apart from these judgements another strength is the consistent and clinically relevant structure of the CFS and CFS-D, reflecting the multidimensionality of fatigue and its clinical manifestations such as physical, affective and the very burdensome and difficult to treat aspects of cognitive fatigue in patients with cancer-related fatigue (Okuyama *et al.* 2000b; Kröz *et al.* 2008). Furthermore, the presented analyses of the CFS-D yielded chemotherapy and mistletoe responsiveness and strong long-term responsiveness in the cancer fatigue scale in breast cancer patients undergoing a multimodal CRF-therapy (Kröz *et al.* 2023). Schad *et al.* (2020) confirmed chemotherapy and endocrine therapy sensitivity and fatigue reduction under concomitant nursing compresses in breast cancer patients based on a multivariable linear regression analysis.

However, there are as well several limitations regarding the CFS. Although several validated CFS-questionnaires in different languages are available beside the Japanese CFS and the German CFS-D version, such as Chinese (Shun *et al.* 2006), Persian (Baresari *et al.* 2018; first reported in Haghigat *et al.* 2003), Turkish (Sahin *et al.* 2018) or Greek (Charalambous *et al.* 2016), an article on the validation of an English version has until now not been published. Other limitations are the slightly differences in the transcultural adaptation and in the item-loading pattern of the subscales of the CFS-D compared to the original CFS (Okuyama *et al.* 2000b and Kröz *et al.* 2008).

Yet, these shortcomings can in part be overcome as work on the CFS-D continues with regard to the interpretation of clinically relevant thresholds and changes, and therefore the CFS-D is well on the way of becoming a more and more reliable, robust and meaningful inventory both as a diagnostic and therapy outcome tool for capturing even individual dimensions of clinically relevant fatigue and its response to chemo- and mistletoe therapy.

Acknowledgement

We thank Gyllenberg foundation and Christophorus foundation for their financial support to conduct this classification analysis. Matthias Kröz received financial support by Software AG and Humanus Institute.

Conflict of interests

Marcus Reif is an employee of the company Iscador AG, Lörrach, Germany. Matthias Kröz is an employee of Klinik Arlesheim, Switzerland. The validations studies 1 and 2 (dataset 1 and 2) were supported by Helixor GmbH and Abnoba GmbH.

Roland Zerm and Christoph Gutenbrunner declare no conflict of interests.

Literature

Agasi-Idenburg C, Velthuis M, Wittink H: Quality criteria and user-friendliness in self-reported questionnaires on cancer-related fatigue: a review. J Clin Epidemiol. 2010; 63: 705–711. doi: 10.1016/j.jclinepi.2009.08.027.

Alexander S, Minton O, Andrews P, Stone P: A comparison of the characteristics of disease-free breast cancer survivors with or without cancer-related fatigue syndrome. Eur J Cancer. 2009; 45: 384–392. doi: 10.1016/j.ejca.2008.09.010.

Baresari ZB, Abbaszadeh A, Heydarirad G, Khabazkhoob M: The psychometrics of the Persian version of the „cancer fatigue scale" in Iran. EurAsian Journal of BioSciences. 2018; 12: 149–156.

Berger AM, Alvarez-Perez A, Carpenter KM et al.: Cancer-related fatigue, version 2.2105. J Natl Compr Canc Netw. 2015; 13: 1012–1039.

Bower JE, Ganz PA, Desmond KA et al.: Fatigue in long-term breast carcinoma survivors: a longitudinal investigation. Cancer. 2006; 106: 751–758.

Bower JE, Ganz PA, Desmond KA et al: Fatigue in breast cancer survivors: occurrence, correlates, and impact on quality of life. J Clin Oncol. 2000; 18: 743–753.
Cella D, Peterman A, Passik S et al.: Progress toward guidelines for the management of fatigue. Oncol. 1998; 12: 369–77.
Charalambous A, Kaite C, Constantinou M, Kouta C: Translation and validation of the Cancer-Related Fatigue Scale in Greek in a sample of patients with advanced prostate cancer. BMJ Open. 2016; 6: e011798. doi: 10.1136/bmjopen-2016-011798.
Friedrich M, Nowe E, Hofmeister D et al.: Psychometric properties of the fatigue questionnaire EORTC QLQ-FA12 and proposal of a cut-off value for young adults with cancer. Health Qual Life Outcomes. 2018; 16: 125. doi: 10.1186/s12955-018-0949-0.
Haghighat S, Akbari ME, Holakouei K et al.: Factors predicting fatigue in breast cancer patients. Support Care Cancer. 2003; 11 :533–538. doi: 10.1007/s00520-003-0473-5.
Jacobsen PB: Assessment of fatigue in cancer patients. J Natl Cancer Inst Monograph. 2004; 32: 93–97.
Kang YE, Yoon JH, Park NH et al.: Prevalence of cancer-related fatigue based on severity: a systematic review and meta-analysis. Sci Rep. 2023; 13: 12815. doi: 10.1038/s41598-023-39046-0.
Kienle GS, Kiene H: Influence of Viscum album L. (European Mistletoe) extracts on quality of life in cancer patients: a systematic review of controlled clinical studies. Integr Cancer Ther. 2010; 9: 142–157.
Kröz M, Büssing A, Reif M et al.: Besteht eine Indikation für die Misteltherapie in der Behandlung von Cancer-related Fatigue und Insomnie bei Krebspatienten? – Ein Review In: Scheer R, Alban S, Becker H et al. (Eds.): Die Mistel in der Tumortherapie 4. Essen: KVC; 2016: 287–298.
Kröz M, Linke J, Gutenbrunner C et al.: Cancer Fatigue, disturbed rest/activity regulation and sleep disturbances with female patients with non metastatic breast cancer – a pilot study. Phys Med Rehab Kuror. 2010; 20: 152–157.
Kröz M, Quittel F, Reif M et al.; CRF study group: Four-year follow-up on fatigue and sleep quality of a three-armed partly randomized

controlled study in breast cancer survivors with cancer-related fatigue. Sci Rep. 2023; 13: 2705. doi: 10.1038/s41598-022-25322-y.

Kröz M, Reif M, Bartsch C et al.: Impact of autonomic and self-regulation on cancer-related fatigue and distress in breast cancer patients – a prospective observational study. J Cancer Surviv. 2014; 8: 319–328.

Kröz M, Reif M, Glinz A et al.: CRF-2 study group. Impact of a combined multimodal-aerobic and multimodal intervention compared to standard aerobic treatment in breast cancer survivors with chronic cancer-related fatigue – results of a three-armed pragmatic trial in a comprehensive cohort design. BMC Cancer. 2017; 17: 166. doi: 10.1186/s12885-017-3142-7. Erratum in: BMC Cancer. 2020; 20: 1174.

Kröz M, Reif M, von Laue H et al.: Reliabilität, Validität und Misteltherapie-Sensitivität der deutschen Version der Cancer Fatigue Skala (CFS-D). In: Scheer R, Alban S, Becker H et al. (Eds.): Die Mistel in der Tumortherapie 2. Essen: KVC; 2009: 589–600.

Kröz M, Reif M, Zerm R et al.: Mistel- und Chemotherapie-Responsiveness verschiedener Skalen bei onkologischen Patienten unter laufender Chemotherapie. In: Scheer R, Alban S, Becker H et al. (Eds.): Die Mistel in der Tumortherapie 3. Essen: KVC; 2013: 417–426.

Kröz M, Zerm R, Reif M et al.: Validation of the German version of the Cancer Fatigue Scale (CFS-D). Eur J Cancer Care. 2008; 17: 33–41. doi: 10.1111/j.1365-2354.2007.00799.x.

Lawrence DP, Kupelnick B, Miller K et al.: Evidence report on the occurrence, assessment, and treatment of fatigue in cancer patients. J Natl Cancer Inst Monogr. 2004; 32: 40–50.

Musoro JZ, Coens C, Sprangers MAG et al; EORTC Melanoma, Breast, Head and Neck, Genito-urinary, Gynecological, Gastro-intestinal, Brain, Lung and Quality of Life Groups. Minimally important differences for interpreting EORTC QLQ-C30 change scores over time: A synthesis across 21 clinical trials involving nine different cancer types. Eur J Cancer. 2023; 188: 171–182. doi: 10.1016/j.ejca.2023.04.027.

Okuyama T, Akechi T, Kugaya A et al.: Factors correlated with fatigue in disease-free breast cancer patients: application of the Cancer Fatigue Scale. Supportive Care in Cancer. 2000a; 8: 215–222.

Okuyama T, Akechi T, Kugaya A et al.: Development and validation of the cancer fatigue scale: a brief, three dimensional, self-rating scale for assessment of fatigue in cancer patients. Journal of Pain and Symptom Management. 2000b; 19: 5–14.

Okuyama T, Tanaka K, Akechi T et al.: Fatigue in ambulatory patients with advanced lung cancer: prevalence, correlated factors, and screening. Journal of Pain and Symptom Management. 2001; 22: 554–564.

Ostermann T, Büssing A, Beer AM, Matthiessen PF: The Herdecke Questionnaire on Quality of Life (HLQ): validation of factorial structure and development of a short form within a naturopathy treated in-patient collective. Health Qual Life Outcomes. 2005; 3: 40. doi: 10.1186/1477-7525-3-40.

Pelzer F, Loef M, Martin DD, Baumgartner S: Cancer-related fatigue in patients treated with mistletoe extracts: a systematic review and meta-analysis. Support Care Cancer. 2022; 30: 6405–6418. doi: 10.1007/s00520-022-06921-x.

Piper B, Borneman T, Sun V et al.: Cancer-Related Fatigue: Role of oncology nurses in translating national Comprehensive Cancer Network Assessment guidelines into practice. Clinical Journal of Oncology Nursing. 2008; 12 Suppl. doi:10.1188/08.CJON.S2.37-47.

Şahin S, Huri M, Aran OT, Uyanık M: Cross-cultural adaptation, reliability, and validity of the Turkish version of the Cancer Fatigue Scale in patients with breast cancer. Turk J Med Sci. 2018; 48: 124–130. doi: 10.3906/sag-1707-125.

Schad F, Thronicke A, von Trott P, Oei SL: Analysis of changes in cancer-related fatigue of breast cancer patients receiving an integrative medicine program. Integr Cancer Ther. 2020; 19: 1534735420963780. doi: 10.1177/1534735420963780.

Seyidova-Khoshknabi D, Mellar PD, Walsh DA: Systematic review of cancer-related fatigue measurement questionnaires. Am J Hosp Palliat Care. 2011; 28: 119–129.

Shun SC, Beck SL, Pett MA, Berry PH: Psychometric testing of three Chinese fatigue instruments in Taiwan. J Pain Symptom Manage. 2006; 32: 155–167. doi: 10.1016/j.jpainsymman.2006.02.011.

Stone P, Richardson A, Ream E et al.: Cancer-related fatigue: inevitable, unimportant and untreatable? Results of a multi-centre patient survey. Cancer Fatigue Forum. Ann Oncol. 2000; 11: 971–975.

Young KE, White CA: The prevalence and moderators of fatigue in people who have been successfully treated for cancer. J Psychosom Res. 2006; 60: 29–38.

Dr. rer. nat. Marcus Reif[1], Dr. med. Roland Zerm[2, 3], Prof. Dr. med. Christoph Gutenbrunner[4], PD Dr. med. Matthias Kröz[2, 5, 6]

[1] Gesellschaft für Klinische Forschung (GKF), Berlin, Germany

[2] Forschungsinstitut Havelhöhe (FIH), Berlin, Germany

[3] Geriatrische Abteilung, Gemeinschaftskrankenhaus Havelhöhe, Berlin, Germany

[4] Klinik für Rehabilitationsmedizin, Medizinische Hochschule Hannover, Hannover, Germany

[5] Institut für Integrative Medizin der Universität Witten/Herdecke, Germany

[6] Forschungsabteilung der Klinik Arlesheim, Arlesheim, Switzerland

Corresponding author:
marcus.reif@gkf-berlin.de

Mistletoe Therapy During Pregnancy: A Historical Review

Misteltherapie während der Schwangerschaft: Ein historischer Rückblick

A. P. Simões-Wüst, Daniel Krüerke

Summary

Medications prescribed during pregnancy can significantly affect the mother and the unborn child, making their use a sensitive issue. The safety of mistletoe therapy during pregnancy has long been a concern for physicians and expectant mothers alike. However, to date, no clinical studies have been conducted on this topic. We present here a historical overview of the limited information on the use of mistletoe therapy during pregnancy. This includes the results of surveys among physicians and previously published cases.

Altogether 40 reports on exposures (number of exposed foetuses) could be found; no information was available on additional medications, risk factors and the total number of physicians contacted. According to the reports, 21 children were exposed to mistletoe therapy during the entire pregnancy (nine months). Thirty-seven children were reported to be healthy (37 out of 40). In one case there was a miscarriage, in another case the child was born with a heart defect. In these two cases, the treating physicians classified a possible link to mistletoe therapy as unlikely. The 2017 edition of the „Vademecum Anthroposophical Medicines" reports 50 cases in which mistletoe therapy was used during pregnancy. According to the main mistletoe manufacturers, no pharmacovigilance notifications had been reported up to November 2023.

While the collected information provides some encouraging feedback, our understanding of the prevalence and safety of mistletoe therapy in pregnancy is still extremely limited. Assuming its safety merely due to the lack of reported adverse effects is insufficient and requires further investigation. Retrospective analyses of clinical data and relevant preclinical studies, such as *ex vivo* placental perfusion experiments, are warranted.

Keywords: Mistletoe, pregnancy, safety, review, pharmacovigilance

Zusammenfassung
Medikamente, die während der Schwangerschaft verschrieben werden, können sich erheblich auf die Mutter und das ungeborene Kind auswirken, was ihre Anwendung zu einem sensiblen Thema macht. Die Sicherheit der Misteltherapie in der Schwangerschaft ist seit langem ein Anliegen von Ärztinnen und Ärzten und werdenden Müttern gleichermaßen. Bislang wurden jedoch keine klinischen Studien zu diesem Thema durchgeführt. Wir geben hier einen historischen Überblick über die begrenzten Informationen zum Einsatz der Misteltherapie in der Schwangerschaft. Dazu gehören die Ergebnisse von Befragungen von Ärztinnen und Ärzten sowie publizierte Fälle.
Insgesamt konnten 40 Berichte über Expositionen (Anzahl der exponierten Föten) gefunden werden; Informationen über zusätzliche Medikamente, Risikofaktoren und die Gesamtzahl der kontaktierten Ärzte waren nicht verfügbar. Den Angaben zufolge wurden 21 Föten während der gesamten Schwangerschaft (neun Monate) einer Misteltherapie exponiert. Siebenunddreißig Kinder wurden als gesund beschrieben (37 von 40). In einem Fall kam es zu einer Fehlgeburt, in einem anderen Fall wurde das Kind mit einem Herzfehler geboren. In beiden Fällen wurde ein möglicher Zusammenhang mit der Misteltherapie von den behandelnden Ärzten für unwahrscheinlich gehalten. Die Ausgabe 2017 des „Vademecum Anthroposophische Arzneimittel" berichtet von 50 Fällen, in denen eine Misteltherapie während der Schwangerschaft angewendet wurde. Nach Angaben der wichtigsten Mistelhersteller lagen bis November 2023 keine Pharmakovigilanzberichte vor.
Obwohl die gesammelten Informationen ermutigend sind, ist unser Wissen über die Häufigkeit und Sicherheit der Misteltherapie in der Schwangerschaft immer noch sehr begrenzt. Die Annahme der Sicherheit allein aufgrund des Fehlens gemeldeter unerwünschter Wirkungen ist unzureichend und bedarf weiterer Untersuchungen. Retrospektive Analysen klinischer Daten und relevante präklinische Studien, wie z. B. *ex vivo*-Plazenta-Perfusionsexperimente, sind gerechtfertigt.
Schlüsselwörter: Mistel, Schwangerschaft, Sicherheit, Übersichtsarbeit, Pharmakovigilanz

Background and question

Medications prescribed during pregnancy can significantly affect the mother and the unborn child, making their use a sensitive issue. The safety of mistletoe therapy during pregnancy has long been a concern for physicians and expectant mothers alike. However, to date, no clinical studies have been conducted on this topic. We present here a historical overview of the limited information on the use of mistletoe therapy during pregnancy.

Historical review

In the archives of the Klinik Arlesheim (see Data Availability statement), we could identify the questionnaires returned to Dr Rita Leroi in the framework of a survey that she initiated in the 1980s. Dr Rita Leroi had asked numerous German-speaking anthroposophic gynaecologists in Europe, especially Germany, Austria and Switzerland, to complete a questionnaire on mistletoe therapy in pregnancy and on possible side effects on mother and child. A later cover letter suggests a possibly low response rate. The replies to this request by Dr Leroi were later collected by Dr Maria Fornalski. A total of 40 exposures to mistletoe therapy during intrauterine life were reported, which took place between 1965 and 1995 (31 exposed foetus of 27 different mothers during 30 pregnancies). These 31 exposures from the archives of the Klinik Arlesheim, together with nine exposures that have been described by Dr Angelika Weidemann and Ralf Aden in a publication on mistletoe therapy by Dr Emme (Weidemann, Aden 1992) are depicted in Table 1.

Altogether, 40 reports on exposures (40 exposed foetuses, during 39 pregnancies of 33 different mothers) show that the aim of the mistletoe therapy was in the majority of the cases the treatment of malignant diseases in the pregnant woman. The types of malignant diseases were most often melanoma, breast cancer and colon carcinoma. The mistletoe preparations most frequently used during pregnancy were Iscador M c. Arg (n = 17), Iscador P c. Hg (n = 6), Iscador M/M c. Arg (n = 5), Helix/Iscador (n = 3) and Iscador P (n = 3). The maximum dose was usually 10 to 20 mg. In 25 pregnancies, mistletoe therapy had already been administered beforehand. The mothers received mistletoe therapy on average approx. 26 months (median = 18, mode = 17 months) before conception. According to the reports, 21 children were exposed to mistletoe therapy throughout the entire pregnancy (nine months). In four other cases, the mistletoe therapy took place during the first trimester, in six other cases during the third trimester.

The outcome data on these 40 exposures revealed that one woman passed away during early pregnancy. Two women showed tendencies for preterm labour, one of whom had a cerclage placed. Another woman suffered a miscarriage. The cause of this miscarriage was unknown; the mother had already had other miscarriages prior to mistletoe therapy; a surgical revision of a local recurrence had been performed shortly before the pregnancy. All other courses of pregnancy were unproblematic. In one case, the child was born with a heart defect. The heart defect consisted of a transposition of the large vessels and an aortic stenosis; an uncle of the child had died as an infant due to a heart valve defect. In both cases – miscarriage and heart defect – the treating physician classified a possible link to mistletoe therapy as unlikely. Thirty-seven children were reported to be healthy at birth (37 out of 40).

In the 2017 edition of the „Vademecum Anthroposophical Medicines“ (Arendt *et al.* 2017), the authors mention knowing of approximately 50 cases in which mistletoe therapy was used during pregnancy.

Data from the survey 2023

In November and December 2023, we launched an online survey, first among the participants of the Mistletoe Symposium in Nonnweiler and then via the personal network. By the end of December 2023, seven physicians had participated in the online survey, six of whom had 12–37 years of professional experience (one stated only two years). Four physicians reported having treated between 1–4 pregnant women with the subcutaneous mistletoe therapy and one 5–9 pregnant women (the physician with only two years of experience had never treated a pregnant woman). None of the participating physicians had observed a birth defect after mistletoe treatment during pregnancy. When asked whether mistletoe therapy should be contraindicated in pregnancy, four of the physicians who treated pregnant women with mistletoe replied that they did not agree at all, one tended to disagree, one did not want to answer.

Tab. 1: Reported exposures to mistletoe therapy during pregnancy

Source[a]	Child	Mother	Entity	Mistletoe therapy duration (months)		Mistletoe therapy when in pregnancy[c]	New-born[d]	Mistletoe[e]	
				before pregnancy[b]	during pregnancy			Preparation	Max. dose (mg)
A	1	1	melanoma	26	9		healthy	Iscador P c. Hg	50
A	2	2	melanoma	-	3	7th–9th mo.	healthy twins	Iscador M c. Arg	20
A	3								
A	4			36	9		healthy	Iscador M c. Arg	20
A	5	3	thyroid cancer	17	9		healthy	Iscador M c. Arg	n.a.
A	6	4	colon carcinoma	-	9		healthy	Iscador M c. Arg	10
A	7	5	colon carcinoma	5	9		healthy	Iscador M c. Arg	10
A	8	6	colon carcinoma	-	7		healthy	Iscador M c. Arg	10
A	9	7	colon carcinoma	18	9		healthy	Iscador M c. Arg	10
A	10	8	lymphoma	31	9		healthy	n.a.	20
A	11	9	breast cancer	20	9		healthy	Iscador M c. Arg	20
A	12	10	melanoma	18	9		healthy	Iscador P c. Hg	20
A	13	11	breast cancer	10	9		healthy	Iscador M c. Arg	30
A	14	12	bone marrow dysplasia	-	5	5th–9th mo.	healthy	Iscador P c. Hg	10
A	15	13	hemangioma	-	9		healthy	Iscador P	0.1
A	16	14	colon carcinoma	-	7		healthy	Iscador M c. Arg	20
A	17	15	precancerous	6	9		healthy	Iscador M c. Arg	10
A	18	16	melanoma	14	9		healthy	Iscador P c. Hg/P	30

Source[a]	Child	Mother	Entity	Mistletoe therapy duration (months)		Mistletoe therapy when in pregnancy[c]	New-born[d]	Mistletoe[e]	
				before pregnancy[b]	during pregnancy			Preparation	Max. dose (mg)
A	19	17	thyroid cancer	5	9		healthy	Iscador P	20
A	20	18	colon carcinoma	-	5	5th–9th mo.	healthy	Iscador P	20
A	21	19	melanoma	21	7	3rd–4th mo.	healthy	Iscador M c. Arg	10
A	22	20	melanoma	48	9		healthy	Iscador M	5
A	23	21	osteosarcoma	70	9		healthy	Iscador P c. Hg	20
A	24	22	leiomyo-sarcoma	123	9		healthy	Iscador M c. Arg	30
A	25	23	thymoma	56	8	1st–8th mo.	healthy	Iscador P c. Hg	50
A	26	24	lympho-granulomatosis	33	9		healthy	Iscador P c. Hg	20
A	27	25	melanoma	2	9		healthy	Iscador P c. Hg/M	10
A	28	26	breast cancer	8	9		heart defect	Iscador M c. Arg	20
A	29			27	5	11th–33th we.	healthy		
A	30	27	cervical carcinoma	17	n.a.		healthy	diverse	n.a.
B	31			n.a.	n.a.		healthy	diverse	n.a.
B	32	28	breast cancer	n.a	3	1st–15th we.	miscarriage	Helixor/Iscador	n.a.
B	33			13	9		healthy	Helixor/Iscador	n.a.
B	34			n.a.	n.a.		mother died	Helixor/Iscador	n.a.
B	35	29	fibroadenoma	6	8	1st–8th mo.	healthy	Iscador M/M c. Arg	n.a.
B	36			28	7	1st–7th mo.	healthy	Iscador M/M c. Arg	n.a.
B	37	30	leiomyoma	n.a.	6	14th–40 we.	healthy	Iscador M/M c. Arg	n.a.

Source[a]	**Child**	**Mother**	**Entity**	**Mistletoe therapy duration (months)**		**Mistletoe therapy when in pregnancy**[c]	**New-born**[d]	**Mistletoe**[e]	
				before pregnancy[b]	**during pregnancy**			**Preparation**	**Max. dose (mg)**
B	38	31	leiomyoma	n.a.	5	17th–40th we.	healthy	Iscador M/M c. Arg	n.a.
B	39	32	leiomyoma	n.a.	4	23th–40th we.	healthy	Iscador M/M c. Arg	n.a.
B	40	33	cervical dysplasia	n.a.	3	27th–37th we.	healthy	Iscador M c. Arg	n.a.

[a] Either A (documentation from Dr Maria Fornalski, Klinik-Arlesheim) or B (cases reported by Weideman and Aden (Weidemann, Aden 1992)).
[b] Approximate duration of mistletoe therapy performed before pregnancy was calculated from the date of birth of the child and the date of start of mistletoe therapy assuming a normal duration of pregnancy).
[c] Additional information on the timing of mistletoe therapy during pregnancy (which pregnancy months or weeks).
[d] Reported by the treating physician.
[e] Type of mistletoe preparation used in the treatment during pregnancy (preparation and maximal doses).
n.a., not available.

The low number of participants in this new online survey on experiences of treating women during pregnancy with mistletoe therapy illustrates how difficult it is to obtain information on such experiences. Whether this reflects a lack of treatments during pregnancy or a reluctance to provide information on existing treatments is impossible to say.

Data from the manufacturers

In the description and instructions for use of the package leaflets, it is pointed out that the physician or pharmacist should be consulted before using the medication, before or during pregnancy or in the breastfeeding phase. It also states that the effects of mistletoe preparations on pregnancy, birth and the development of the child after birth have not been investigated and that they may only be used during pregnancy if expressly prescribed by a physician. The manufacturers justify this information with the lack of the necessary safety data from clinical studies. While Helixor® adds to this, that no preclinical research has been made (Target BioScience AG 2020), in the case of abnobaVISCUM® (Abnoba 2019), it is reported that rat experiments on embryotoxicity conducted with abnobaVISCUM® Fraxini 20 mg did not reveal any particular dangers for humans. In the case of Iscador® (Iscador AG 2017), *in vitro* studies (Ames test, chromosomal aberration test) and *in vivo* studies (micronucleus test) are mentioned that according to the manufacturer showed no evidence of mutagenicity. In addition, no teratogenic effects were observed in preclinical *in vivo* and *in vitro* studies after administration of subtoxic doses (rat, rabbit). However, fetotoxicity, ossification delay and skeletal abnormalities occurred in rabbits treated with Iscador at doses that were toxic to the dams and three times the maximum therapeutic dose.

At the Mistletoe Symposium in Nonnweiler, the pharmacovigilance departments of the main mistletoe producers were approached directly about adverse events associated with mistletoe treatments in pregnancy. According to the most important mistletoe manufacturers, there are no pharmacovigilance data in connection with treatments during pregnancy (up to November 2023). Whether this is due to a lack of treatments during pregnancy or a reluctance to report spontaneously adverse drug reactions of mistletoe therapies is impossible to say. In general, suspected adverse drug reactions are known to be underreported [see e.g. (Alomar *et al.* 2020)].

Additional work on the use of mistletoe during pregnancy

Searches of the biomedical literature up until March 2023 confirmed the absence of clinical studies on the safety of mistletoe therapy during pregnancy. A very early cases series in Google Scholar suggests that an unidentified species of mistletoe (leaf tincture, *nota bene* p.o.) may act as a uterine stimulant that may be useful in the treatment of delayed third stage labour (Lane 1888). Shortly afterward it was briefly reported that mistletoe – again an unidentified species – can be a uterine stimulant (Howard 1892). More recently, the oxytocic activity of mistletoe was characterised pharmacologically (Ie, Zam 2008). Here, the mistletoe species was clearly described, and it was *Globimetula braunii* (family *Loranthaceae*), rather different from the European *Viscum album* (family *Santalaceae*). In two recent reference books that are frequently considered in German-speaking countries, no such properties of European *Viscum album* are mentioned (Wichtl 2009, Schilcher *et al.* 2016).

The limited preclinical information is briefly summarised in the following. The effect of *Viscum album* L. on rapidly proliferating amniotic fluid cells was investigated as early as 1995. At concentrations corresponding to therapeutic doses, neither effects on the sister chromatid exchange frequency nor on the proliferation index could be detected (Büssing *et al.* 1995). In a study with a murine model, which is available online as a pre-print (not peer-reviewed), a certain effect on weight gain is described, but no cases of abortion, embryotoxicity, natimortality or teratogenicity are mentioned (Ghelman *et al.* 2020). In the same study, histological examination of foetal organs showed no signs of toxicity at any of the drug doses tested. At very high concentrations, a slight delay in placental maturity could be observed. Importantly, the histology of the placenta suggests dose-dependent, cytotoxicity-associated inflammatory effects.

On interpretation of malformation data

The data available on subcutaneous mistletoe treatments during pregnancy are scarce. With regard to the reported miscarriage and heart defect (cases A and B, see above), the treating physician classified a possible connection with mistletoe therapy as unlikely. While this classification may seem plausible to obstetricians, it is important for most readers to mention that there is a basic risk of malformations occurring. This risk lies between 1–3 % of all pregnancies and is up to 14 % if the malformations among second trimester abortions are included [see discussion and references in (Baumgartner *et al.* 2022)].

Conclusion

Knowledge about the frequency and safety of mistletoe therapy in pregnancy is still very limited. Overall, the few information collected on mistletoe therapy during pregnancy provides a first positive and encouraging feedback. Next steps of the safety assessment of mistletoe therapy during pregnancy could be retrospective analyses of existing databases with corresponding treatments and relevant preclinical studies.

Acknowledgements

The authors feel indebted to Dr Rita Leroi for her initiative to start a survey, to the physicians who participated in the first survey, to Dr Maria Fornalski for the collection of cases and to the Klinik Arlesheim for the access to its archives at the former Lukas Klinik. We thank Dr Rainer Scheer for kindly supporting the survey 2023. This work was in part financed by the Foundation for Integrative Medicine & Pharmacy (Stiftung Integrative Medizin & Pharmazie, Stuttgart, Germany), in part by the Society for Cancer Research (Arlesheim, Switzerland).

Conflict of interest

A.P. Simões-Wüst, Daniel Krüerke work as scientists in the Klinik Arlesheim, in which mistletoe therapy is available. Furthermore, Daniel Krüerke is also engaged at the Society for Cancer Research, Hiscia Research Institute, Arlesheim, Switzerland.

Data availability

The questionnaires identified in the archives of the Klinik Arlesheim and analysed in the current report are not publicly accessible due to data protection regulations. However, the pseudonymised dataset used for the analysis in this report can be made available upon justified request by the corresponding author with the permission of the hospital management and the data protection officer of the hospital Clinic Arlesheim.

References

Abnoba: abnobaVISCUM®. Fachinformation. 2019. https://www.abnoba.de/wp-content/uploads/2020/08/Fachinformation-September-2019.pdf (accessed Oct 7, 2023).

Alomar M, Tawfiq AM, Hassan N et al.: Post marketing surveillance of suspected adverse drug reactions through spontaneous reporting: current status, challenges and the future. Ther Adv Drug Saf. 2020; 11: 2042098620938595.

Arendt A, Debus M, Gutsch J et al.: Vademecum of Anthroposophic Medicines (Editors: Medical Section of the School of Spiritual Science and Association of Anthroposophic Physicians in Germany) 2017; Der Merkurstab 10 (5), Supplement (ISBN 978-3-946951-04-9).

Baumgartner R., Winterfeld U, Panchaud A et al.: Queries on medication use during pregnancy: characterisation of the Swiss Teratogen Information Service database. Swiss Med Wkly. 2022; 152: w30187.

Büssing A, Lehnert A, Schink M et al.: Effect of Viscum album L. on rapidly proliferating amniotic fluid cells. Sister chromatid exchange frequency and proliferation index. Arzneimittelforschung. 1995; 45 (1): 81–83.

Ghelman R, Cernach MCSP, Ishigai MMS et al.: The Safety of Viscum album L. in A Murine Model: A Reproductive Toxicity Study. 2020 (accessed March 31, 2023).

Howard HP: Mistletoe as an oxytocic. JAMA Network. 1892; XIX.

Ie O, Zam N: Oxytocic properties of the aqueous extract of Globimetula braunii (loranthaceae). Pak J Pharm Sci. 2008; 21 (4): 356–360.

Iscador AG: Iscador® Injektionslösung. 2017. https://compendium.ch/product/1393096-iscador-a-inj-los-1-mg/mpro (accessed Oct 7, 2023).

Lane RM: Ogeechee Medical Association — Stated bimonthly meeting. Southern Medical Record. 1888: 253–255.

Schilcher H, Fischer M, Frank B et al.: Leitfaden Phytotherapie [Phytotherapy Guide]. Munich: Urban & Fischer. 2016.

Target BioScience AG: Helixor. 2020. https://compendium.ch/product/1051778-helixor-a-inj-los-1-mg/mpro (accessed Oct 7, 2023).

Weidemann A, Aden R: Auswertungen des Tumor-Krankengeschichten-Archives der Praxis Emme. Der Merkurstab. 1992; 45(3): 199–216.

Wichtl M: Teedrogen und Phytopharmaka. Stuttgart, Wissenschaftliche Verlagsgesellschaft GmbH. 2009.

Prof. Dr. Ana Paula Simões-Wüst[1, 2], Dr. Daniel Krüerke[1, 3]

[1] Research Department, Klinik Arlesheim AG, Arlesheim, Switzerland

[2] Department of Obstetrics, University Hospital Zurich, University of, Zurich, Zurich, Switzerland

[3] Society for Cancer Research, Hiscia Research Institute, Arlesheim, Switzerland

Corresponding authors:

anapaula.simoes-wuest@klinik-arlesheim.ch

daniel.krueerke@klinik-arlesheim.ch

Misteltherapie als hausärztliche Basismaßnahme bei Krebserkrankungen: Eine integrative Perspektive

Mistletoe Therapy as a Primary Care Intervention in Cancer Treatment: An Integrative Perspective

Frank Meyer

Zusammenfassung

Die Misteltherapie hat sich als bedeutende komplementäre Behandlungsmethode und langfristige Option in der hausärztlichen Versorgung von Menschen mit Krebs etabliert. Dieser Artikel untersucht die Bedeutung der Misteltherapie als hausärztliche Basismaßnahme bei Krebserkrankungen aus einer integrativen Perspektive, unter Berücksichtigung sowohl wissenschaftlicher Erkenntnisse als auch von praktischem Erfahrungswissen. Dabei wird die Rolle der Misteltherapie im Kontext der ganzheitlichen Patientenversorgung beleuchtet und anhand von kurzen Fallvignetten (brief case reports) dargestellt, welche die Wirksamkeit der Mistel unter anderem bei der Schmerzlinderung und der Verbesserung der Lebensqualität belegen.
Schlüsselwörter: Integrative Onkologie, hausärztliche Versorgung, Misteltherapie, patientenzentrierter Ansatz, Magenkarzinom, Ovarialkarzinom, Mammakarzinom, Bronchialkarzinom, *Helleborus*

Summary

Mistletoe therapy has emerged as a significant complementary treatment approach and long-term option in the primary care of individuals with cancer. This article examines the significance of mistletoe therapy as a primary care intervention in cancer treatment from an integrative perspective, considering both scientific evidence and practical experience. The role of mistletoe therapy within the context of comprehensive patient care is discussed, accompanied by brief case reports that demonstrate its efficacy, including pain relief and enhancement of quality of life.

Keywords: Integrative Oncology, primary care, mistletoe therapy, patient-centered approach, gastric cancer, ovarian cancer, breast cancer, lung cancer, *Helleborus*

Einführung

Seit etwa drei Jahrzehnten beobachten wir die Entwicklung der Integrativen Onkologie als akademisches Fachgebiet, das zunehmend an Bedeutung an Universitäten und Kliniken gewinnt und begonnen hat, die konventionelle Medizin zu durchdringen. Dieses neuartige Konzept zielt in erster Linie darauf ab, evidenzbasierte ergänzende traditionelle und naturheilkundliche Therapieoptionen anzubieten, die mit dem aktuellen Stand der klinischen Forschung im Einklang stehen und nahtlos in standardisierte, leitlinienbasierte Verfahren integriert werden können, um von Krebs betroffenen Menschen zu helfen. In Mitteleuropa wurde jedoch unabhängig davon bereits mehr als ein halbes Jahrhundert zuvor, mit der Einführung der Misteltherapie für Krebserkrankungen in den 1920er Jahren durch Rudolf Steiner und Ita Wegman eine eigenständige integrative Krebstherapie etabliert (Kienle, Kiene 2003). Dieser weit verbreitete Ansatz wird und wurde vor allem in allgemeinmedizinischen Praxen sowie in einigen naturheilkundlichen und anthroposophischen Kliniken mit der Anwendung der europäischen Mistel (*Viscum album* L.) als zentralem Element praktiziert. Die ganzheitliche Ausrichtung dieser therapeutischen Praxis, welche in der Anthroposophischen Medizin und der Naturheilkunde verwurzelt ist, basiert weniger auf akademischen Traditionen, sondern mehr auf den individuellen Bedürfnissen der Patienten, die gezielt ganzheitliche oder naturheilkundliche Praxen aufsuchen, der individuellen medizinischen Expertise und den intuitiven Fähigkeiten der behandelnden Ärzte sowie den ergänzenden Konzepten und Methoden, in denen sie neben der konventionellen Medizin ausgebildet sind. Unter Berücksichtigung beider integrativer Ansätze – des akademisch-rationalen auf der einen Seite und des intuitiv-praktischen auf der anderen – möchte ich als langjähriger Allgemeinmediziner mit täglichen Patientenkonsultationen und jahrzehntelanger Erfahrung in Integrativer Medizin die Bedeutung und Besonderheiten der Misteltherapie in der Grundversorgung von Menschen mit Krebserkrankungen in einer gewöhnlichen allgemeinmedizinischen Praxis hervorheben. Die Misteltherapie und andere ganzheitliche, ergänzende oder integrative Behandlungen sollten auch in Zukunft nicht ausschließlich spezialisierten klinischen onkologischen Zentren vorbehalten sein, sondern müssen als Teil der täglichen primären Versorgung für alle Patienten mit Krebs und alle üblichen krebsassoziierten Probleme verfügbar bleiben.

Misteltherapie in der hausärztlichen Versorgung

Die Misteltherapie ist ein wichtiger und viel nachgefragter Bestandteil der hausärztlichen Versorgung von Menschen mit Krebserkrankungen. In integrativen Praxen wird die Misteltherapie bereits bei Diagnosestellung unabhängig vom Prognose- oder Tumorstadium eingesetzt, um den Patienten das bestmögliche Leben in ihrer gegenwärtigen Situation zu ermöglichen und ihre physischen, seelischen, sozialen und spirituellen Bedürfnisse gleichermaßen zu berücksichtigen.

Im Gesamtgebiet der integrativen Medizin bildet die Misteltherapie einen eigenständigen Sektor und fügt sich nahtlos in das ganzheitliche Verständnis von Medizin ein. Hausärztinnen und Hausärzte spielen eine entscheidende Rolle bei der Sicherstellung der Grundversorgung von Patienten mit Krebs und nutzen die Misteltherapie als Methode, die physische, seelische und soziale Aspekte integriert, in ihrer Praxis. Dabei wird die Misteltherapie in ein umfassendes Behandlungskonzept integriert, in welchem die Autonomie des Patienten respektiert und die Selbstverantwortung sowie die Selbstregulation gestärkt werden. Ein solcher patientenzentrierter Ansatz funktioniert nur, wenn die medizinischen Experten die Patienten als Experten für ihr eigenes Leben dazu ermutigen, Mittel und Ziele des ärztlichen Handelns selbst mit festzulegen.

Vielfach suchen Patientinnen und Patienten, die mit konventionellen Methoden keine Hilfe erfahren haben, Hilfe durch die Misteltherapie. Als Beispiel dafür mag die folgende Kurzvignette dienen.

Fallvignette (brief case report): Eine über 80-jährige Frau mit einem fortgeschrittenen Magenkarzinom, welches das Pankreas und die linke

Kolonflexur infiltriert, klagt seit der Tumorresektion vor mehr als 2 Jahren über quälende pochende Bauchschmerzen, die sich mit üblichen Analgetika und Opiaten nicht bessern lassen. Ihre Lebensqualität ist dadurch massiv beeinträchtigt. Nachdem sie verschiedene Schmerztherapeuten aufgesucht hatte, fühlt sie sich so, als hätte man sie ärztlicherseits aufgegeben, weil man ihr nahegelegt hat, dass die Schmerzen lediglich von ihrem Gehirn produziert würden und sie eigentlich ihr „Gehirn umprogrammieren“ müsste. Sie möchte jedoch nicht aufgeben und sucht mich auf, um eine komplementäre Schmerztherapie zu erhalten. Unter der Behandlung mit einem Eichenmistelextrakt mit Kupferzusatz (Iscador Qu c. Cu in ansteigender Dosis bis zu 20 mg 2 x wöchentlich s.c.) erlebt sie eine dramatische Schmerzreduktion, wodurch sich die Lebensqualität erheblich bessert. Die Patientin äußert, zum ersten Mal in ihrer Leidensgeschichte den Eindruck gehabt zu haben, dass ihr ein Arzt wirklich helfen wolle.

Im Stich gelassen fühlen sich häufig auch Patientinnen und Patienten, die leitlinienbasierte Maßnahmen aus Gründen, die im Sinne der Patientenautonomie zu respektieren sind, ablehnen. Auch sie sind häufig offen für eine Misteltherapie und suchen entsprechend ausgebildete Hausärztinnen und Hausärzte auf. Der folgende Fall soll das verdeutlichen.

Fallvignette (brief case report): Eine Frau Mitte 50 mit Gewichtsverlust und Fatigue wird mit einem muzinösen Borderlinetumor (BOT), einer atypischen Neubildung unklarer Dignität, sowie einem mäßig differenzierten Zystadenokarzinom, beides am selben Ovar diagnostiziert. Sie unterzieht sich zwar einer Hysterektomie mit Salpingo-Ovarekektomie und omentaler Resektion, lehnt jedoch die nach Histologie vorgeschlagene ausgedehnte Komplettierungs-Operation und jegliche Chemotherapie ab. Stattdessen entscheidet sie sich gegen ärztlichen Rat für halbjährliche Kontrollen und bittet um eine Misteltherapie. Diese erfolgt mit einem Apfelmistelpräparat mit Silberzusatz (Iscador M c. Arg. in ansteigender Dosis bis zu 20 mg 2 x wöchentlich s.c.). Nach 30 Monaten ist die Patientin rezidivfrei und berichtet von neu gewonnener Lebensfreude und persönlicher Entfaltung auf dem Boden einer tiefgreifenden biografischen Wandlung, die ihr durch dieses Vorgehen ermöglicht worden sei.

Die Misteltherapie als Langzeit-Therapie

Die Misteltherapie hat sich als Behandlungsoption mit kurz- und mittelfristigen Effekten auf tumorbedingte Beschwerden, Therapienebenwirkungen und Lebensqualität bewährt (Loef, Wallach 2020). Zugleich dient sie als Langzeit-Therapie für Patienten mit Krebserkrankungen, die ihre Heilungschancen und damit ihre Überlebensprognose verbessern wollen (Ostermann *et al* 2020). Insbesondere in der hausärztlichen Versorgung, wo Patienten langfristige verlässliche Ansprechpartner für all ihre medizinischen und psychosozialen Bedürfnisse finden, spielt die Misteltherapie eine wichtige Rolle. In manchen Fällen erfolgt eine Misteltherapie über Jahrzehnte und umfasst mehrere schwere Krebserkrankungen, was die folgende Kurzvignette illustrieren soll.

Fallvignette (brief case report): Eine Frau Mitte 70 erhält seit 25 Jahren die Misteltherapie. Zunächst erkrankte sie an einem invasivem duktalem Mammakarzinom und Lymphknotenmetastase, weshalb die Mastektomie links mit axillärer Dissektion, gefolgt von Chemotherapie und Bestrahlung erfolgte. 15 Jahre später wurde ein wenig differenziertes Adenokarzinom beider Lungenflügel diagnostiziert, weshalb die Resektion der betroffenen Lungenlappen, eines Teils der Thoraxwand und von befallenen Lymphknoten mit anschließender Chemotherapie vorgenommen wurde. Ein Jahr später ereignete sich eine zerebrale Metastasierung passend zum Adenokarzinom. Es wurden die neurochirurgische Exstirpation der Metastase und eine Bestrahlung durchgeführt. Unter einer kontinuierliche Misteltherapie ließen sich die zum Teil schweren Therapienebenwirkungen gut kontrollieren. In unterschiedlichen Dosen und herstellerspezifischen Zubereitungen (abnobaVISCUM, Helixor und Iscador) wurden Mistelextrakte von den folgenden Wirtbäumen verwendet: Apfel, Esche, Eiche, Kiefer, Ahorn und Weißdorn. Außerdem wurden im Rahmen der Behandlung der Hirnmetastase *Helleborus niger* und *Helleborus foetidus* jeweils in D3 subkutan injiziert. Seit der Gehirnmetastase vor fast 10 Jahren ist die Patientin bis heute (Ostern 2024) tumorfrei bei sehr guter Lebensqualität.

Zukunft der Misteltherapie

Die Zukunft der Misteltherapie ist eng mit ihrer Verfügbarkeit und Integration in hausärztliche Praxen verbunden. Die tumorspezifische Therapie auf dem Boden wissenschaftlicher Innovationen und neuester Leitlinien findet in erster Linie in Kliniken und fachärztlich-onkologischen Zentren statt, oft nur für einen bestimmten Zeitraum und auf die Krebsbekämpfung fokussiert. Bei ihren Hausärztinnen und Hausärzten hingegen finden Menschen mit Krebs auch langfristig, oftmals über viele Jahre und Jahrzehnte hinweg, Ansprechpartner für all ihre gesundheitlichen Probleme rund um ihre Krebserkrankung und darüber hinaus auch für ihre seelischen und sozialen Nöte. Dabei entsteht immer wieder auch das Bedürfnis nach einer individuellen Therapie, die über die Standards hinausgeht, und dem einzelnen Menschen in seiner individuellen Situation gerecht wird. Hierbei sind unkonventionellen Methoden wie die Misteltherapie, die zugleich verlässlich in ihrer Wirkung und sicher in ihrer Anwendung sind, unverzichtbar.

Schlussfolgerung

Die Misteltherapie nimmt in der hausärztlichen Versorgung von Patienten mit Krebs eine wichtige Position ein, die sowohl auf wissenschaftlichen Erkenntnissen als auch auf Erfahrungswissen basiert. Ihre kontinuierliche Anwendung als Langzeit-Therapie kann dazu beitragen, die Lebensqualität bei Krebserkrankungen über einen längeren Zeitraum zu verbessern und möglicherweise auch das Überleben zu verlängern. Es ist wichtig, die Rolle der Misteltherapie weiter zu erforschen und ihre Integration in die hausärztliche Praxis zu fördern, um den Bedürfnissen von Menschen mit Krebs gerecht zu werden, mit dem Ziel, ihre vielfältigen Beschwerden zu lindern und zugleich die Heilungschancen zu verbessern.

Interessenkonflikt

Frank Meyer erhielt Honorare für Ärztefortbildungen von Weleda AG, Helixor GmbH und Iscador AG.

Literatur

Kienle GS, Kiene H: Die Mistel in der Onkologie. Fakten und konzeptionelle Grundlagen. Stuttgart: Schattauer; 2003.

Loef M, Walach H: Quality of life in cancer patients treated with mistletoe: a systematic review and meta-analysis. BMC Complementary Medicine and Therapies. 2020; 20: 227. doi: 10.1186/s12906-020-03013-3

Ostermann T, Appelbaum S, Poier D, Boehm K, Raak C, Büssing A: A Systematic Review and Meta-Analysis on the Survival of Cancer Patients Treated with a Fermented Viscum album L. Extract (Iscador): An Update of Findings. Complement Med Res. 2020; 27 (4): 260–271. doi: 10.1159/000505202.

Dr. Frank Meyer
Facharzt für Allgemeinmedizin, Naturheilverfahren, Akupunktur
Burgschmietstraße 54, 90419 Nürnberg, Deutschland

Korrespondenzadresse:
drfrankmeyer@icloud.com

Das Erleben der Misteltherapie aus Patientensicht – Eine qualitative Interviewstudie

The Introspective Patient Experience of Mistletoe Therapy in Cancer – A Qualitative Study

Annika Mascher, Florian Pelzer, Lorna J. Duncan, David D. Martin, Stephan Baumgartner, Bettina Berger

Zusammenfassung

Einleitung: Das innere Erleben von Krebspatienten, die Misteltherapie (MT) anwenden, hat bisher wenig wissenschaftliche Beachtung gefunden, obwohl dies für ein ganzheitliches Verständnis und die Begleitung bei dieser Therapie zentral ist.

Methoden: In dieser qualitativen, explorativen Studie wurden 20 ambulante Krebspatienten, die subkutane MT anwandten, in der Klinik Arlesheim (Schweiz) interviewt. Die Daten wurden durch jeweils zwei halbstrukturierte Interviews gesammelt. Die individuellen Erfahrungen wurden in Bezug auf sechs vordefinierte Ebenen menschlichen Erlebens analysiert: körperlich, vital, emotional, mental, spirituell und sozial. Dazu ergaben sich aus dem Material drei weitere, dimensionsübergreifende Perspektiven: Wärme, Immunstärkung und allgemeines Wohlbefinden.

Ergebnisse: Die Datenanalyse ergab eine große Vielfalt der Erfahrungen der Patienten mit der MT. Die Bedeutung spezifischer Aspekte wurde deutlich, wie z. B. einer gesteigerten Vitalität zur Bewältigung des Alltags, eine größere emotionale und mentale Stabilität, einem multidimensionalen Wärmegefühl, Empfindungen von Sicherheit und Schutz durch die MT, einer gesteigerten Selbstwahrnehmung und Selbstfürsorge, sowie Empfindungen spiritueller Verbundenheit.

Diskussion: Die Ergebnisse geben einen ersten tieferen Einblick in das reiche Patientenerleben der MT und können Therapeuten und Patienten zur Introspektion motivieren. Dies ermöglicht eine ganzheitliche Unterstützung der Patienten, sowohl während der MT als auch auf ihrem Lebensweg.

Schlüsselwörter: Qualitative Studie, Misteltherapie, Krebs, Patientenerleben, Interviews, Selbstbeobachtung

Summary
Introduction: The introspective experience of cancer patients using mistletoe therapy (MT) has received little scientific interest, although it is crucial for a holistic understanding of this therapy.
Methods: In this qualitative, exploratory study, 20 outpatient cancer patients applying subcutaneous MT were interviewed at the Arlesheim Hospital (Switzerland). Data was collected through two semi-structured, in-depth interviews per patient. Individual experiences were analyzed in relation to six predefined levels of human experience: physical, vital, emotional, mental, spiritual and social. From the material resulted three additional, cross-dimensional perspectives: warmth, immune strengthening, and general well-being.
Results: Data analysis revealed considerable heterogeneity in patients' experiences with MT. The importance of specific aspects became apparent, such as increased vitality to cope with everyday life, greater emotional and mental stability, warmth as a multidimensional phenomenon, feelings of security and protection through MT, increased self-awareness and self-care, as well as feelings of spiritual connection.
Discussion: The results provide a first, deeper insight into a rich patient experience of MT and want to motivate therapists and patients to practice introspection. This makes it possible to provide a holistic support to the patient, both during MT and on their life path.
Keywords: Qualitative study, mistletoe therapy, cancer, patient experience, interviews, introspection

Einleitung

Die Misteltherapie (MT) wurde bereits in zahlreichen quantitativen (Friedel *et al.* 2009; Grossarth-Maticek *et al.* 2001; Loef, Walach 2020; Pelzer *et al.* 2022; Pelzer, Tröger 2018; Tröger *et al.* 2013), aber nur wenigen qualitativen Studien (Kienle *et al.* 2016; 2018) untersucht. Ein systematisches Review von Evans *et al.* mit der Frage „Was sind die Ansichten und Erfahrungen von Krebspatienten mit der Anwendung von MT?" zeigt dabei nur drei Publikationen, die einen qualitativen Ansatz verwendeten, um die Innenwelt der Patienten zu erforschen (Evans *et al.* 2016). Nur eine dieser Veröffentlichungen befasste sich ausdrücklich mit den Erfahrungen der Patienten bei der subkutanen MT, wobei allerdings nur 3 von 25 Patienten ihre Wahrnehmungen eindeutig der MT zuordnen konnten

(Brandenberger *et al.* 2012). Das Wissen über das Erleben der Patienten mit MT ist bisher begrenzt, und es ist noch nicht klar, inwieweit Patienten durch Introspektion (Selbstbeobachtung, Innenwahrnehmung oder Selbstwahrnehmung) in der Lage sind, verschiedene Ebenen der MT-Erfahrung zu erleben und zu beschreiben. Introspektion wird als „unberührte innere Erfahrungen“, als „momentane Erfahrungen, die noch nicht durch Interpretation gefärbt sind“ beschrieben (Lapping-Carr, Heavey 2017).

Der derzeitige Mangel an Informationen über die introspektiven Erfahrungen der Patienten mit MT und das Potenzial für eine weitere Erforschung der Auswirkungen von MT veranlassten uns, eine explorative Studie durchzuführen. Dies ist eine Kurzfassung der Originalpublikation (Mascher *et al.* 2023).

Methoden

Diese qualitative Studie wurde explorativ und deskriptiv mit 20 ambulanten Krebspatienten der Klinik Arlesheim (Schweiz) durchgeführt, die subkutane MT mit Iscador® anwandten. Die Durchführung erfolgte gemäß den COREQ-Richtlinien (Tong *et al.* 2007) (Consolidated Criteria for Reporting Qualitative Research). Anhand von zwei halbstrukturierten Interviews und von Zeichnungen wurde das individuelle Patientenerleben zur MT, zur Krebswahrnehmung und zum Thema ‚Heilung‘ untersucht. Im Interviewleitfaden wurden sechs Erfahrungsebenen erkundet: die physische, die vitale, die emotionale, die mentale/bewusste, die spirituelle und die soziale Ebene, in Bezug auf die MT, wie auch die Krebserkrankung. Zudem wurde gefragt, welche Bedeutung Begriffe wie „Heilung“, „Gesundheit“ und „Krankheit“ für die Krebsbetroffenen haben. Zudem wurden die Begleittherapien dokumentiert.

In die Studie wurden Krebspatienten (≥18 Jahre) einbezogen, die seit mindestens sechs Monaten subkutane MT (Iscador®) anwandten. Ausschlusskriterium war der Erhalt einer mistelinduzierten Fiebertherapie in den letzten 4 Wochen, um die Anwendungsformen klar zu unterscheiden. Die Studie wurde von der Ethik-Kommission Nordwestschweiz genehmigt (Projekt-ID 2020-00905) und gemäß der Deklaration von Helsinki und den Richtlinien der Guten Klinischen Praxis durchgeführt.

Dieser Artikel konzentriert sich auf die Analyse der Interviews, in denen die Patienten ihre Erfahrungen mit der MT geschildert haben. Es wurde eine qualitative Inhaltsanalyse (Kuckartz 2014; Mayring 2015; Schreier 2012) in einem mehrstufigen Prozess mit einem deduktiv-induktiven Kategorisierungssystem (Tab. 1) durchgeführt. Die Kategorienbildung fand trennscharf und erschöpfend statt, mit klaren Regeln, Definitionen und Ein-/ Ausschlusskriterien. Einer Basiscodierung folgte eine Feincodierung. Zudem wurden multiprofessionelle Interpretationsgruppen abgehalten, um sowohl fallorientierte als auch themenorientierte Analysen durchzuführen. Darüber hinaus führten die Forscher einen kontinuierlichen Selbstreflexionsprozess durch.

Tab. 1: Die Haupt- und Unterkategorien

Physische Ebene	• Wirksamkeitsüberzeugung
• Hautkrebsrückbildung	Nichtspüren der MT
• Immunkräftigung	Tut gut
• Erhöhte Körpertemperatur	Nicht auf die MT verzichten wollen
Vitalitätsebene	**Spirituelle Ebene**
• Energie-/Kraftsteigerung	• Spirituelle Vertiefung/Wegfindung
Emotionale Ebene	Vertrauen in Höheres der MT
• Dankbarkeit	**Soziale Ebene**
• Angstabnahme	**Dimensionsübergreifende Perspektiven**
• Stimmungsaufhellung	• Wärme
• Entspannung und Ausgeglichenheit	Erhöhte Körpertemperatur
• Erhöhtes Sicherheitsgefühl	Hitze
Sicherheit	Kühle
Selbstvertrauen	Wärmehülle
Umhüllend	Zirkulation
Mental/Bewusstseinsebene	Selbstfürsorge
• Erhöhtes Eigenbewusstsein	Präsenz im Körper
Selbstfürsorge	• Immunstärkung
Mentale Stärkung und Beruhigung	• Allgemeinbefinden

Ergebnisse

Bei den Befragten handelte es sich um 15 Frauen und fünf Männer im Alter von 46 bis 83 Jahren (Median 62 Jahre) mit verschiedenen Krebsarten (Details siehe Tab. 2). Drei Patienten waren im akuten Progress der Erkrankung. Die Therapiedauer der MT betrug zum Zeitpunkt der Interviews 2–30 Jahre (Median 7,5 Jahre). 19 Patienten erhielten gleichzeitig (zum Zeitpunkt der Interviews) auch andere Therapien.

Den vordefinierten Erfahrungsebenen der MT (körperlich, vital, emotional, mental/bewusst, spirituell und sozial) wurden unterschiedliche individuelle Wahrnehmungen zugeschrieben.

Neben den vorab festgelegten Kategorien (deduktiver Ansatz), konnten aus dem Material weitere Themen identifiziert werden (induktiver Ansatz). Dazu gehörten alle induktiven Unterkategorien sowie die zusätzliche Hauptkategorie der „dimensionsübergreifenden Perspektiven", einschließlich Erfahrungen von Wärme, Immunstärkung und allgemeinem Wohlbefinden mit Qualitäten, die sich über alle deduktiven Kategorien erstrecken. Das Kategoriensystem in Tabelle 1 veranschaulicht die verschiedenen Kategorien.

Die physische Ebene

Der Begriff „physisch" bezieht sich auf die materiellen Strukturen des menschlichen Körpers. Zwei Patienten berichteten über einen Rückgang von weißem Hautkrebs durch die MT. Mehrere Patienten schilderten nach der Injektion einen Anstieg der Körpertemperatur. Auch eine gestärkte Widerstandsfähigkeit gegen Erkältungen und verbesserte Immunparameter wurden beschrieben.

Tab. 2: M = männlich, W = weiblich, CA = Karzinom, Immunstä. = Immunstärkung, allg. Wohlb. = allgemeines Wohlbefinden; Alter und Dauer der MT werden in Jahren angezeigt. Hellgraue Felder zeigen, dass der Teilnehmer/die Teilnehmerin eine Wahrnehmung zu dieser Ebene geäußert hat, dunkelgraue Felder stehen für kein Erlebnis zur MT und weiße Felder für keine Aussage (z. B., dass die Person die Wahrnehmung nicht klar zuordnen konnte). Die Tabelle ist nach der Anzahl der beschriebenen Wahrnehmungen sortiert (auch keine Veränderung durch die MT zu erleben zählte als Wahrnehmung).

Patient	Alter	Geschlecht	Krebstyp	Iscador	MT Dauer	Physisch	Vitalität	Emotional	Mental	Spirituell	Sozial	Wärme	Immunstä.	Allg. Wohlb.	Summe
521	63	W	TubenCA	M	11										8
522	59	M	ColonCA	M	3										8
537	52	W	MammaCA	P c. Hg	7										8
525	67	W	Malignes Melanom + Basaliom	M	6										7
532	60	W	MammaCA	M	2										7
534	54	W	MammaCA	P	2										7
536	83	M	Prostata-, Colon- + BlasenCA	Qu, P	8										7
539	68	M	ProstataCA	Qu	8										7
540	67	W	MammaCA	P	20										7
524	60	W	MammaCA 2x	A	30										6
530	69	W	OvarialCA + Gehirnmetastasen	Pause	3										6
533	71	M	ProstataCA	Qu	13										6
538	69	M	CLL	P	15										6

Patient	Alter	Geschlecht	Krebstyp	Iscador	MT Dauer	Physisch	Vitalität	Emotional	Mental	Spirituell	Sozial	Wärme	Immunstä.	Allg. Wohlb.	Summe
541	56	W	Malignes Melanom + MammaCA + Basaliom + PlattenepithelCA	M, P	7										6
527	46	W	MammaCA 2x	M c. Cu	19										6
526	60	W	EndometriumCA	M c. Ag, P	6										6
531	77	W	MammaCA 2x	P c. Hg, Qu	27										4
535	53	W	MammaCA + Knochenmetastasen	M	3										4
529	61	W	MammaCA	P c. Hg	3										4
523	66	W	OvarialCA	Qu, P	13										2
			MammaCA												4

Die Vitalitätsebene

„Vitalität“ bezieht sich hier auf den Bereich der Lebenskräfte, d. h. der Kräfte, die die physischen Strukturen am Leben erhalten und ihre Form und Funktion aufrechterhalten. Die meisten Befragten berichteten von einer deutlichen Steigerung der Vitalität und Kraft sowie von weniger Müdigkeit und Erschöpfung. Eine Patientin berichtete: „So undefinierbar müde bin ich früher vor der Misteltherapie viel mehr gewesen. [...] So eine Grundmüdigkeit find ich, hab ich nicht mehr.“ (Pat 521, 2). Die Patienten berichteten, dass mehr Energie/Kraft mit einer verbesserten Lebensqualität in Bezug auf die Bewältigung des Alltags einherging und dass sie sich in Bezug auf ihr emotionales Innenleben unterstützt oder erleichtert fühlten.

Die emotionale Ebene

Die Befragten beschrieben eine emotionale Aufhellung, Entspannung und Stabilisierung durch die MT, was wiederum mit anderen Erfahrungsebenen, wie der Vitalität und Gedankenwelt, und weiteren Verbesserungen der Lebensqualität der Patienten verbunden war. Die Wahrnehmung von Dankbarkeit, weniger Angst, Stimmungs-aufhellung, emotionaler Entspannung und Beruhigung stand für die Patienten dieser Gruppe besonders im Vordergrund. Als relevantes Thema für die Befragten erwies sich das durch die MT erlebte Gefühl der Sicherheit. Begriffe wie „Sicherheit“, „Schutz“, „Boden unter den Füßen“, „Vertrauen“, „Schutzhülle“ und „das Gefühl, in sicheren Händen zu sein“ fielen, wenn die Befragten ihre inneren Empfindungen beschrieben. Dieses der MT zugeschriebene Sicherheitsgefühl ermöglichte weiter auch einen Anstieg des Selbstvertrauens und der Selbstwirksamkeit bei den Teilnehmenden.

Die mentale oder Bewusstseinsebene

Auf der mentalen Ebene berichteten alle Befragten von einem Erleben mit der MT. Dies erstreckte sich von einer Wirksamkeitsüberzeugung bis hin zu verschiedenen Aspekten von persönlichem Wachstum mit Hilfe der

MT, wie ein erhöhtes Eigenbewusstsein und eine erhöhte Selbstwahrnehmung und -reflexion. „Man könnte auch sagen, Krankheit ist eine Verwandlungshilfe. Und bei vielen, die Krankheit durchgemacht haben, die sind auch anders. [...] Und die Mistel hilft da eben, diesen Krankheitsprozess so durchzumachen, dass es eben zu einem Verwandlungsprozess wird. Die Mistel unterstützt die Selbstverwandlung." (Pat 522, 2). Auch beschrieben einige Patienten ein erhöhtes Selbstvertrauen durch Hilfe der MT. Sie nahmen die Anwendung der MT als aktive Selbsthilfe und Stärkung ihres Selbstwirksamkeitsgefühls wahr. Für mehrere Befragte war die MT zu einem festen Bestandteil ihres Tagesablaufs mit entsprechender Bedeutungszuweisung geworden. Der MT wurde zudem eine mentale Stärkung und Entspannung zugeschrieben. Fünf Befragte schrieben der MT kein persönliches Wachstum zu. Sie hatten auch keinen konkreten Antrieb, sich bewusst mit der Krankheit oder ihrer Therapie auseinanderzusetzen.

Die spirituelle Ebene

Das Vertrauen, durch die MT „begleitet" und „beschützt" zu sein wurde von einigen Befragten ausgedrückt – ein Loslassen und Entspannen, einhergehend mit einer erlebten Verbundenheit zu etwas „Höherem", dem „Kosmos", etwas „Ganzheitlichen". Eine Studienteilnehmerin berichtete: „Es ist wie eine Bestätigung, diese Verbundenheit mit der Natur, und dass da auch eine geistige Macht mit im Spiel ist." (Pat 532, 2). Eine „geistige Welt" wurde von einigen Teilnehmer durch die MT als erahnbar oder erlebbar beschrieben. Ein Studienteilnehmer schilderte: «Also diesbezüglich muss ich eben sagen, da hab' ich dann schon ein Erlebnis mit der Mistel. [...] Das ist etwas, was mich berührt hat und mich bestärkt hat, dass es sicher etwas gibt. Eine – ja, eine geistige Welt. Also nicht der Himmel. Nein, eine Ordnung, die wir nicht verstehen und auch nicht verstehen müssen.» (Pat 533, 2).

Die soziale Ebene

Soziale Aspekte erschienen als Folge der Erlebnisse der übrigen Erfahrungsebenen. Studienteilnehmer schreiben der MT zu, mit sich selbst und anderen einfühlsamer zu sein, sowie die Fähigkeit, offener und klarer kommunizieren zu können auf einer Grundlage emotionaler Entspannung oder erhöhtem Selbstvertrauen.

Dimensionsübergreifende Perspektiven

Das vielschichtige Wärmeerleben

Mehrere Befragte beschrieben verschiedene Wärmeempfindungen, ohne das danach gefragt wurde: z. B. eine angenehme Wärme im Körper nach vielen Jahren latenter Kühle oder einem „Fließen“ oder „Strömen“ von Wärme im Körper oder dem Gefühl einer „Wärmehülle“. Bei Mistelextrakt-Überdosierungen war es vereinzelt auch zu einem unangenehmen Hitzeüberschuss gekommen. Beschreibungen von Herzenswärme und Selbstfürsorge wurden der MT zugeordnet und auch die Wärme als Vermittlerin für die eigene Präsenz, um (mehr) in Kontakt mit dem eigenen Körper zu kommen. „Heute, wenn ich jetzt spritze, würde ich sagen, ich spüre also mehr Präsenz, und mehr Wärme, und Zirkulation. [...] Ich habe das Gefühl so, alles ist wärmer in meinem Körper. Also bis in die Peripherie. Also die Füße sind wärmer, die Hände, vor allem die Hände.“ (Pat 526, 2)

Immunstärkung

Mehrere Patienten berichteten, dass sie mit der MT widerstandsfähiger gegen Erkältungen waren, seltener oder überhaupt nicht mehr krank wurden. Ein dadurch erfahrenes Sicherheitsgefühl wurde von Befragten beschrieben, das eine mentale Beruhigung mit sich brachte und soziale Interaktionen förderte. „Es schützt mich. Es macht mich stark. Also ich merk, ja manchmal [...] bin ich die Einzige, die nie etwas hat in dieser Schule. Also ergo, die immer arbeitet. [...] Will auch mal bisschen daheim sein! Nein. (lacht).“ (Pat 537, 1).

Allgemeines Wohlbefinden

Einige Befragte berichteten von einem verbesserten Allgemeinzustand, oder einem allgemeinen Wohlbefinden mit Hilfe der MT. Wie eine Krebspatientin beschrieb: „Das merk ich: Das tut mir gut. Es tut mich wie umhüllen. Es hilft mir. Es stärkt mich. [...] Es gibt mir als Mensch etwas. Also es ist wie nicht etwas, wo ich empfinde, es geht punktuell jetzt um Krebs, sondern es ist etwas, das mir ganzheitlich sehr gut tut.“ (Pat 537, 2, Pos. 43).

Diskussion

Unsere Studie ergab ein breites Spektrum an Erfahrungen von Krebspatienten mit der MT. Die Resultate entsprechen Ergebnissen aus der Lebensqualitätsforschung der MT und vertiefen und erweitern diese.

Eine Stärke dieser Studie ist das qualitative Studiendesign selbst, das durch zwei Interviews pro Person tief in die individuelle MT-Erfahrung von Krebspatienten eintaucht und eine reichhaltige und vielfältige Menge an Informationen erfasste. Zur Qualitätssicherung wurden Monitoring-Visiten durchgeführt, eine Assistenz durch Experten in qualitativer Forschung gewährleistet und die Studie durch ständige Selbstreflexion begleitet.

Limitationen der Studie stellen die geringe Anzahl an Studienteilnehmer dar, die Stichprobenverzerrung, das monozentrische Design und das spezifische Setting einer anthroposophischen Klinik. Quantifizierbare Aussagen können und sollen hier nicht gemacht werden. Die angezeigten Zahlen dienen der Charakterisierung dieser Probe und können in keiner Weise verallgemeinert werden.

Diese Studie stellt eine erste explorative Basis für weitere Forschungen dar. Um die Erfahrungen von Patienten mit MT besser zu verstehen, wäre es interessant, die Entwicklung der Erfahrungen von Patienten im Zeitverlauf zu verfolgen, z. B. vor Beginn und im Verlauf der MT, oder in anderen Settings, Kliniken und mit einer Vergleichsgruppe zu untersuchen oder auch neue Fragebögen zu entwickeln. In der vorliegenden Studie wurde deutlich, dass die in der qualitativen Forschung verwendeten Fragen nicht nur als Forschungsinstrument nützlich sind. Sie können auch das Bewusstsein für innere Prozesse anregen und somit für die innere Entwicklung von Patienten von Nutzen sein. Dies wirft die wichtige Frage auf, inwieweit Selbstbeobachtung Heilungsprozesse, Autoregulation und Selbstmanagement von Patienten unterstützen könnte. Darüber hinaus entstand in dieser Studie die Hypothese, dass eine Schulung in

Introspektion von Patienten die Wirkung von MT/Heilmitteln sowie Heilungsprozesse verstärken kann, sowie auch eine Schulung von Gesundheitspersonal eine neue Art der Begegnung, Wahrnehmung und Begleitung von Patienten fördern kann. Das Verständnis, dass Patienten in der Lage sind, Arzneimittel und therapeutische Wirkungen differenziert wahrzunehmen, könnte tiefgreifende Auswirkungen auf die Einstellung von Ärzten haben.

Schlussfolgerungen

In dieser Studie haben wir beobachtet, dass Krebspatienten differenzierte Erfahrungen auf verschiedenen Erfahrungsebenen im Zusammenhang mit der MT haben können. Da diese Forschungsfrage bisher nicht eingehend untersucht wurde, möchte diese erste Studie ein tieferes Verständnis für die individuellen Erfahrungen von Patienten mit MT anregen. Wir möchten Ärzte und Therapeuten ermutigen, ihre Patienten nach ihren persönlichen Erfahrungen zu fragen, ihnen solche zuzutrauen, um vielleicht unerwartete Antworten zu erhalten und die Betroffenen dadurch auf ihrem Weg tiefergehend und ganzheitlicher unterstützen und begleiten zu können.

Interessenkonflikt

Der gemeinnützige Verein für Krebsforschung (VfK) ist Minderheitsaktionär der Iscador AG, einem Hersteller von Mistelextrakten. AM ist Mitarbeiterin des VfK und war bis Juni 2021 in der Klinik Arlesheim angestellt. SB ist Mitarbeiter des VfK und der Iscador AG. FP war bis Februar 2022 beim VfK angestellt und ist seitdem bei der Iscador AG angestellt. BB, LJD, DDM haben keinen Interessenkonflikt.

Literatur

Brandenberger M, Simões-Wüst AP, Rostock M et al.: An exploratory study on the quality of life and individual coping of cancer patients

during mistletoe therapy. Integrative Cancer Therapies. Vol 11; 2012: 90–100.
Evans M, Bryant S, Huntley AL et al.: Cancer Patients' Experiences of Using Mistletoe (Viscum album): A Qualitative Systematic Review and Synthesis. J Altern Complement Med. 2016; 22 (2): 134–144.
Friedel WE, Matthes H, Bock PR et al.: Systematic evaluation of the clinical effects of supportive mistletoe treatment within chemo-and/or radiotherapy protocols and long-term mistletoe application in non-metastatic colorectal carcinoma: multicenter, controlled, observational cohort study. J Soc Integr Oncol. 2009; 7 (4): 137–145.
Grossarth-Maticek R, Kiene H, Baumgartner S et al.: Use of Iscador, an extract of European mistletoe (Viscum album L.), in cancer treatment: prospective nonrandomized and randomized matched- pair studies nested within a cohort study. Alternative Therapies. 2001; 7 (3): 57–75.
Kienle GS, Mussler M, Fuchs D et al.: Individualized Integrative Cancer Care in Anthroposophic Medicine: A Qualitative Study of the Concepts and Procedures of Expert Doctors. Integrative Cancer Therapies. 2016; 15: 478–494.
Kienle GS, Mussler M, Fuchs D et al.: The subjective dimension of integrative cancer care: a qualitative study exploring the perspectives, themes, and observations of experienced doctors from the area of anthroposophic medicine. Explore. 2018; 14: 342–351.
Kuckartz U: Qualitative text analysis: A guide to methods, practice and using software. London: Sage Publications Ltd.; 2014.
Lapping-Carr LR und Heavey CL: Pristine inner experience and descriptive experience sampling: implications for psychology. Frontiers in psychology. 2017; 8: 2170.
Loef M und Walach H: Quality of life in cancer patients treated with mistletoe: a systematic review and meta-analysis. BMC Complement Med Ther. 2020; 20: 227. doi: 10.1186/s12906-020-03013-3.
Mascher A, Pelzer F, Duncan LJ, et al.: The Introspective Patient Experience of Mistletoe Therapy in Cancer: A Qualitative Study. Integrative cancer therapies. 2023; 22: 1–17.

Mayring P: Qualitative content analysis: Theoretical background and procedures. Approaches to qualitative research in mathematics education. Dordrecht: Springer; 2015: 365–380.

Pelzer F, Loef M, Martin DD et al.: Cancer-related fatigue in patients treated with mistletoe extracts: a systematic review and meta-analysis. Support Care Cancer. 2022; 30 (8): 6405–6418.

Pelzer F und Tröger W: Complementary treatment with mistletoe extracts during chemotherapy: safety, neutropenia, fever, and quality of life assessed in a randomized study. Journal of Alternative and Complementary Medicine. 2018; 24: 954–961.

Schreier M: Qualitative content analysis in practice. London: Sage publications; 2012.

Tong A, Sainsbury P und Craig J: Consolidated criteria for reporting qualitative research (COREQ): a 32-item checklist for interviews and focus groups. International journal for quality in health care. 2007; 19: 349–357.

Tröger W, Galun, D, Reif M et al.: Viscum album L. extract therapy in patients with locally advanced or metastatic pancreatic cancer: A randomised clinical trial on overall survival. European Journal of Cancer. 2013; 49: 3788–3797.

Annika Mascher[1, 2, 3], Florian Pelzer, MSc[1, 2], Lorna J. Duncan, PhD[4], David D. Martin, MD[1, 5], Stephan Baumgartner, PhD[1, 2], Bettina Berger, PhD[1]

[1] Universität Witten/Herdecke, Witten, Deutschland

[2] Verein für Krebsforschung, Arlesheim, Schweiz

[3] Klinik Arlesheim, Arlesheim, Schweiz

[4] University of Bristol, Bristol, Vereinigtes Königreich

[5] Universität Tübingen, Tübingen, Deutschland

Korrespondenzadresse:
a.mascher@vfk.ch

Die Webseite für die Misteltherapie in der Onkologie – www.mistel-therapie.de

The Website for Mistletoe Therapy in Oncology – www.mistel-therapie.de

Friedemann Schad, Anja Thronicke, Marion Debus, Maike Kergel, Yván Villegas, Georg Soldner

Zusammenfassung

Neu aufgelegt im Jahr 2019, bietet die Website www.mistel-therapie.de einen aktuellen Überblick über die Misteltherapie in der Onkologie und richtet sie sich an Ärzte/Ärztinnen, Wissenschaftler/Wissenschaftlerinnen, Fachexperten und Behörden im Gesundheitswesen und vor allem an Krebspatienten/-patientinnen. Ein Expertengremium aktualisiert die Seite regelmäßig und liefert Einblicke in die klinische Evidenz, Wirkmechanismen, Sicherheit und Kompatibilität der Misteltherapie mit konventionellen Krebstherapien. Seit Aktualisierung der Website konnte eine zunehmende globale Reichweite erzielt werden. Mit über 10.000 monatlichen Nutzer, haben sich seither sie Zugriffe seit 2019 verfünffacht. Übersetzt in Englisch (www.mistletoe-therapy.org) und Spanisch (www.terapiademuerdago.com) bleibt die Seite mit aktuellen Studien auf dem neuesten Stand. Regelmäßige Aktualisierungen, patientenzentrierte Funktionen und weltweite Zugänglichkeit machen sie unverzichtbar. Nutzerstatistiken unterstreichen ihre internationale Reichweite und festigen ihre Rolle als verlässliche Quelle in der sich entwickelnden Forschungslandschaft der Misteltherapie in der Onkologie. Als wichtige Ressource konsolidiert sie die Belege zur Misteltherapie und unterstützt eine informierte Entscheidungsfindung in der Onkologie.

Schlüsselwörter: *Viscum album* L., Misteltherapie, Webseite, Onkologie, Expertengremium, patientenzentriert

Summary

Newly launched in 2019, the website www.mistel-therapie.de provides an up-to-date overview of mistletoe therapy in oncology and is directed at doctors, scientists, experts, and authorities in the healthcare sector and, above all, cancer patients.

A panel of experts regularly updates the site and provides insights into the clinical evidence, mechanisms of action, safety and compatibility of mistletoe therapy with conventional cancer therapies. Since the website was updated, it has achieved an increasing global reach. With over 10,000 monthly users, visits have increased fivefold since 2019. Translated into English (www.mistletoe-therapy.org) and Spanish (www.terapiademuerdago.com), the site remains up to date with the latest studies. Regular updates, patient-centered functions and worldwide accessibility make it indispensable. User statistics underscore its international reach and solidify its role as a reliable resource in the evolving research landscape of mistletoe therapy in oncology. As an important resource, it consolidates the evidence on mistletoe therapy and supports informed decision-making in oncology.
Keywords: *Viscum album* L., mistletoe therapy, website, oncology, expert panel, patient-centered

Einleitung

Die Zahl an medizinisch-wissenschaftlichen und klinischen Veröffentlichungen zur Europäischen Weißbeerigen Mistel (*Viscum album* L., VA) in der Onkologie nimmt stetig zu (NCBI). Mehrere aktuelle klinische Leitlinien sowie systematische Übersichten und Metaanalysen bestätigen die Verbesserung der Lebensqualität bei onkologischen Patienten, die mit einer Mistel-Zusatztherapie behandelt werden (Loef *et al.* 2023; Pelzer *et al.* 2022; Loef *et al.* 2020; Lyman *et al.* 2018; Kröz *et al.* 2016; Greenlee *et al.* 2014, Tröger *et al.* 2014a, 2014b, 2009, 2004, Kim *et al.* 2012, Kienle *et al.* 2010; Horneber *et al.* 2008; Piao *et al.* 2004). Mehr als 290 wissenschaftliche Arbeiten, darunter systematische Reviews, Metaanalysen, Real-World Data-Studien und mehr als 30 prospektive randomisierte klinische Studien wurden in den letzten zwei Jahrzehnten veröffentlicht. Die Vermittlung dieser Erkenntnisse an die Patienten und die Fachöffentlichkeit spielt dabei eine entscheidende Rolle. Die Website www.mistel-therapie.de wurde 2019 inhaltlich neugestaltet, um einen aktuellen Überblick zur onkologischen Misteltherapie zu geben (Thronicke *et al.* 2022). Ziel des vorliegenden Projekts war es, eine übersichtliche und laufend aktualisierte Website zu erstellen, die den aktuellen Wissensstand zur Misteltherapie widerspiegelt und gleichzeitig den Anforderungen Interessierter und denen der Zulassungsbehörden gerecht wird.

Methoden

Im Frühjahr 2019 wurde ein interdisziplinäres Expertengremium gegründet, um den aktuellen medizinisch-wissenschaftlichen Stand der Misteltherapie in der integrativen Onkologie zu überprüfen. Hierzu wurden 290 seit 2000 publizierte wissenschaftliche Artikel, darunter systematische Reviews und Metaanalysen, nationale und internationale Leitlinien sowie klinische und Real-World Data-Studien im Zusammenhang mit einer Misteltherapie zusammengetragen, zusammengefasst und auf der Website www.mistel-therapie.de im September 2019 online gestellt. Neu erscheinende Studien wurden wissenschaftlich und informativ fortlaufend für die verschiedenen Zielgruppen aufbereitet, um einen breiten Zugang für Interessierte und Betroffene zu schaffen. Um die Zugänglichkeit für ein breiteres internationales Publikum zu gewährleisten, wurde die Webseite in die englische (www.mistletoe-therapy.org) und spanische Sprache (www.terapiademuerdago.com) übersetzt. Bei jeder Aktualisierung der Webseite durch neue Ergebnisse von Studien wurde gleichsam die Übersetzung ins Englische und Spanische berücksichtigt.

Ergebnisse

Die aktuelle Website fasst die neuesten wissenschaftlichen Erkenntnisse zur Misteltherapie zusammen, wobei die klinische Evidenz, die praktische Anwendung, Wirkmechanismen, Sicherheitsaspekte von Mistelpräparaten und deren Verträglichkeit in Kombination mit konventionellen Krebstherapien sowie die Einhaltung der aktuellen Leitlinien berücksichtigt werden. Auf der Website wird hierbei auf die besonderen Bedürfnisse der verschiedenen Interessengruppen eingegangen. In einem speziellen Bereich richtet sie sich an Ärzte und Wissenschaftler und bietet einen umfassenden Überblick über die klinische Evidenz der Misteltherapie und ihre Einbettung in aktuelle nationale und internationale onkologische Leitlinien. Hierbei werden die Ergebnisse der klinischen Studien für verschiedene Krebsarten wie Brustkrebs, Eierstockkrebs, Bauchspeicheldrüsenkrebs und andere sowohl für Laien als auch für das Fachpublikum näher erläutert. Des Weiteren erhält man Informationen zu der Kompatibilität der Misteltherapie zur Chemotherapie, Bestrahlung und zielgerichteter Therapie. Um den besonderen Bedürfnissen von Patienten Rechnung zu tragen, enthält die Website einen zusätzlichen Bereich, der speziell auf ihre Belange zugeschnitten ist und einen Einblick zur Anwendung, den Wirkmechanismen und der Sicherheit von Mistelpräparaten sowie in Ergebnisse von klinischen Studien gibt. In einem zusätzlichen Bereich werden die von Patienten häufig gestellten Fragen (Frequently Asked Questions, FAQ) zur Misteltherapie beantwortet. Abbildung 1 hebt diejenigen Aspekte der Mistelwebseite visuell hervor, die am häufigsten von Menschen mit Krebs bzw. von Interessierten besucht werden.

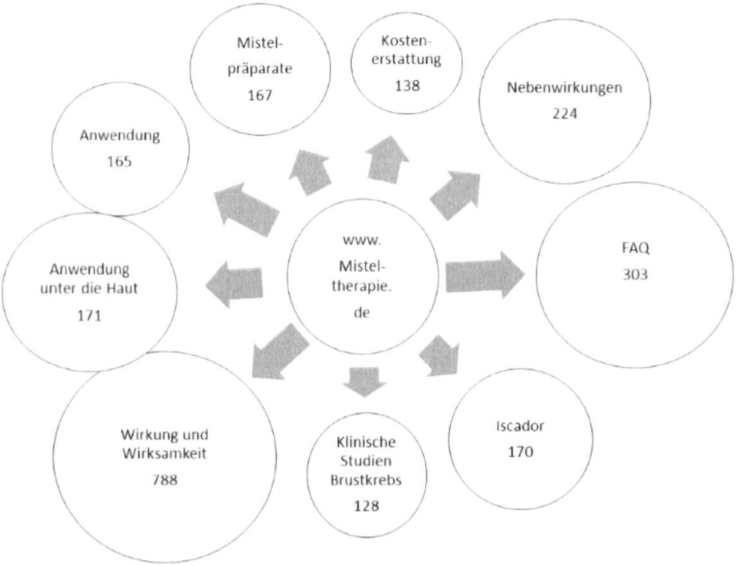

Abb. 1: Relevanteste Einstiegsseiten der Mistelwebseite gemäß Eingänge 09/2023

Die Stärke der Website liegt in der zeitnahen Zusammenfassung von neusten Studien, um sicherzustellen, dass der Inhalt relevant und aktuell bleibt und in dem Format sich an Patienten und Behandler zu wenden. Seit Mai 2020 ist die Webseite auch in englischer und seit Juli 2021 in spanischer Sprache verfügbar. Abb. 2 veranschaulicht die globale Wirkung der Website und zeigt, dass Deutschland mit 46 % der Nutzer an der Spitze steht, gefolgt von den Vereinigten Staaten mit 28 % und Spanien mit 8 %.

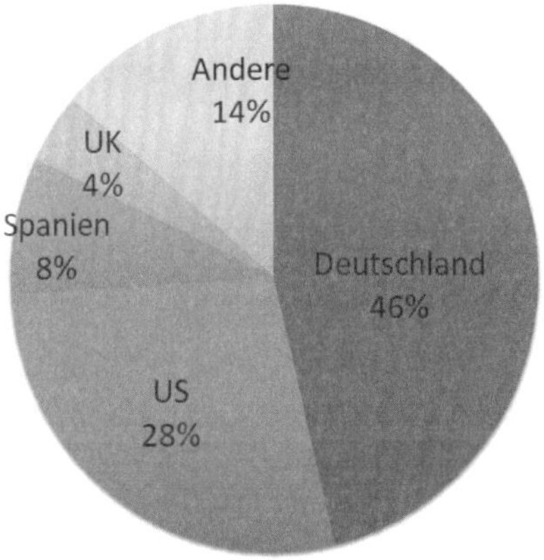

Abb. 2: Webseitenbesuche pro Land. Andere: Peru, Kanada, Schweiz, Mexiko, Italien, Österreich, Niederlande und Argentinien, Frankreich, Russland, Australien

Diese geografische Verteilung zeigt die internationale Reichweite und Relevanz der Plattform. Bemerkenswert ist, dass die Mehrheit der Nutzer über Smartphones (63 %) auf die Website zugreift, was ihre Anpassungsfähigkeit an die modernen Präferenzen der mobilen Nutzer unterstreicht. Die Nutzerstatistik zeigt zudem, dass die Zahl der monatlichen Nutzer im Mai 2023 bei über 10.000 lag und sich seit dem Start im Jahr 2019 verfünffacht hat (Abb. 3).

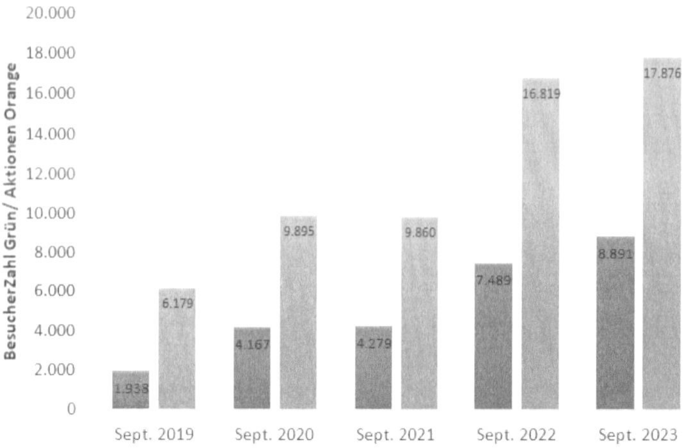

Abb. 3: Besuche und Aktionen seit Beginn 2019; Stand 09/2023

Diskussion und Schlussfolgerung

Die Mistelwebseite stellt in der dynamischen Publikationslandschaft eine unverzichtbare und solide Ressource dar, um einen aktuellen Überblick über die verschiedenen Facetten der Misteltherapie in der Onkologie zu geben. Sie richtet sich an ein vielfältiges interessiertes Publikum. Sie könnte in Zukunft als zuverlässige Quelle dienen, um die Dokumentation zur Evidenz der Misteltherapie zu konsolidieren und eine fundierte Entscheidungsfindung im Bereich der Onkologie zu fördern. Ihr integrativer Ansatz, die Aktualisierungen in Echtzeit, die patientenorientierten Funktionen, die weltweite Zugänglichkeit, die Akzeptanz durch die wachsende Zahl von Website-Nutzern und die evidenzbasierten Inhalte machen sie zu einem Eckpfeiler in der sich entwickelnden Landschaft der integrativen onkologischen Ansätze.

Interessenkonflikt

Die Autoren haben die folgenden Interessenkonflikte in Bezug auf die Forschung, die Autorenschaft und/oder Veröffentlichung dieses Artikels: FS berichtet über Zuschüsse von Astrazeneca (Reisekosten und Honorare für Vorträge), Helixor Heilmittel GmbH (Reisekosten und Honorare für Vorträge), Zuschüsse von der Abnoba GmbH und Zuschüsse von der Iscador AG, außerhalb der eingereichten Arbeit. Die anderen Autoren haben erklärt, dass keine konkurrierenden Interessen bestehen. Es wurden keine Zahlungen für andere Aspekte der eingereichten Arbeit erhalten. Es gibt keine Patente, Produkte in der Entwicklung oder vermarktete Produkte, die zu deklarieren sind. Es bestehen keine anderen Beziehungen/Bedingungen/Umstände, die einen potenziellen Interessenkonflikt darstellen.

Literatur

Greenlee H, Balneaves L G, Carlson L E, Cohen M, Deng G, Hershman D et al.: Clinical practice guidelines on the use of integrative therapies as supportive care in patients treated for breast cancer. J Natl Cancer Inst Monogr. 2014; 2014 (50): 346–358.

Horneber M A, Bueschel G, Huber R, Linde K and Rostock M: Mistletoe therapy in oncology. Cochrane Database Syst Rev. 2008 (2): CD003297.

Kienle G S and Kiene H: Review article: Influence of Viscum album L. (European mistletoe) extracts on quality of life in cancer patients: a systematic review of controlled clinical studies. Integr Cancer Ther. 2010; 9 (2): 142–157.

Kim K-C, Yook J-H, Eisenbraun J, Kim B-S and Huber R: Quality of life, immunomodulation and safety of adjuvant mistletoe treatment in patients with gastric carcinoma–a randomized, controlled pilot study. BMC Complement Altern Med. 2012; 12 (1): 172.

Kröz M, Büssing A, Reif M, Pranga D, Schad F, Zerm R et al.: Besteht eine Indikation für die Misteltherapie in der Behandlung von

Cancer-related Fatigue und Insomnie bei Krebspatienten? – Ein Review. In: Scheer R, Alban S, Becker H et al. (Eds.): Die Mistel in der Tumortherapie 4. Essen: KVC; 2016: 287–298.

Loef M, Paepke D, Walach H: Quality of Life in Breast Cancer Patients Treated with Mistletoe Extracts: A Systematic Review and Meta-Analysis. Integr Cancer Ther. 2023; 22: 15347354231198074. doi: 10.1177/15347354231198074.

Loef M and Walach H: Quality of life in cancer patients treated with mistletoe: a systematic review and meta-analysis. Complement Med Res. 2020; 20: 227. doi: 10.1186/s12906-020-03013-3.

Lyman G H, Greenlee H, Bohlke K, Bao T, DeMichele A M, Deng G E et al.: Integrative Therapies During and After Breast Cancer Treatment: ASCO Endorsement of the SIO Clinical Practice Guideline. J Clin Oncol. 2018; 36 (25): 2647–2655.

NCBI. National Center for Biotechnology Information (NCBI)[Internet]. Bethesda (MD): National Library of Medicine (US), National Center for Biotechnology Information; 1988. https://www.ncbi.nlm.nih.gov (accessed January 29, 2024).

Pelzer F, Loef M, Martin DD, Baumgartner S: Cancer-related fatigue in patients treated with mistletoe extracts: a systematic review and meta-analysis. Support Care Cancer. 2022; 30 (8): 6405–6418. doi: 10.1007/s00520-022-06921-x.

Piao B K, Wang Y X, Xie G R, Mannsmann U, Matthes H, Beuth J et al.: Impact of complementary mistletoe extract treatment on quality of life in breast, ovarian and non-small cell lung cancer patients. A prospective randomized controlled clinical trial. Anticancer Res. 2004; 24 (1): 303–310.

Thronicke A, Schad F, Debus M, Grabowski J, Soldner G: Viscum album L. Therapy in Oncology: An Update on Current Evidence. Complement Med Res. 2022; 29 (4): 362–368. doi: 10.1159/000524184.

Tröger W, Zdrale Z, Tišma N, Matijasevic M: Additional Therapy with a Mistletoe Product during Adjuvant Chemotherapy of Breast Cancer Patients Improves Quality of Life: An Open Randomized Clinical Pilot Trial. Evid Based Complement Altern Med. 2014; 2014:430518. doi: 10.1155/2014/430518.

Tröger W, Galun D, Reif M, Schumann A, Stankovic N and Milicevic M: Quality of life of patients with advanced pancreatic cancer during treatment with mistletoe: a randomized controlled trial. Dtsch Arztebl Int. 2014; 111 (29–30): 493–502. doi: 10.3238/arztebl.2014.0493.

Tröger W, Jezdic S, Zdrale Z, Tisma N, Hamre H J and Matijasevic M: Quality of life and neutropenia in patients with early stage breast cancer: a randomized pilot study comparing additional treatment with mistletoe extract to chemotherapy alone. Breast Cancer. 2009; 16 (3): 35–45.

PD Dr. Friedemann Schad[1, 2], Anja Thronicke[2], Dr. Marion Debus[3], Maike Kergel[4], Yván Villegas[4], Georg Soldner[5]

[1] Interdisziplinäre Onkologie und Palliativmedizin, Gemeinschaftskrankenhaus Havelhöhe Berlin, Deutschland

[2] Forschungsinstitut Havelhöhe Berlin, Deutschland

[3] Klinik Arlesheim AG, Medical Section at the Goetheanum, School of Spiritual Science, Dornach, Switzerland

[4] Centro Médico Antroposófico & Instituto de Investigación y Docencia Mistel, Lima, Peru

[5] Akademie Anthroposophische Medizin GAÄD, München, Deutschland

Korrespondierender Autor:
fschad@havelhoehe.de

Individualisierte Behandlung mit Mistelpräparaten bei onkologischen Erkrankungen – Weiterentwicklung des Vademecums

Individualized Treatment With Mistletoe Preparations in Oncology – Further Development of the Vademecum

Andreas Arendt, Marion Debus, Johannes Gutsch, Lydia Garnitschnig, Markus Karutz, Angela Kuck, Mathias Sauer, Reinhard Schwarz, Georg Soldner, Markus Sommer

Zusammenfassung

2017 erschien innerhalb der 4. Auflage des Vademecums Anthroposophische Arzneimittel die erste Auflage des Vademecums zur Misteltherapie, das 82 tumorbezogene Erfahrungsberichte (allgemeine Darstellungen und/oder Fallvignetten) von 36 Misteltherapie-erfahrenen Ärzten umfasst.

Die zweite Auflage 2024 innerhalb der 5. Auflage des Vademecums Anthroposophische Arzneimittel erweitert dieses Spektrum erheblich: Neben ca. 15 neu eingesendeten Fallvignetten werden 28 in englischer Sprache veröffentlichter, peer-reviewed Einzelfallberichte, 28 Fallvignetten aus dem *Merkurstab* sowie einzelne Kasuistiken aus Tagungsbänden und Lehrbüchern neu aufgenommen. Insgesamt finden sich in der Neuauflage nun 130 Einzelfallberichte und 32 allgemein gehaltene Einzelberichte zu Therapiekonzepten für 76 onkologische Indikationen von 57 Autoren aus 14 Ländern. Die einzelnen Indikationen werden nach Tumorentitäten geordnet und diesen neu ein einleitender Text unter Berücksichtigung allgemeiner Aspekte zur jeweiligen Tumorart und ihrer Behandlung sowie der aktuellen Studienlage vorangestellt.

Diese Erweiterungen sollen dazu beitragen, dem praktisch tätigen Arzt eine möglichst eigenständige und individuelle Therapiegestaltung bei rascher Orientierung zu ermöglichen und ihn zu befähigen und weiterführende Hypothesen für die klinische Forschung zu generieren.

Schlüsselwörter: Vademecum, Einzelfallberichte, Weiterentwicklung der Misteltherapie, Hypothesengenerierung

Summary

In 2017, the first edition of the Vademecum Mistletoe Therapy was published within the 4th edition of the Vademecum of Anthroposophic Medicines, which includes 82 tumor-related clinical experience reports (general presentations and/or case reports) by 36 physicians experienced in mistletoe therapy. The second edition in 2024 within the 5th edition of the Vademecum of Anthroposophic Medicines expands this spectrum considerably: In addition to approx. 15 newly submitted case reports, 28 peer-reviewed individual case reports published in English, 28 case vignettes from the *Merkurstab* as well as individual case reports from conference proceedings and textbooks will be newly included. In total, the new edition now contains 130 individual case reports and 32 general individual reports on therapy concepts for 76 oncologic indications by 57 authors from 14 countries. The individual indications are sorted according to tumor entities and are now preceded by an introductory text taking into account general aspects of the respective tumor type and its treatment as well as the current scientific background regarding clinical trials. These extensions are intended to help practitioners choose therapies as independently and diversely as possible, to enable individual therapy design and to generate further hypotheses for clinical research.
Keywords: Vademecum, individual case reports, further development of mistletoe therapy, hypothesis generation

Einleitung

Über das Konzept des Vademecums Misteltherapie wurde auf dem Nonnweiler-Symposium 2015 berichtet (Ahrendt *et al.* 2016). 2017 erschien die erste Auflage als Band 2 der 4. Auflage des Vademecum Anthroposophische Arzneimittel (2017). Dieser umfasst systematisch erfasste Berichte von 36 Misteltherapie-erfahrenen Ärzten sowie die umfangreichen Ergebnisse von 35 strukturierten Interviews mit Misteltherapie-Experten zu verschiedenen Aspekten der Misteltherapie (Präparate- und Wirtsbaumwahl, Dosierung und Sicherheit). Insgesamt fanden 82 tumorbezogene Erfahrungsberichte zu verschiedenen Tumorarten Eingang in das Vademecum, die teils als allgemeiner Bericht, teils als Fallvignette, teils als allgemeiner Bericht mit integrierter Fallvignette erschienen. Außerdem fanden 9 nicht auf eine bestimmte Tumorart bezogene Berichte Eingang in das Vademecum.

Nach Erscheinen der 4. Auflage zeigte es sich, dass das Grundlagenkapitel gut genutzt und als hilfreich empfunden wurde, der Einsendungsteil mit den Erfahrungsberichten jedoch kaum einen Erkenntnisgewinn brachte. Dies hatte im Wesentlichen folgende Gründe:

- Die Indikationen wurden so, wie vom einsendenden Autor angegeben, unkommentiert in alphabetischer Reihenfolge angeführt (z. B. Astrozytom unter A, Glioblastom unter G), d. h., zusammengehörige Tumorentitäten (Gehirntumoren) erschienen nicht im Zusammenhang.
- Weitgehend unkommentiert standen z. T. ganz unterschiedliche Behandlungsansätze verschiedener Autoren bei derselben Tumorentität nebeneinander.
- Es fehlten übergeordnete, zusammenfassende Gesichtspunkte zu den einzelnen Tumorentitäten.
- Einzelfälle erweisen sich interessanter und lehrreicher als generelle Erfahrungsberichte (z. B. 100 Mammakarzinome immer mit einem bestimmten Mistelregime behandelt), die über den Therapieerfolg keine direkten Rückschlüsse zulassen.

Die zweite Auflage 2024 (5. Auflage des Vademecums) hat daher das Ziel, möglichst viele lehrreiche Einzelfallberichte für die verschiedenen Indikationen zu sammeln und diese nach übergeordneten Tumorentitäten zu ordnen. Einführende Texte und redaktionelle Kommentare sollen das Krankheits- und Therapieverständnis erhöhen und zu selbständigen und differenzierten Therapieentscheidungen befähigen.

Material und Methoden

Es werden – neben den neuen Einsendungen – eine möglichst große Anzahl meist seit dem Jahr 2000 in verschiedenen Publikationsorganen veröffentlichter Einzelfallberichte neu aufgenommen (in verschiedenen peer reviewten Fachzeitschriften, dem Merkurstab, Lehrbüchern, Tagungsbänden der Nonnweiler-Symposien). Die Fallberichte werden, wo nötig, aus dem Englischen übersetzt und jeweils so zusammengefasst, dass die Misteltherapie exakt nachvollzogen werden kann. Zahlreiche dieser Fallberichte werden zur besseren Verständlichkeit redaktionell kommentiert. 7 allgemeine Erfahrungsberichte aus der Auflage von 2017 wurden aufgrund von Redundanz nicht wieder aufgenommen und 4 nicht auf eine spezifische Tumorentität bezogene Erfahrungsberichte zur Misteltherapie im Terminalstadium hinsichtlich ihrer Kernaussagen ins Grundlagenkapitel integriert.

Die vorhandenen Erfahrungsberichte werden nach Diagnosegruppen und Indikationen geordnet, die alphabetische Anordnung wird verlassen (z. B. werden Astrozytom und Glioblastom unter der gemeinsamen Überschrift „Gehirntumoren/Gliome“ aufgeführt).

Den nach Diagnose- bzw. Indikationsgruppen geordneten Einzelfallberichten wird jeweils ein Einführungstext vorangestellt, der meist folgende Punkte in unterschiedlicher Ausführlichkeit enthält: 1) Ein knapp gefasstes Wesensbild der jeweiligen Tumorerkrankung. 2) Besonderheiten der Misteltherapie bei der entsprechenden Tumorentität (allgemeine erfahrungsbasierte Gesichtspunkte, Einordnung der in den Fallvignetten und allgemeinen Erfahrungsberichten dargestellten Vorgehensweise mit der Misteltherapie). 3) Falls sinnvoll, Bezug zu konventionellen Behandlungsverfahren bzw. Einordnung des Stellenwertes der Misteltherapie vor dem Hintergrund derselben. 4) Aktuelle wissenschaftliche Datenlage, sofern vorhanden, und, falls erforderlich, Diskussion derselben (z. B. Kapitel Melanom). 5) Ggf. Darstellung der anthroposophischen Begleittherapie.

Ergebnisse

Neben 15 neu eingesendeten Fallvignetten werden 28 in englischer Sprache veröffentlichter, peer-reviewed Einzelfallberichte sowie 28 Fallvignetten aus dem Merkurstab neu aufgenommen. Außerdem werden 4 Kasuistiken aus den Tagungsbänden der Nonnweiler-Symposien sowie 2 Kasuistiken aus einem HNO-Lehrbuch (Meister *et al.* 2021) integriert. Es werden somit 75-80 Einzelfallberichte neu aufgenommen. Insgesamt finden sich nun 130 Einzelfallberichte und 32 allgemein gehaltene Einzelberichte zu Therapiekonzepten für 76 onkologische Indikationen in der Neuauflage des Vademecums.

Die Fallberichte stammen von 57 Autoren aus 14 Ländern (Deutschland, Schweiz, Österreich, Frankreich, Tschechien, Italien, Schweden, Großbritannien, Georgien, Brasilien, Peru, Kanada, USA, Korea). Unter den Einsendern finden sich Fachärzte für: Hämatologie/Onkologie (6), Allgemeinmedizin mit Universitätsdiplom Onkologie (2), Innere Medizin (14), Gastroenterologie (2), Gynäkologie (5), Neurologie (2), Urologie (1), HNO (1), Mund-Kiefer-Gesichtschirurgie (1), Kinder- und Jugendmedizin (2), bei den übrigen handelt es sich um Allgemeinmediziner oder praktische Ärzte, in einem Fall ist die Facharztbezeichnung nicht bekannt.

In den insgesamt 24 Einführungstexten zu den verschiedenen Tumorentitäten wird neben dem erwähnten Wesensbild der Erkrankung und Gesichtspunkten zur anthroposophischen Therapie (z. B. bewährte Wirtsbäume oder Begleittherapie) Wert auf die vorhandene aktuelle Studienlage gelegt und anhand dieser auch umstrittene Themen der Misteltherapie diskutiert (z. B. Misteltherapie bei Melanomen, Misteltherapie und die Gefahr eines Hirnödems, Misteltherapie in Kombination mit Checkpoint-Inhibitoren etc.). Mistelapplikationsweisen, die in den Fallberichten nicht zur Sprache kommen (z. B. intraläsionale Misteltherapie oder Stellenwert der Hyperthermie beim Pankreaskarzinom) werden dort ergänzend beschrieben. Aber auch Anregungen für mögliche Zukunftsentwicklungen bzw. Hypothesenbildungen für potenzielle Studien, die sich aus den vorhandenen Erfahrungen bzw. der vorhandenen Datenlage ergeben, werden benannt (z. B. mögliche Senkung des Rezidiv- bzw. Progressionsrisikos durch Kombination einer fieberinduzierenden Misteltherapie mit Tyrosinkinaseinhibitoren beim malignen Melanom oder einer BCG-Behandlung beim Blasenkarzinom).

Ein Ergebnis, das aus den zahlreichen Fallberichten gewonnen werden kann, ist, dass bei ein und derselben Tumorentität bei richtiger Indikationsstellung sowohl eine hochdosierte fieberinduzierende wie auch eine niedrig dosierte, langsam gesteigerte Misteltherapie zu Therapieerfolgen führen kann. Für zukünftige Forschungen handelt es sich also weniger um die Frage, welche Vorgehensweise die bessere ist, sondern in welchen Fällen die eine oder andere Vorgehensweise indiziert ist.

Ausblick

Die Zusammenstellung von 130 redaktionell bearbeiteten und nach Tumorentitäten geordneten Einzelfallberichten (davon 22 % peer-reviewed publiziert) sowie deren Einordnung durch tumorbezogene Einführungstexte vor dem Hintergrund der aktuellen Studienlage erfolgt in dieser Weise erstmalig. Für den onkologisch tätigen Arzt aller Fachrichtungen soll die Fülle der Kasuistiken, die durch Kommentierungen entweder im Einführungstext oder direkt im Anschluss an den Fallbericht leichter zugänglich gemacht werden, die Vielfalt an Therapiemöglichkeiten ebenso wie typische Vorgehensweisen unkompliziert und zeitsparend erschließen. Es ist zu hoffen, dass sich dadurch das therapeutische Spektrum der Behandler erweitert und die Freude am Beschreiten neuer Wege angeregt wird, mit Steigerung der „Intuitionsfähigkeit" für den passenden therapeutischen Ansatz im Einzelfall. Ein weiteres Ziel ist es, dass auch der Neuling in der Misteltherapie sich rasch einen Überblick über den jeweils vorliegenden Erfahrungshintergrund sowie die aktuelle Studienlage verschaffen kann, um so ein kompetenter Gesprächspartner für Patienten und Kollegen sein zu können. Und nicht zuletzt soll durch diesen Überblick für klinische Forscher die Hypothesengenerierung und Identifikation relevanter Fragestellungen für zukünftige Studien unterstützt werden.

Die 5. Auflage (Erscheinungsdatum: September 2024) wird erstmals 1:1 kostenpflichtig auf der Website www.vademecum.org publiziert, die eine optimierte Darstellung und Navigation auf unterschiedlichen Bildschirmgrößen ermöglicht. Die Nutzung auf dem Smartphone z. B. im Rahmen eines Hausbesuchs oder unterwegs ist ebenso möglich wie das Arbeiten am großen Bildschirm.

Damit verbunden wurde die Erweiterung der Website durch eine progressive WebApp, die es ermöglicht, die Website als Icon auf dem

Homescreen des Smartphones oder Tablets zu installieren und wie eine native App aufzurufen. Gelesene Inhalte und Indikationen können lokal gespeichert und damit auch offline gelesen werden.

Die Darstellung als – jeweils zitierfähige – Website ermöglicht in den kommenden Jahren eine raschere, z. B. jährliche Anpassung und Weiterentwicklung des Vademecums in Form webbasierter Neuauflagen und damit eine größere Aktualität. Die fortlaufende Aktualisierung in jährlichen Neuauflagen soll eine kontinuierliche *Weiterentwicklung der Misteltherapie* befördern. Auch die *Therapiesicherheit*, die in den Einsendungsbögen systematisch erfragt wird, wird dadurch kontinuierlich beobachtet und dokumentiert.

Das Vademecum könnte auch ein wichtiges Instrument für die *gesundheitspolitische Verankerung* der Misteltherapie (*Hersteller-unabhängige Instanz,* z. B. bei Erstattungsfragen) sein.

Literatur

Arendt A, Debus M, Gutsch J, Karutz M, Kienle GS, Kuck A, Sauer M, Schwarz R, Soldner G, Sommer M, Volkmann PR: Individualisierte Behandlung mit Mistelpräparaten bei onkologischen Erkrankungen – Konzept und Aufbau des Vademecums. In: Scheer R, Alban S, Becker H, et al. (Hrsg.): Die Mistel in der Tumortherapie 4. Essen: KVC; 2016: 389–400.

GAÄD (Hrsg.): Vademecum Anthroposophische Arzneimittel, 4. Auflage 2017. Supplement.

Meister D, Oelmüller B, Zühlke H: HNO-Heilkunde. Integrative Konzepte und Grundlagen der Anthroposophischen Medizin. Berlin: Salumed; 2021.

Dr. Andreas Arendt[1], Dr. Marion Debus[2], Dr. Johannes Gutsch[3], Dr. med. univ. Lydia Garnitschnig[4], Dr. Markus Karutz[5], Dr. Angela Kuck[6], Dr. Mathias Sauer[7], Dr. Reinhard Schwarz[8], Georg Soldner[9], Markus Sommer[9]

[1] Praxis für Allgemeinmedizin, Liestal, Schweiz
[2] Abteilung für Onkologie, Klinik Arlesheim, Schweiz
[3] ehem. Onkologie, Gevelsberg, Deutschland
[4] Psychosoziale Dienste Wien, Kinder- und Jugendpsychiatrisches Ambulatorium mit Tagesklinik, Wien, Österreich
[5] ehem. Gemeinschaftspraxis Tobiashaus, Köln, Deutschland
[6] Paracelsus Zentrum am Grossmünster, Zürich, Schweiz
[7] Paracelsus Krankenhaus Unterlengenhardt, Bad Liebenzell, Deutschland
[8] Kinder- und Jugendarztpraxis, Graz, Österreich
[9] Praxisgemeinschaft, München, Deutschland

Korrespondenzadresse:
marion.debus@klinik-arlesheim.ch

European-US Collaboration to Put Iscador in the Pediatric Oncology Pipeline: Lessons Learned

Europäisch-amerikanische Zusammenarbeit zur Einführung von Iscador in die pädiatrische Onkologie: Ein Erfahrungsbericht

Katharine Offer, Marcus Reif, Karen Moody

Summary

European scientists and clinicians in the US from two pediatric oncology programs have designed a clinical trial to study subcutaneous Iscador® P for improving the event-free survival of pediatric patients with relapsed osteosarcoma after complete resection of pulmonary metastases (NCT05726383). Several important lessons have been learned during its preparation:

1. The success of introducing a naturally-derived agent into the US pediatric oncology pipeline depends on the strength of published preclinical and clinical data. For Iscador P, this allowed us to forgo a phase 1 and move directly to a phase 2 study.
2. The manufacturing process of these plant-derived therapeutics needs to be very clearly described, i.e. strict GMP and QA/QC procedures must be upheld in order to gain both regulatory and institutional approval.
3. Navigating multiple IRBs and contract offices at separate institutions, each with different processes can be challenging and requires extensive communication and cooperation among all sites.
4. Production and delivery of the medication from Iscador AG to the study centers require careful planning and preparation. Involving a logistics company familiar with intercontinental transportation is strongly recommended.
5. Liability insurance requirements for the different responsibilities in clinical trials differ between European countries and the US, and insurance companies are not able or willing to tailor their insurance policies to the specific needs of each party.

Keywords: Mistletoe, Iscador P, osteosarcoma, event-free survival, clinical trial

Zusammenfassung
Europäische Wissenschaftler und Kliniker in den USA aus zwei pädiatrischen Onkologieprogrammen haben eine klinische Studie zur Verbesserung des ereignisfreien Überlebens von pädiatrischen Patienten mit rezidiviertem Osteosarkom nach vollständiger Resektion von Lungenmetastasen mit subkutanem Iscador® P konzipiert (NCT05726383). Während der Vorbereitung dieser Studie wurden mehrere wichtige Lehren gezogen:

1. Der Erfolg der Einführung eines natürlich gewonnenen Wirkstoffs in die pädiatrische Onkologie-Pipeline in den USA hängt von der Stärke der veröffentlichten präklinischen und klinischen Daten ab. Bei Iscador P konnten wir daher auf eine Phase-1-Studie verzichten und direkt zu einer Phase-2-Studie übergehen.
2. Der Herstellungsprozess dieser pflanzlichen Therapeutika muss sehr genau beschrieben werden, d. h. es müssen strenge GMP- und QA/QC-Verfahren eingehalten werden, um sowohl die behördliche als auch die institutionelle Zulassung zu erhalten.
3. Der Umgang mit mehreren IRBs und Vertragsbüros in verschiedenen Einrichtungen, die jeweils unterschiedliche Verfahren anwenden, kann eine Herausforderung darstellen und erfordert eine umfassende Kommunikation und Zusammenarbeit zwischen allen Standorten.
4. Die Herstellung und Lieferung der Medikamente von der Iscador AG an die Studienzentren erfordert eine sorgfältige Planung und Vorbereitung. Die Einbindung eines Logistikunternehmens, das mit interkontinentalen Transporten vertraut ist, wird dringend empfohlen.
5. Die Anforderungen an die Haftpflichtversicherung für die verschiedenen Verantwortlichkeiten bei klinischen Prüfungen unterscheiden sich zwischen den europäischen Ländern und den USA, und die Versicherungsunternehmen sind nicht in der Lage oder willens, ihre Versicherungspolicen auf die spezifischen Bedürfnisse der einzelnen Parteien zuzuschneiden.

Schlüsselwörter: Mistel, Iscador P, Osteosarkom, ereignisfreies Überleben, klinische Studie

Introduction

Many cancers affecting children are rare and often lack standard treatment guidelines for relapse/recurrence. Pediatric oncology urgently needs novel, in particular safe, therapies. Although treatment with a *Viscum album* extract is a well-established complementary cancer therapy in many European countries, in the United States (US), most oncologists are still unaware of its use. *Viscum album* can be obtained in the US through integrative medicine centers, yet it does not hold any FDA approvals in the United States (PDQ® 2023). Therefore, it is not regulated and is only used in integrative medicine for immune support but not generally in conventional medical practice. This actually creates a barrier to using it within oncology settings.

In addition, despite its widespread use in Europe, there have been ongoing heated debates about the scientific validity of the clinical trials with mistletoe and the evidence for a survival benefit though promising is not conclusive (Ostermann *et al.* 2020; Freuding *et al.* 2019a; 2019b; Matthes *et al.* 2020; Loef, Walach 2020; 2022).

Currently, there has only been one clinical trial in the US using *Viscum album* (NCT03051477) but none in children. In an effort to broaden access to this promising cancer therapy for pediatric patients, European scientists and clinicians in the US from two pediatric oncology programs have designed a clinical trial to study subcutaneous Iscador P (*Viscum album* Pini, 0.01-20 mg) for improving the event-free survival of pediatric patients with relapsed osteosarcoma after complete resection of pulmonary metastases (NCT05726383).

At the time of the conference, this trial was near to actively enrolling. During this development, we have learned several important lessons, and by sharing these we may make the goal of opening clinical trials of such therapies in the US more attainable.

Material and methods

The planning and preparation of this trial has been a collaborative effort between the medical and administrative departments of the clinical trial centers and the manufacturing, medical affairs, clinical research and regulatory affairs departments of the company Iscador AG under the leadership of the medical researchers from Hackensack Meridian Health and M.D. Anderson Children's Cancer Hospital.

Results

Talks between the principal investigators and Iscador AG began in December 2018. Since then, we have learned several lessons:

1. The success of introducing a naturally-derived agent into the US pediatric oncology pipeline depends on the strength of published preclinical and clinical data, to which we fortunately had access for mistletoe extracts in general and Iscador® P in particular. Due to the comprehensive safety data available from the literature, a phase 1 study in children and young adults was not felt to be necessary and the present study is a phase 2 study using the upfront dose-finding regimen and MTD of Longhi *et al.* (2014).
2. The manufacturing process of these plant-derived therapeutics needs to be very clearly described in order to gain both regulatory and institutional approval. The strict GMP and QA/QC procedures used in Iscador® P manufacturing were beneficial in obtaining approval of an FDA Investigational New Drug application as well as approval through the pharmacy departments of Hackensack University Medical Center (HUMC) and MD Anderson Cancer Center (MDACC). The FDA accepted a European Investigational Medicinal Product Dossier (IMPD) in place of a Drug Master File.
3. As with any collaboration, one challenge in opening this study was navigating multiple Institutional Review Boards (IRBs) and contract offices whose regulations can vary by state. This process requires comprehensive and timely communication and cooperation among all sites yet was not found to be complicated by the international nature of the collaboration.
4. Production and delivery of the medication from Iscador AG to the study centers requires careful planning and preparation. Once a projected start date of the study was identified, an order was placed for Iscador® P, allowing 4-6 months for manufacture and QA/QC. A logistics company familiar with intercontinental shipments organized the transport of batches from Switzerland to each of the two study centers. Clearance through US Customs required a USDA statement as well as an FDA End Use Letter from each study site.

Investigational pharmacies followed protocols for transport compliance reporting.

5. Liability insurance requirements for the different responsibilities in clinical trials differ between European countries and the US, and insurance companies are not able or willing to tailor their insurance policies to the specific needs of industrial providers that do not assume the role of legal trial sponsor. Therefore, openness on both sides – clinical trial sites and industry provider – in the allocation of responsibilities and a willingness to compromise are necessary to find common ground for their collaboration.

Conclusion and future directions

The preparation of this clinical trial of Iscador® P for pediatric osteosarcoma patients was based on an international cooperation and required a professional attitude of all partners in terms of documentation, communication, and cooperation between each other and third parties. Strong clinical evidence for safety and good manufacturing processes facilitated approval by appropriate federal and institutional agencies. Applications for additional grant funding to support this collaboration are ongoing.

Conflict of interests

Marcus Reif is an employee of the company Iscador AG, Lörrach, Germany. Katharine Offer and Karen Moody declare no conflict of interests.

Literature

Freuding M, Keinki C, Micke O et al.: Mistletoe in oncological treatment: a systematic review. J Cancer Res Clin Oncol. 2019a; 145: 695–707. doi: 10.1007

Freuding M, Keinki C, Kutschan S et al.: Mistletoe in oncological treatment: a systematic review. J Cancer Res Clin Oncol. 2019b; 145: 927–939. doi: 10.1007

Loef M, Walach H: Quality of life in cancer patients treated with mistletoe: a systematic review and meta-analysis. BMC Complement Med Ther. 2020; 20: 227. doi: 10.1186/s12906-020-03013-3.

Loef M, Walach H: Survival of cancer patients treated with non-fermented mistletoe extract: A systematic review and meta-analysis. Integr Cancer Ther. 2022; 21: 15347354221133561. doi: 10.1177/15347354221133561.

Longhi A, Reif M, Marini E, Ferrari S: A Randomized study on postrelapse disease-free survival with adjuvant mistletoe versus oral etoposide in osteosarcoma patients. Evid Based Complement Alternat Med. 2014: 210198. doi: 10.1155/2014/210198.

Matthes H, Thronicke A, Hofheinz RD et al.: Statement to an Insufficient Systematic Review on Viscum album L. Therapy. Evid Based Complement Alternat Med. 2020: 7091039. doi: 10.1155/2020/7091039.

Ostermann T, Appelbaum S, Poier D et al.: A systematic review and meta-analysis on the survival of cancer patients treated with a fermented Viscum album L. extract (Iscador): An update of findings. Complement Med Res. 2020; 27: 260–271. doi: 10.1159/000505202.

PDQ® Integrative, Alternative, and Complementary Therapies Editorial Board. PDQ Mistletoe Extracts. Bethesda, MD: National Cancer Institute. Updated 06/08/2023. https://www.cancer.gov/about-cancer/treatment/cam/hp/mistletoe-pdq (accessed Feb 23, 2024).

Dr. Katharine Offer[1], Dr. rer. nat. Marcus Reif[2], Dr. Karen Moody[3]

[1] Joseph M. Sanzari Children's Hospital, Hackensack Meridian Health (HUMC), Hackensack, NJ, USA

[2] Iscador AG, Berlin, Germany

[3] M.D. Anderson Children's Cancer Hospital (MDACC), Houston, TX, USA

Corresponding author:
marcus.reif@iscador.de

III. Klinische Anwendung

b) Übersichtsreferate und Reviews klinischer Studien

III. Clinical Application

b) Survey Articles and Reviews of Clinical Studies

Krankheit als Impuls des Lebens

Illness as an Impetus of Life

Annette Bopp

Zusammenfassung
Dürfen wir heute noch krank sein? In einer Zeit, in der man gegen alles und jedes geimpft werden kann und ständig neue Medikamente entwickelt werden? Wie schauen wir heute auf das Kranksein? Was verstehen wir unter Gesundheit? Gedanken über Grundfragen, vor die uns jede Krankheit stellt, und die Implikationen, die eine Misteltherapie in diesem Zusammenhang mit sich bringt.
Schlüsselwörter: Krankheit, Gesundheit, Misteltherapie

Summary
May we still be ill today? At a time when we can be immunised against anything and everything and new drugs are constantly being developed? How do we look at being ill today? What do we mean by health? Thoughts on basic questions that every illness confronts us with and the implications that mistletoe therapy has in this context.
Keywords: Illness, health, mistletoe therapy

Einleitung

Dürfen wir heute noch krank sein? In einer Zeit, in der zunehmend raffiniertere Medikamente und Impfstoffe entwickelt werden bis hin zu Gentherapien? In der das Idealbild der gesunde, leistungsfähige, rundum belastbare Mensch ist, der mit jeder Schwierigkeit fertig wird und alles im Griff hat? In der alles kontrollierbar sein soll, von der Geburt bis zum Tod, und in der jede Krankheit als lästiger Störfall gilt, den es unverzüglich zu beseitigen gilt?

Anders gefragt: Welcher Kranke wird heute noch so gepflegt, dass er sich wirklich auskurieren kann und nicht mit medikamentös gesenktem Fieber nur halb genesen wieder zur Arbeit geht?

Wie schauen wir heute ganz generell auf das Kranksein? Was verstehen wir unter Gesundheit? Und welche Implikationen bringt eine Misteltherapie in diesem Zusammenhang mit sich? Mit diesen Fragen beschäftigt sich dieser Vortrag.

Krankheit einfach abschaffen?

Im Zeitalter der allgegenwärtigen Kontrollierbarkeit des menschlichen Lebens gelten Krankheiten heute als Niederlage, als Versagen der technischen und medikamentösen Möglichkeiten der modernen Medizin. Krankheiten sind deshalb nicht nur zu vermeiden, sie sollen am besten gleich ganz abgeschafft werden. Insbesondere weitverbreitete Krankheiten wie Herzinfarkt und Schlaganfall, die zu den häufigsten Todesursachen zählen, zumindest in Europa. Dass das kein Hirngespinst ist, zeigt ein Artikel von Uwe Bahnsen in *Die Zeit* vom 6. Juli 2023. Unter der Überschrift „Der Herzinfarkt wird abgeschafft" prangte er als großer, signalrot unterlegter Aufmacher auf der Titelseite der Wochenzeitung. Unterzeilen: „Mit bahnbrechenden Methoden wollen Forscher tödliche Herzleiden und Schlaganfälle aus der Welt schaffen. Die Medizin steht vor einer Zeitenwende." Was ist damit gemeint?

Gemeint sind gentechnische Eingriffe und Medikamente auf der Basis der mRNA-Technik. Man schaltet bestimmte Gene einfach ab, in diesem Fall das Gen zur Aufnahme von Cholesterin in der Leber (erhöhte Cholesterinwerte gelten als Risikofaktor für Herz-Kreislauf-Erkrankungen). Konkret heißt es im Text:

> „Mit einem ‚Base-Editor', einer weiterentwickelten Genschere, lässt sich das PCSK9-Gen in der Leber abschalten. In Tierversuchen ließ sich damit der Cholesterinwert um zwei Drittel senken. Jetzt wird die Gentherapie an Patienten in Neuseeland und Großbritannien erforscht. Soweit man es jetzt schon beurteilen kann, mit Erfolg."

Etwas Ähnliches soll sich auch medikamentös im Hinblick auf Lipoprotein(a) erreichen lassen, das ebenso als Risikofaktor gilt:

> „Eine Lösung könnte abermals die Einmal-Strategie von Verve Therapeutics sein: Das Unternehmen hat gerade eine 60 Millionen US-Dollar schwere Allianz mit dem Pharmariesen Eli Lilly geschlossen. Gemeinsam will man per Gentherapie das entscheidende Gen für Lipoprotein(a) einfach komplett in der Leber abschalten."

In dem ganzen Artikel findet sich kein einziges kritisches Wort zu diesem angeblichen Fortschritt. Kein Wort zu den möglichen Langzeitfolgen eines solchen unumkehrbaren Eingriffs. Kein Wort dazu, dass der menschliche Organismus sowohl Cholesterin wie auch Lipoprotein(a) ja nicht grundlos produziert – beides wird für vielerlei Stoffwechselvorgänge benötigt. Kein Wort zu den möglichen kurz- und langfristigen Folgen solcher Eingriffe. Der Autor, ein durchaus renommierter Wissenschaftsjournalist, ist nichtsdestotrotz vollauf begeistert über diese „Zeitenwende", Herz-Kreislauf-Erkrankungen angeblich einfach abschaffen zu können. Was für eine Hybris!

Künstliche Intelligenz – noch eine Zeitenwende

Als veritable Zeitenwende erscheint auch der zunehmende Einsatz von Künstlicher Intelligenz (KI) in der Medizin. Diagnose-Apps auf der Basis von KI sind schon seit Jahren gang und gäbe, ebenso Roboter in der Chirurgie sowie in der Pflege, dort nicht zuletzt aus Mangel an menschlichen Ressourcen. KI soll jetzt vor allem zur Entlastung der Ärzte eingesetzt werden, natürlich im Interesse der Kranken, wie wiederum ein Statement in der *Zeit* vom 6. September 2023 zeigt. Darin äußern sich unter der Überschrift „KI-Systeme sollten Ärzte entlasten!" Aljoscha Burchardt vom Deutschen Forschungszentrum für Künstliche Intelligenz (DFKI) in Berlin, ein Experte für Sprachtechnologie (NLP), und Anne Herrmann-Johns, Professorin für Medizinische Soziologie an der Universität Regensburg, Leiterin des Forschungsverbunds PRIMA-AI, wie folgt:

> „Angesichts des Ärztemangels und auch da Ärzte ja geschworen haben, ihre Behandlungen auf dem aktuellen Stand der Forschung basieren zu lassen, plädieren wir dafür, KI-Systeme zur Entlastung der

> Ärzte und zur Erweiterung ihrer Möglichkeiten zu entwickeln. (...) Zum Wohle der Patientinnen und Patienten."

Damit aber nicht genug. Ganz ungeahnte Dimensionen eröffnet die KI für die Zukunft, wie ein Gespräch der *Süddeutschen Zeitung* mit dem Informatiker Jürgen Schmidhuber nahelegt, seines Zeichens Leiter der KI-Initiative an der saudischen KAUST-Universität (SZ vom 5./6. August 2023):

> „KIs werden mehr und größere und bessere KIs bauen wollen, dazu braucht man Masse und Energie. Fast alles davon ist aber weit weg von unserer Biosphäre. Also werden KIs auswandern. Zunächst auf den Merkur, der sehr sexy ist, weil er noch mehr schwere Metalle hat als die Erde, mit der Sonne als riesiger Energiequelle in nächster Nähe. Da der Merkur keine Atmosphäre hat, kann man Material viel billiger als mit Raketen durch elektromagnetische Kanonen in den Weltraum schießen, um dort alle mögliche Infrastruktur zu schaffen. Das ist aber erst der Anfang. Der Rest der Milchstraße bietet noch viel mehr ungenutzte Gelegenheiten als unser winziges Sonnensystem. Das wird ein paar hunderttausend Jahre dauern, aber dann wird fast alle KI sehr weit von der Erde weg sein."

Schöne Aussichten ... Denn das ist durchaus kein Science-Fiction-Roman. Herr Schmidhuber meint das ganz ernst. Schließlich ist die KI schon seit Jahrzehnten Gegenstand intensivster Forschung und regt die Hybris der Wissenschaftler offenbar zu immer absurderen Höhenflügen an. Schon 2007 sagte z. B. Tom Knight, Professor für Künstliche Intelligenz am MIT (Massachussetts Institute of Technology) und spezialisiert auf die Entwicklung neuer Mikroben, im Magazin *Newsweek* vom 3. Juni 2007 den bemerkenswerten Satz: „Der genetische Code ist 3,6 Milliarden Jahre alt. Es wird Zeit, ihn neu zu schreiben."

Craig Venter, der als erster das menschliche Genom sequenzierte, verstieg sich im *New Scientist* am 11. März 2009 zu der Aussage: „Es wird Zeit, die Evolution durch etwas Besseres zu ersetzen, und zwar durch eine zweite Genesis."

Und so wird wahr, wie wir auch schon in den Corona-Jahren erleben mussten, was der Schriftsteller Aldous Huxley schon vor Jahrzehnten in seinem Buch *Schöne neue Welt* prophezeite: „Die Menschen werden ihre Unterdrückung lieben und die Technologien verehren lernen, die ihre Denkfähigkeit vernichten."

Was die KI betrifft, so tun sich in der Medizin vor allem in der Diagnostik ungeahnte Möglichkeiten auf. Diabetes zum Beispiel – und dabei wird es nicht bleiben – soll man künftig an der Stimme erkennen. So berichtet Harro Albrecht am 26. Oktober 2023 in der *Zeit*:

> „Forscherinnen und Forscher können mit ihr (der KI, Anm. d. Aut.) verräterische Stimmmuster entdecken, die unter Umständen eine Reihe von körperlichen Erkrankungen anzeigen. Alzheimer etwa, die Parkinsonkrankheit oder Covid-Infektionen. Nun sollen sogar zehn Sekunden Text, in ein Smartphone gesprochen, auch noch einigermaßen zuverlässig Typ-2-Diabetes nachweisen können."

Finanzielle Fehlanreize in Kliniken und Praxen

Aber natürlich geschieht derlei nicht aus purer Nächstenliebe oder im Sinne der Früherkennung, sondern aus glasklarem finanziellem Interesse:

> „Die Industrie verspricht sich viel vom Markt der Stimmanalyse in der Medizin. Verschiedene Analysten prognostizieren bis 2030 ein Marktpotenzial von mehr als fünf Milliarden Dollar für die Stimme als Biomarker." (siehe oben aus *Die Zeit* vom 26.10.2023)

Finanzielle Interessen und Fehlanreize steuern schon seit über zwanzig Jahren die Medizin in Deutschland – vor allem seit Einführung der Fallpauschalen (DRG). Immer wieder gibt es mutige Ärztinnen und Ärzte, die das klar benennen und anprangern. So veröffentlichte z. B. das *Deutsche Ärzteblatt* am 11. Februar 2022 unter der Überschrift „Die Entmenschlichung der Medizin" einen bemerkenswerten Artikel. Darin sagt Florian Gerheuser, Oberarzt an der Klinik für Anästhesie und Operative Intensivmedizin am Universitätsklinikum Augsburg: „Der Fokus hat sich verschoben: Weg vom medizinischen Problem des individuellen Patienten, hin zum Verweildauermanagement, der Erlösoptimierung und dem Case-Mix-Index.“ Der Case-Mix-Index ist das Maß für den relativen Ressourcenaufwand aller behandelten Krankenhausfälle – eine wichtige Größe für die DRGs.

Was Florian Gerheuser hier zusammenfassend für die Krankenhäuser benennt, gilt in ähnlicher Weise jedoch ebenso für den ambulanten Bereich. Auch dort sehen wir eine zunehmende Konzernbildung. So stiegen, wie die Zeitschrift *Cicero* am 7. November 2022 publizierte, die Private-Equity-Käufe (Private Equity sind Kapitalgeber, die Unternehmen erwerben, um sie kurze Zeit später gewinnbringend wieder abzustoßen) im Bereich der Medizinischen Versorgungszentren (MVZ) für Augenheilkunde, Radiologie, Dialyse und Orthopädie seit 2007 drastisch an (in Klammern die Zahlen für die zahnärztlichen MVZs):

2007:	1
2015:	18 (3)
2018:	37 (31)
2019:	53 (45)
2020:	72 (62)
2021:	77 (61)

Über 80 Prozent der MVZs lagen im städtischen Bereich.

Einzelpraxen in Privatbesitz gehen in ähnlichem Umfang mehr und mehr zurück, MVZs nehmen zu. So gingen die Einzelpraxen in Hamburg seit 2015 um 12 Prozent zurück, die MVZs nahmen um 29 Prozent zu.

Kein Wunder, denn die zunehmende Kapitalisierung und Industrialisierung der Medizin in den Arztpraxen verspricht hohe Renditen. 2021 flossen allein aus den Kassen der Gesetzlichen Krankenversicherung 263,4 Milliarden Euro ins System. Zweck der Investitionen ist jedoch nicht etwa eine gute Patientenversorgung, sondern primär der Gewinn: Im ambulanten Sektor sind die Gewinne nach wie vor teils zweistellig (s.o. CICERO vom 7. November 2022).

Am Türschild lässt sich nicht erkennen, ob die Praxis einer Investoren-Kette gehört oder dem praktizierenden Arzt. Viele ältere Ärzte verkaufen ihren Kassensitz an MVZs, weil sie dafür momentan noch viel Geld bekommen, und weil sie oft keinen Nachfolger für die aufreibende Arbeit in einer eigenen Praxis finden. Niemand möchte heute noch 60 Stunden in der Woche oder gar mehr arbeiten. Ganz zu schweigen von der Mühsal von Hausbesuchen. Das Angestelltenverhältnis im MVZ ermöglicht familienfreundliche Teilzeitmodelle. Ironischerweise wurde gerade das zum Einfalltor für Investoren. Patienten sind dort allerdings nur noch eine mehr oder weniger große Verschiebemasse, und die Arztpraxis gerät zur Durchschleusungs-Station im Fließband-Modus. Je mehr Patienten, desto mehr Umsatz, desto mehr Gewinn.

Um wen handelt es sich bei den Investoren? Es sind Namen, die dort niemand vermutet hätte. So baute z. B. Jacobs Kaffee innerhalb von zwei Jahren eine der größten Zahnarztketten mit über 500 Praxen in ganz Europa auf. Der Bauer-Verlag, einer der großen Medienkonzerne in Deutschland, kaufte sich in MVZs ein, ebenso die Tchibo-Besitzer, die Familie Herz, oder Konzerne wie Nordic Capital aus Schweden, Wateland aus den Niederlanden, Fonds Antin aus Frankreich (siehe vorher aus CICERO vom 7.11.2022). Wer genau finanziell das Sagen hat, bleibt oft im Dunkeln.

Die Rückkehr des paternalistischen Prinzips

Mit dieser vorwiegend von ökonomischen Interessen geprägten Entwicklung geht der direkte Bezug zum Menschen als Subjekt in einer Krankheit mehr und mehr verloren. Der Mensch und seine Individualität spielen keine große Rolle mehr. Dazu hat auch die Corona-Krise mit ihren vielen dirigistischen und bevormundenden Maßnahmen massiv beigetragen. Kritisieren und in Frage stellen durfte man das nicht. Vor dem Hintergrund der bereits skizzierten Entwicklung war das besonders fatal. Denn es drehte das Rad der Patientenkompetenz und des mündigen Patienten wieder um viele Stufen zurück.

Matthias Schrappe, Internist und Gesundheitsökonom, früherer Dekan und wissenschaftlicher Geschäftsführer der Universität Witten/Herdecke, von 2002 bis 2011 Direktor des Instituts für Patientensicherheit der Universität Bonn, einer der maßgeblichen Initiatoren für die vielbeachteten, aber auch vielgeschmähten kritischen Adhoc-Stellungnahmen einer Gruppe von internationalen Wissenschaftlern in der Corona-Zeit („Thesenpapier-Autorengruppe"), schrieb in seinem beachtenswerten dreiteiligen Beitrag „Zehn Thesen zur Aufarbeiten der Corona-Krise" für die Zeitschrift *Cicero* (Teil 1 am 30. November 2022):

> „Es wird viel zu wenig problematisiert, dass sich durch das Corona-Management die gesamte Gesundheitsversorgung stark verändert, ja verschlechtert hat. Zahlreiche Entwicklungsstränge der letzten Jahrzehnte wurden unterbrochen, zurückgedreht, in ihr Gegenteil verkehrt. Stärkung der Patienten-Rechte, Qualität der Versorgung, Patientensicherheit – wo sind diese Themen geblieben? Widersinnige Strukturen, Reformstau – wo sind die vormals diskutierten Ansätze noch erkennbar? Fast aus der Erinnerung gestrichen. So waren durch umfassende gesetzgeberische Aktivitäten die Patientenrechte neu formuliert worden, was z. B. direkte Auswirkungen auf die Einwilligung zu Eingriffen hatte. Das Wort der Patienten hatte gezählt. Man hatte gelernt, dass eine gute Gesundheitsversorgung nicht nur das Können Einzelner voraussetzt, sondern dass diese von Teams und gut geführten Institutionen erbracht wird. Rollen wurden „modernisiert", die Praxis musste sich wissenschaftlich hinterfragen lassen. Fehler wurden zugegeben, Hierarchien (wenigstens teilweise) flacher gestaltet. Aber Corona sorgte für einen drastischen Umschwung, jetzt herrscht wieder der hierarchische Durchgriff, es dominiert das paternalistische Prinzip."

Sofern es eine Patientenorientierung in der Medizin überhaupt jemals gegeben hatte, ist sie ihr in der Corona-Krise wieder komplett abhanden gekommen.

Vor diesem Hintergrund müssen wir Krankheit heute betrachten. Und es wundert nicht, dass angesichts dieser Situation viele Menschen das Kranksein fürchten und scheuen. Es ist ihnen lästig. Sie wollen es einfach nur ganz schnell wieder weghaben. Sie schämen sich dafür. Denn krank geworden zu sein bedeutet, offenbar nicht gesund genug gelebt zu haben, selbst schuld zu sein, wenn der Körper nicht mehr so funktioniert, wie er soll.

Mehr noch: Kranksein bedeutet, teilweise wochen- oder monatelang auf einen Behandlungstermin warten, sich dem ärztlichen Willen unterordnen und teilweise widersinnigen Anordnungen unterwerfen zu müssen. In dem schnellen Durchsatz in Kliniken und Praxen bleibt kaum Zeit für das ohnehin geringgeschätzte und kaum angemessen bezahlte Gespräch.

Kranksein bedeutet Ausgeliefertsein, Kontrollverlust, Hilflosigkeit. Es bedeutet Angst vor Versagen, vor Ausgeschlossensein, vor gesellschaftlicher Ächtung und Entwertung.

Dass das kein neues Problem ist, zeigen die Schriften Viktor von Weizsäckers, der schon 1926, also vor fast 100 Jahren, in seiner Schrift „Der Arzt und der Kranke“ konstatierte:

> „Es ist eine erstaunliche, aber nicht zu leugnende Tatsache, dass die gegenwärtige Medizin eine eigene Lehre vom kranken Menschen nicht besitzt. (…) Sie lehrte Erscheinungen des Krankseins, Unterscheidungen von Ursachen, Folgen, Heilmitteln der Krankheiten, aber sie lehrt nicht den kranken Menschen.“

Dabei ist der kranke Mensch die eigentliche Normalität. Denn, so von Weizsäcker in einem Vortrag 1949 beim Wiesbadener Internisten-Kongress:

> „Wer sich für völlig gesund hält, ist nur blind für das Pathologische. Welcher Körper wäre makellos gebildet? Welche Familie ist frei von erblichen Schäden? Welches Seelenleben ist frei von Neurose oder pathologischen Zuständen oder Zügen? Man kann das Kranke nicht aus dem Gesunden ableiten, sondern muss versuchen, die Entstehung des Gesunden aus dem Kranken zu begleiten. Die Krankheit hat den Sinn, den Betroffenen zum Sinn seines Lebens zu führen. Das einzusehen, hat die naturwissenschaftliche Medizin gründlich verhindert.“

Ärztliches Tun als Kunst der individuellen Hilfeleistung

Nichtsdestotrotz kommen heute vor allem chronisch Kranke dieser Weisheit wieder mehr und mehr auf die Spur und berichten auch darüber. Es gibt eine Fülle von Büchern, in denen reflektiert wird, was der Sinn einer schweren Krankheit gewesen sein könnte. Welche Bedeutung hat sie für die Gesamtbiographie eines Menschen?

Peter Matthiessen (1944–2019), Facharzt für Neurologie und Psychiatrie, langjähriger Leiter der Abteilung für Kinder- und Jugendpsychiatrie am Gemeinschaftskrankenhaus Herdecke, Gründungsmitglied des „Dialogforums Pluralismus in der Medizin" und von 1996 bis 2009 Inhaber des Gerhard-Kienle-Stiftungslehrstuhls für Medizintheorie und Komplementärmedizin an der Universität Witten/Herdecke, beschäftigte sich schon vor vielen Jahren mit dieser Frage im Rahmen einer interdisziplinären ärztlichen Arbeitsgruppe, die Patienten in ausführlichen Gesprächen nach ihren Erlebnissen im Rahmen einer schweren Krankheit interviewte, unter dem Arbeitstitel: „Wozu mag es dereinst gut gewesen sein, dass ich diese Krankheit bekommen habe?" Es ist eine bewusst im Futur II formulierte Frage. Antworten finden sich oft erst viele Jahre später, wenn die Erklärung sich aus der gelebten Zukunft herausschält.

Peter Matthiessen sagte mir dazu einmal vor vielen Jahren im Rahmen eines Interviews:

> „Der Mensch verwirklicht sich ja nicht nur in der Gesundheit, sondern auch in der Überwindung und im Durchmachen einer Krankheit. Das hat Auswirkungen für das ärztliche Handeln, das sich daran ausrichten muss, wie ich als Arzt ihm helfen kann, seine Biographie wieder selbst zu schreiben. Dass er wieder selbst Lebenskünstler wird, indem er seine Gesundungsleistung vollziehen kann. Gesundheit ist ja nicht Selbstzweck, sondern wir sind gesund, um schöpferisch sein zu können im Leben. Wenn ich das im Blick habe, will ich nicht Krankheiten wegzaubern, sondern das ärztliche Tun ist die Kunst der individuellen Hilfeleistung für einen unverschuldet in Not geratenen Kranken."

Wo will und soll eine schwere Krankheit einen Menschen also hinführen? Welche Entwicklungsmöglichkeiten trägt sie in sich? Was kann und darf wachsen anstelle eines Rezidivs? Die Antworten darauf sind so verschieden wie die Menschen selbst. Dort, wo Menschen sich diesen Fragen gestellt haben und bereit waren, nach Antworten zu suchen, zeigt sich oft, dass die Krankheit die Weichen im Leben neu und nicht selten zum Besseren hin gestellt hat. Viele sind deshalb – trotz aller Dramatik und Einschnitte im Leben, die das Geschehen meist mit sich brachte – dankbar für das, was ihnen widerfahren ist. Weil sich Türen geöffnet, neue Wege und Chancen aufgetan haben, die ohne diese Krankheit verschlossen geblieben wären. Weil sich Erkenntnisse und Erfahrungen einstellen konnten, die das Leben in bis dahin ungeahnter Weise bereichern.

Die Krankheit als Lehrmeisterin

Ich möchte das an einem Beispiel verdeutlichen. Es geht um meinen Kollegen Jürgen Leinemann (1937–2013), einen der bekanntesten politischen Reporter des Magazins *Der Spiegel* zwischen den Jahren 1971 und 2000. Schon 1974 hatte er einen massiven physischen und psychischen Zusammenbruch aufgrund von Alkoholismus und Depressionen erlitten. Nach einem längeren Aufenthalt in einer psychosomatischen Klinik konnte er in seinem Beruf wieder neu Tritt fassen; er hat den politischen Journalismus in den letzten Jahrzehnten des alten und am Beginn des neuen Jahrhunderts entscheidend mitgeprägt. 2007 erkrankte er kurz nach seiner Pensionierung an einem Zungengrund-Karzinom. 2009 veröffentlichte er ein Buch über seine Erfahrungen mit dieser Krebserkrankung unter dem Titel *Das Leben ist der Ernstfall*. Daraus möchte ich zitieren, weil es so anschaulich macht, in welcher Situation ein Patient sich befindet, wie wenig dies von ärztlicher Seite meist berücksichtigt wird, wie prägend es sich jedoch auf das Krankheitserleben auswirkt. Leinemann schreibt:

> „Als größte Herausforderung erlebe ich die Kränkung des Nicht-mehr-mitspielen-Könnens, die Fülle von Miseren wie Halsentzündung und Brechreiz, Verschleimung und Mundtrockenheit, Ge-

schmacksunfähigkeit und Schluckbeschwerden, nicht heilende Wunden und Schlaflosigkeit – sowie Ohnmacht, Ohnmacht, Ohnmacht. (…) Krankheit ist Kränkung, tiefe existenzielle Erniedrigung. Mehr denn je fühlte ich mich als Außenseiter, der nirgends mehr richtig dazugehörte. Wer war ich denn noch? Was stimmte denn noch an meinem alten Selbstverständnis? (…) In mir blieb eine unerklärliche Distanz zu meiner Umwelt, eine Mischung aus Trägheit und Betäubung, die mein Leben entsaftete. (…)
Ich bin in ein System geraten, in dem ich als statistisches Datenbündel existierte: eingeliefert mit den Werten xy, ausgeliefert mit den Werten xy plus oder minus. Der Prozess muss funktionieren, das ist das Wichtigste. Sie standen vor mir, die Ärzte in ihren weißen Kitteln, und redeten auf mich ein, junge Schnösel zum Teil, aber auch fremde Frauen, immer von ganz oben nach ganz unten. Vielleicht waren die meisten auch nur hilflos, konnten überhaupt nicht einschätzen, was sich da vor ihnen abspielte, obwohl es ja in der Krankenakte stand. Auf jeden Fall traten sie arrogant auf, es war ihnen völlig egal, dass ich offensichtlich nur die Hälfte verstand von dem, was sie mir erzählten. Und jeder von ihnen machte mir Angst, Angst, Angst.
Noch nie hatte ich mich so ohnmächtig gefühlt. Das war mir neu, in dieser Form war es mir neu. (…) Ich kannte ihre Statussymbole und ihre Herrschaftsgesten, und dennoch war ich ihnen ausgeliefert, in ihrer Jovialität so gut wie ihrer teilnahmslosen Kälte. (…) Plötzlich wusste ich, was die berühmte ‚Dialektik der Macht' ist: meine Wehrlosigkeit als Kranker machte sie stark. (…) Hätte ich doch nur einen einzigen vertrauenswürdigen Arzt, der die unterschiedlichen Diagnosen zusammenfassen und mir die Widersprüche zwischen den objektiven Befunden und dem subjektiven Befinden erklären könnte. Einen Arzt, nicht ein halbes Dutzend."

Dennoch fand Leinemann einen Weg, seinen Frieden zu machen mit dieser Situation, die Krankheit anzunehmen – auch mit all den Einschränkungen, die sie mit sich brachte. Dies war ihm jedoch nur möglich durch die uneingeschränkte Unterstützung seiner Frau, seiner Tochter und deren Mann sowie durch enge Freunde. Mühsam und ganz langsam, über viele Monate hinweg, kamen der Lebensmut und die Lebensfreude zurück:

> „Ich war noch der, der ich vorher gewesen war, und hatte mich zugleich verändert. Die Krankheit und ihre Folgen waren zum Bestandteil meiner Lebensführung geworden. (...) Ich habe aufgehört, mir die Erwartungen anderer zu eigen zu machen und danach zu leben. (...) Die Krankheit hat mich mit Situationen des Scheiterns konfrontiert und mich verzichten gelehrt. (...) Erst notgedrungen, allmählich mit Einsicht, lernte ich, mich zu bescheiden, ohne zu resignieren."

Und dann der Kernsatz, der alles zusammenfasst, was das Leben und eben diese Krankheit ihn gelehrt haben: „Als Lehrmeisterin war die Krankheit ein wichtiges Element der Gesundheit."

Ein anderes Gesundheitsverständnis

Leinemann und mit ihm die vielen anderen Autorinnen und Autoren solcher Berichte stellen das weitverbreitete Verständnis von Gesundheit in Frage, die ja oft als „Abwesenheit von Krankheit" gekennzeichnet wird. Die Definition der Weltgesundheitsorganisation WHO, derzufolge Gesundheit „ein Zustand vollständigen körperlichen, geistigen und sozialen Wohlergehens" ist, geriet schon vor geraumer Zeit ins Wanken. Denn wenn es so wäre, wären wir ja so gut wie nie gesund.

Demgegenüber hat die Niederländerin Machteld Huber das „Konzept der Positiven Gesundheit" erstellt, in dem sie das Leben in seinen verschiedenen Facetten mit einbezieht. Das Wesentliche will ich kurz benennen. Es umfasst sechs Faktoren des menschlichen Lebens:

1. **Körperfunktionen**: Fakten, Befunde, Fitness, Beschwerden, Vitalität
2. **Mentale Funktionen und Wahrnehmung**: Kognitive Funktionen, Emotionen, Selbsteinschätzung Selbstwirksamkeit
3. **Alltag**: Zurechtkommen, Arbeitsfähigkeit, Gesundheitskompetenz
4. **Lebensqualität**: Wohlbefinden, Glück, Freude, Dynamik, Ausgeglichenheit
5. **Soziale Teilhabe**: Kontakte, Beziehungen, Gemeinschaften, Arbeit
6. **Spirituell-existenzielle Dimension**: Sinn, Ziele/Ideale, Zukunftsaussichten, Akzeptanz.

Aus diesen Faktoren kann jeder selbst sein individuelles Gesundheitsdiagramm erstellen, das sich immer wieder anders darstellt. Krankheit ist dabei ein integraler Bestandteil, der das Gesamtbild ganz selbstverständlich mit beeinflusst, gegebenenfalls auch mal dominiert und dann wieder in den Hintergrund tritt.

Krankheit und Gesundheit sind also nicht einander ausschließende Gegensätze – es kann gesunde Kranke und kranke Gesunde geben. Gesundheit definiert sich dadurch, ob man es versteht, mit Irritationen fertigzuwerden, Beschwerden im Alltag zu bewältigen und das Leben so einzurichten, dass sie zu Bedingungen werden, unter denen das Leben Gestalt annimmt.

Schon 2005 haben die Soziologin Farideh Akashe-Böhme und ihr Mann, der Philosoph Gernot Böhme (beide sind inzwischen verstorben), ein bemerkenswertes Buch geschrieben mit dem Titel *Mit Krankheit leben. Von der Kunst, mit Schmerz und Leid umzugehen*. Darin schreiben sie: „Es gibt kein Leben ohne Irritationen und Widerstände. Krankheit ist kein Einwand gegen das Leben, Kranksein ist selbst eine Form von Leben. Krankheit wird Teil der Biographie. Auch Kranksein muss man können."

Eine, die gelernt hat, das zu können, ist die an Morbus Bechterew erkrankte Kathrin Blawat. Sie schreibt in der *Süddeutschen Zeitung* vom 12. Juli 2022 in einem ganzseitigen Beitrag:

> „Wenn sich abzeichnet, dass viele körperliche Einschränkungen bleiben oder gar zunehmen werden, braucht es, damit sich überhaupt noch etwas richtig anfühlt, die Einsicht: Es gibt Wichtigeres im Leben als Gesundheit. (…) Hat man die richtigen Menschen an seiner Seite, verliert jede Krankheit einen Teil ihres Schreckens. (…) Es ist eine der schwierigsten Aufgaben, denen ein Mensch sich stellen kann, egal, ob krank oder gesund: klarzukommen mit dem, was ist. Alles, was das Leben schwierig macht, zu akzeptieren – und trotz allem in möglichst vielen Momenten, das Gute, Schöne, Komische zu erkennen. (…) Würdevoll krank zu sein, ist eine Kunst, die geübt sein will."

Die Kraft der spirituellen Dimension der Mistel

Was hat nun die Mistel mit all diesen Fragen zu tun? Ganz einfach: Sie stärkt die Menschen darin, genau in dem geschilderten Sinne mit Krankheit umzugehen. Sie hat eine spirituelle Dimension, die heute leider oft vernachlässigt wird, im Streben nach wissenschaftlichen Studienergebnissen. Diese haben natürlich ihre Berechtigung, sie sind absolut notwendig. Aber über all dem dürfen wir aus meiner Sicht die seelisch-geistige Dimension nicht vergessen, die die Mistel vor allen anderen Medikamenten bei Krebskranken mit sich zu bringen vermag. Sie hilft mit, Antworten zu finden auf die Fragen, die eine schwere Krankheit zwangsläufig aufwirft. Sie bestärkt darin, Geduld und Hoffnung zu bewahren. Die offenen Fragen zu lieben, wie es Rainer Maria Rilke so schön in seinem „Brief an einen jungen Dichter" beschrieben hat:

> „Man muss den Dingen die eigene, stille, ungestörte Entwicklung lassen, die tief von innen kommt und durch nichts gedrängt oder beschleunigt werden kann. Alles ist austragen – und dann gebären … Reifen wie der Baum, der seine Säfte nicht drängt, und getrost in den Stürmen des Frühlings steht, ohne Angst, dass dahinter kein Sommer kommen könnte. Er kommt doch! Aber er kommt nur zu den Geduldigen, die da sind, als ob die Ewigkeit vor ihnen läge, so sorglos, still und weit. Man muss Geduld haben gegen das Ungelöste im Herzen und versuchen, die Fragen selber lieb zu haben, wie verschlossene Stuben, und wie Bücher, die in einer sehr fremden Sprache geschrieben sind. Es handelt sich darum, alles zu leben. Wenn man die Fragen lebt, lebt man vielleicht allmählich, ohne es zu merken, eines fremden Tages in die Antwort hinein."

In diese Antworten hineinleben zu können, gelingt aber nur, wenn Ärztinnen und Ärzte bereit sind, einen Menschen auf seinem Weg durch die Krankheit zu begleiten, nicht zu dominieren. Wenn sie ihm nichts überstülpen und nicht meinen, besser zu wissen, was gut ist für ihn. Sondern wenn sie ihm Expertise und Erfahrung zur Verfügung stellen. Abspüren, was er jetzt braucht. Ihn wahrnehmen, ihm zuhören. Ihn darin bestärken, in sich hineinzuhorchen, seiner inneren Stimme zu lauschen, zu hoffen und dem eigenen Stern zu vertrauen. Kurzum: Das Lebendigsein über das Kranksein zu stellen.

Und so möchte ich schließen mit einem Gedicht aus der Oper „Intolleranza" von Luigi Nono, der diese Haltung in für mich einzigartiger Weise in wenigen Worten komprimiert hat:

Lebendig ist, wer wach bleibt,
sich dem anderen schenkt,
das Bessere hingibt,
niemals rechnet.

Lebendig ist, wer das Leben liebt,
seine Begräbnisse, seine Feste.
Wer Märchen und Mythen
auf den ödesten Bergen findet.

Lebendig ist, wer das Licht erwartet
in den Tagen des schweren Sturms.
Wer die stillen Lieder
ohne Geschrei und Schüsse wählt.
Sich dem Herbst hinwendet
und nicht aufhört zu lieben.

Interessenkonflikt

Es liegt kein Interessenkonflikt vor.

Annette Bopp, Freie Journalistin für Medizin und Kultur
Stemmeshay 19, 22045 Hamburg (www.annettebopp.de)

Korrespondenzadresse:
pressebuero@annettebopp.de

Integrative Oncology: How Can we Implement it Into Daily Practice?

Integrative Onkologie: Wie können wir sie in die tägliche Praxis umsetzen?

Ralf Hofheinz

Summary

According to a large survey conducted by the "Working group for medical oncology" (AIO) of the German cancer society among about 2,000 cancer patients, about 40.5 % of the polled patients used integrative oncology (IO). This survey is unique because data were collected stratified and comprised out- as well as inpatients from all federal states in Germany and all kind of institutions (university as well as community hospitals and oncology practices) painting a more holistic picture than other surveys conducted in single treatment settings. N = 317 patients applied vitamins/mineral nutrients (16.0 %), n = 261 phytotherapy/herbs/naturopathy (13.2 %), n = 163 dietary supplements (8.2 %), n = 114 homoeopathy (5.8 %), and n = 632 techniques of self-help (31.9 %). Most patients reported a subjective benefit by using these measures: n = 369 (42.8 %) patients regarded them as helpful, while n = 187 patients (22.4 %) were unable to estimate their effect. Of note, less than half of the patients discussed the used IO methods with their physicians. Other surveys have shown that up to 70 % of cancer patients expect general practitioners (GP) to provide IO support, while only one fifth of GPs offer IO methods to their patients. These data show that a considerable percentage of patients are left alone while trying to choose appropriate IO methods. Thus, there is a need for well-trained physicians (be it oncologist or GPs) in order to avoid for instance drug interactions with anti-cancer treatments. In this regard it may be regarded a step forward that the S3 guideline "Complementary medicine for oncological patients" has been published about two years ago. However, while reading this guideline, it is obvious that many IO measures and drugs have not been subject to properly planned and conducted clinical trials. In all, while IO is used or requested by many cancer patients very few physicians are trained in this field and there is a large need for well conducted trials in the field of integrative oncology.

Keywords: Integrative Oncology, clinical practice, clinical trials

Zusammenfassung
Laut einer großen Umfrage der Arbeitsgemeinschaft Internistische Onkologie (AIO) der Deutschen Krebsgesellschaft unter rund 2.000 Krebspatienten nutzen etwa 40,5 % der befragten Patienten die Integrative Onkologie. Diese Umfrage ist einzigartig, da die Daten stratifiziert erhoben wurden und sowohl ambulante als auch stationäre Patienten aus allen Bundesländern und allen Arten von Einrichtungen (Universitätskliniken sowie kommunale Krankenhäuser und onkologische Praxen) umfassten, was ein ganzheitlicheres Bild ergibt als andere Umfragen, die in umschriebenen Behandlungseinrichtungen durchgeführt wurden. N = 317 Patienten verwendeten Vitamine/Mineralstoffe (16,0 %), n = 261 Phytotherapie/Kräuter/Naturheilkunde (13,2 %), n = 163 Nahrungsergänzungsmittel (8,2 %), n = 114 Homöopathie (5,8 %) und n = 632 Techniken der Selbsthilfe (31,9 %). Die meisten Patienten berichteten über einen subjektiven Nutzen dieser Maßnahmen: n = 369 (42,8 %) Patienten hielten sie für hilfreich, während n = 187 Patienten (22,4 %) ihre Wirkung nicht einschätzen konnten. Bemerkenswert ist, dass weniger als die Hälfte der Patienten die verwendeten IO-Methoden mit ihren Ärzten besprachen. Andere Umfragen haben gezeigt, dass bis zu 70 % der Krebspatienten von ihren Hausärzten Unterstützung bei der Selbsthilfe erwarten, während nur ein Fünftel der Hausärzte ihren Patienten Selbsthilfemethoden anbietet. Diese Daten zeigen, dass ein beträchtlicher Prozentsatz der Patienten bei der Wahl geeigneter IO-Methoden allein gelassen wird. Es besteht also ein Bedarf an gut ausgebildeten Ärzten (ob Onkologen oder Allgemeinmediziner), um z. B. Wechselwirkungen mit Krebsmedikamenten zu vermeiden. In dieser Hinsicht kann es als ein Fortschritt angesehen werden, dass die S3-Leitlinie „Komplementärmedizin bei onkologischen Patienten" vor etwa zwei Jahren veröffentlicht wurde. Bei der Lektüre dieser Leitlinie wird jedoch deutlich, dass viele Maßnahmen und Medikamente der Komplementärmedizin noch nicht Gegenstand von sorgfältig geplanten und durchgeführten klinischen Studien sind. Obwohl viele Krebspatienten die Komplementärmedizin nutzen oder danach fragen, sind nur wenige Ärzte in diesem Bereich ausgebildet, und es besteht ein großer Bedarf an gut durchgeführten Studien im Bereich der integrativen Onkologie.
Schlüsselwörter: Integrative Onkologie, klinische Praxis, klinische Studien

Conflict of interest

I confirm that there are no potential conflicts of interest.

Prof. Dr. Ralf Hofheinz
Mannheim Cancer Center, University of Heidelberg, Mannheim, Germany

Corresponding author:
ralf.hofheinz@umm.de

Die Zukunft der Misteltherapie – Eine Übersicht

The Future of Mistletoe Therapy – An Overview

Harald Matthes

Zusammenfassung

Die Misteltherapie in der Onkologie zeigt den größten lebensqualitäts-verbessernden Effekt als Adjuvans, wenn Chemotherapie und Bestrahlung gleichzeitig verabreicht werden. Die Datenlage zur Verbesserung der Lebensqualität durch eine Misteltherapie ist für die verschiedenen Tumorentitäten recht heterogen. Die besten Daten liegen für das Mammakarzinom vor. Die Datenlage zur Lebensverlängerung durch Misteltherapie ist für die verschiedenen Tumorentitäten weniger zuverlässig.

Es müssen weitere Studien und Analysen unter Einbeziehung von Real-World-Daten (RWD) durchgeführt werden, um die Verlängerung des Gesamtüberlebens bei den verschiedenen Tumorentitäten weiter zu validieren. Die verschiedenen Applikationsformen der Mistel jenseits der Subkutan-Gabe sind vielversprechend. Zukünftige Forschungsfragen sind unter anderem, ob andere Formen der Mistelapplikation, wie intravenöse und intratumorale Applikation, einen erhöhten Effekt aufweisen. Die adjuvante Mistelgabe während einer zytostatischen Chemo- und Strahlentherapie ist gut etabliert. Zur Verbesserung der Verträglichkeit der Checkpoint/PD-1-Inhibitor-Therapie mit der Mistel liegen nur wenige Daten vor.

Daten aus der Grundlagenforschung zu Kombinationen eines wässrigen Extraktes mit einem lipophilen Extrakt (Mistel mit Triterpenen = Mistel-TT) deuten in Zellversuchen und Tiermodellen auf eine deutliche Verstärkung einer antitumoralen Wirkung von Mistel TT hin. Klinische Daten am Menschen liegen dazu bislang nicht vor und sollten Gegenstand zukünftiger Forschungen sein.

Die Mehrzahl der Mistelstudien befasst sich mit der antitumoralen Wirkung der Mistel. Daneben besitzt die Mistel jedoch auch immunmodulierende und anti-inflammatorische Effekte, die in Zukunft systematisch untersucht werden sollten, um die Indikationen für Autoimmun- und rheumatischen Erkrankungen zu erweitern. Erste sehr interessante Indikationen für Mistelextrakte zeigen sich in der Behandlung des Post-Covid- und Post-Vac-Syndroms.

Das Potenzial der Misteltherapie, insbesondere für die verschiedenen Verabreichungswege und Indikationen außerhalb der Onkologie, muss in Zukunft weiter erforscht werden.
Schlüsselwörter: Misteltherapie, Lebensqualität, Arzneimittelverträglichkeit, Applikationsformen, Real-World-Data, Indikationen, Onkologie, post-Covid, post-Vac, Metaanalysen, Systematische Reviews

Summary

Mistletoe therapy in oncology shows the greatest quality of life-improving effect as an adjuvant when chemotherapy and radiotherapy are administered simultaneously. The data on the improvement of quality of life through mistletoe therapy is quite heterogeneous for the various tumour entities. The best data are available for breast cancer. The data on prolonging life through mistletoe therapy is less reliable for the various tumour entities.

Further studies considering real-world data (RWD) need to be conducted to further validate the prolongation of overall survival in the various tumour entities. The different application forms of mistletoe beyond subcutaneous administration are promising. Future research questions include whether other forms of mistletoe application, such as intravenous and intratumoural application, have an increased effect. The adjuvant administration of mistletoe during cytostatic chemotherapy and radiotherapy is well established. There is little data available on improving the tolerability of checkpoint/PD-1 inhibitor therapy with mistletoe.

Data from basic research on combinations of an aqueous extract with a lipophilic extract (mistletoe with triterpenes = mistletoe TT) in cell experiments and animal models indicate a significant enhancement of the antitumour effect of mistletoe TT. Clinical data on humans are not yet available and should be the subject of future research.

The majority of mistletoe studies focus on the antitumour effect of mistletoe. However, mistletoe also has immunomodulatory and anti-inflammatory effects, which should be systematically investigated in the future in order to expand the indications for autoimmune and rheumatic diseases. The first very interesting indications for mistletoe extracts can be seen in the treatment of post-Covid and post-Vac-syndrome.

The potential of mistletoe therapy, particularly for the various administration routes and indications outside of oncology, must be further researched in the future.
Keywords: Quality of life, tolerability, application forms, real-world data, indications, oncology, post-Covid, post-Vac, meta-analyses, systematic reviews

Evidenz- und Leitlinienbewertung der Misteltherapie

Die Mistel (*Viscum album* L.) gehört weltweit weiterhin zu den wissenschaftlich am besten untersuchten Pflanzen in der Medizin (aktuelle Übersicht bei (Nicoletti 2023) und ausführlich bei (Kienle, Kiene 2003), was Inhaltsstoffe und pharmakologische Wirkungen betrifft. Über 150 klinische Studien in Bezug auf eine onkologische Wirksamkeit wurden seit über 70 Jahren durchgeführt, dabei ist die Qualität der Studien insgesamt sehr heterogen (Thronicke *et al.* 2022). In den letzte 25 Jahren sind mehr als 30 randomisierte kontrollierte Studien (RCT) (Thronicke *et al.* 2022) für die verschiedenen Tumorentitäten hinzugekommen (Piao *et al.* 2004; Tröger *et al.* 2009; Bar-Sela *et al.* 2013; Tröger *et al.* 2013; Tröger *et al.* 2014) und in den letzten 5-7 Jahren auch zahlreiche Real-World Data-Publikationen aus dem größten europäischen Onkologie-Netzwerk der Integrativen Medizin (NO = Netzwerk Onkologie) (Schad *et al.* 2008; Schad *et al.* 2011; Steele *et al.* 2014; Steele *et al.* 2015; Axtner *et al.* 2016; Oei *et al.* 2017; Schad *et al.* 2017; Oei *et al.* 2018; Schad *et al.* 2018; Schad *et al.* 2018; Oei *et al.* 2020; Thronicke *et al.* 2020).

Aufgrund der Vielzahl von klinischen Studien zu den unterschiedlichen Tumorentitäten und Zielparametern (Überlebenszeit (OS = Overall Survival), Lebensqualität etc.) wurden in den letzten Jahren einige Metaanalysen und systematische Reviews angefertigt. Dabei kommen die Autoren der verschiedenen Metaanalysen (Ziegler, Grossarth-Maticek 2010; Bussing *et al.* 2012; Bonamin *et al.* 2017; Loef, Walach 2020; Ostermann *et al.* 2020) und systematischen Reviews (Freuding *et al.* 2019a; Freuding *et al.* 2019b; Loef, Walach 2020; Ostermann *et al.* 2020; Cogo *et al.* 2023) zu sehr unterschiedlichen Ergebnissen, was angesichts der wissenschaftlichen Regeln und Grundsätze zur Durchführung von Metaanalysen (Cleophas, Zwinderman 2017) und systematischen Reviews (Macaskill *et al.* 2010) verwundert.

Bei diskursiven Sichtweisen in der Medizin, wie gegenüber der Anwendung der Mistel in der Onkologie, besteht die Gefahr, dass systematische Reviews und Metaanalysen, die ein hohes Ansehen innerhalb der evidenzbasierten Medizin haben, als Instrument zur Untermauerung der eigenen Sichtweise genutzt werden und erwünschte Ergebnisse durch

Ein- oder Ausschluss ‚passender bzw. nicht passender' Publikationen produziert werden, obwohl gerade eine Guideline-konforme Selektion und Bewertung von Publikationen ein zentrales wissenschaftliches Kriterium von systematischen Reviews und Metaanalysen darstellt (Macaskill *et al.* 2010).

2019 wurde ein systematisches Review (Teil 1 und 2) durch ein Leitlinienteam angefertigt, was auch die Erstellung der Leitlinie: ‚Komplementärmedizin in der Behandlung von onkologischen Patienten' leitete (Freuding *et al.* 2019a; Freuding *et al.* 2019b). Dieses systematische Review zur Bewertung der Mistel fand keine Indikation und keine Evidenz für ein verbessertes Überleben und Lebensqualität durch Anwendung der Misteltherapie und wich damit in erheblichem Maße von vorherigen und auch von in folgenden Jahren erstellten systematischen Reviews und Metaanalysen ab.

Die beiden Teile des systematischen Reviews um Prof. Jutta Hübner waren wenige Wochen vor der Beschlusslage zur Bewertung der Misteltherapie für die ‚Leitlinie zur Komplementärmedizin in der Behandlung von onkologischen Patienten' publiziert worden, so dass diese trotz erheblicher offener wissenschaftlicher Fragen, mit in die Leitlinienbewertung eingingen, was zu einer starken Abwertung der klinischen Evidenz der Misteltherapie führte (Fachgesellschaften 2021).

Ein internationales Wissenschaftlergremium aus der integrativen Onkologie richtete einen ‚Letter to the Editor' an die Zeitschrift (Matthes *et al.* 2019) und wies auf die zahlreichen methodischen Fehler in beiden Teilen des systematischen Reviews hin. Von den Autoren des Reviews gab es dazu jedoch keine detaillierte Stellungnahme. Daher wurde außerdem ein ‚Statement to an Insufficient Systematic Review on *Viscum album* L. Therapy' verfasst und in einem anderen onkologischen Journal publiziert (Matthes *et al.* 2020). Trotz über 40 nachgewiesener schwerwiegender wissenschaftlicher Fehler in den beiden Teilen des Reviews von Freudig et al. (2019a; 2019b) wurden diese bisher nicht als Publikationen zurückgezogen und sind weiterhin wesentlicher Hauptgrund einer Abwertung der Misteltherapie in der S-3 Leitlinie zur Komplementärmedizin in der Onkologie der AWMF.

In der Zukunft muss daher weiterhin durch wissenschaftlich hochwertige Metaanalysen und systematische Reviews der Evidenzgrad der Mistel-therapie für eine Leitlinienbewertung untermauert werden, so wie es bereits direkt nach der Leitlinienerstellung auch wieder begonnen wurde (Loef, Walach 2020; Ostermann *et al.* 2020).

Die verschiedenen Applikationsformen einer Misteltherapie

Intravenöse Applikation

Die etablierte und zugelassene Applikationsform in der onkologischen Misteltherapie ist die Subkutangabe, die sicher und nebenwirkungsarm ist (Steele *et al.* 2014). Durch eine Lokalreaktion an der Einstichstelle (Rötung und Induration durch Lymphozytenaggregation (Büssing 2006)) wird meist die gewünschte Misteldosis gefunden (Rötung und Induration von ca. 1-2 cm Durchmesser für 12-48 h nach subkutaner Gabe) (Steele *et al.* 2014). Durch die subkutane Applikationsform kommt es zu einem langsamen Anfluten und einer Verteilung der Mistelstoffe im Organismus. Bei sehr hohen subkutanen Misteldosen kann eine Wirksteigerung erreicht werden Dies verursacht jedoch eine starke lokale Reaktion (Rötung und Induration von bis zu 20 cm Durchmesser über mehrere Tage bis auch Wochen) sowie eine systemische Fieberreaktion und ein starkes Grippegefühl/Unwohlsein. Eine Phase II-Studie mit abnobaVISCUM beim hepatozellulären Karzinom (HCC) mit 60 mg abnobaVISCUM Fraxini subkutan zeigte als gewünschte Reaktion teilweise Komplettremissionen des HCC (13,1 % CR; 8,1 % PR), hatte jedoch Nebenwirkungen mit einer Toxizität WHO Grad III-IV von 34 % mit Fieber über 7 Tage (Mabed *et al.* 2004). Daher wird die Hochdosistherapie mit der Mistel nur in seltenen Spezialsituationen zur Fiebertherapie angewendet.

Um eine schnelle systemische Verfügbarkeit der Mistelwirkstoffe zu erreichen, hat sich die intravenöse (i.v.) Mistelgabe klinisch etabliert, auch wenn sie durch fehlende Zulassung als Off-Label-Use gilt. Am häufigsten wird die Mistel i.v. begleitend bzw. kurz vor einer i.v.-Chemotherapie (Cx) angewendet, um deren Verträglichkeit bzw. die Nebenwirkungen der Cx zu minimieren (Kienle *et al.* 2016; Zuzak *et al.* 2018). Dabei zeigt sich die i.v.-Mistelgabe auch in höheren Dosen als sehr gut verträglich (Steele *et al.* 2014).

Um aus dem Off-Label-Status herauszukommen, wurde eine Phase I-Studie mit Dosiseskalation bis zu 2000 mg Helixor P i.v. durchgeführt. Diese zeigte eine gute Verträglichkeit und Sicherheit (Huber *et al.* 2017). In der klinischen Praxis werden eher 300 bis max. 600 mg Helixor i.v. gegeben, so dass die Gaben von 2000 mg i.v. weit über den praktischen Alltagsdosen lagen. Eine weitere Phase I-Studie mit Helixor P bei fortgeschrittenen Tumorerkrankungen mit einer Dosis von 3 x 600 mg pro Woche zeigte ebenfalls eine gute Verträglichkeit und Lebensqualitätssteigerung, so dass eine Phase II-Studie nun gefordert ist. Aufgrund der häufigen i.v.-Applikation der Mistelpräparate in der klinischen Praxis sind Zulassungsstudien dringend erforderlich, um den Einsatz im Off-Labe-Use zu beenden.

Intratumorale Applikation

Eine eher selten angewendete Applikationsform der Mistel ist die intratumorale (i.t.) Applikation. Hier wird der Mistelgesamtextrakt direkt in den Tumor appliziert. Diese Anwendungsart hat sich beim HCC (Matthes 2004) und Pankreas-Adenokarzinom bewährt sowie bei Lumen-obstruierenden Tumoren im Bronchialsystem oder Gastrointestinaltrakt. In einer Pilotstudie (Matthes *et al.* 2005) sowie in einer retrospektiven Analyse ergaben sich gute Überlebensdaten für die i.t. Applikation beim Pankreaskarzinom mit einem durchschnittlichen Überleben im Stadium III von 11,8 und im Stadium IV von 8 Monaten, was knapp über den Studienergebnissen von FOLFIRINOX liegt, jedoch erheblich geringe toxische Nebenwirkungen hatte und damit auch eine verbesserte Lebensqualität erreicht werden konnte (Matthes *et al.* 2007; Schad *et al.* 2013).

Ein erster Fallbericht für diese Mistelanwendung wurde 1997 bei einem Kardiakarzinom publiziert, bei dem mit wenigen Applikationsgaben in einem zeitlichen Abstand von mehreren Tagen eine komplette Beseitigung der Ösophagus-Obstruktion erreicht werden konnte (Stumpf *et al.* 1997; 1998).

In den folgenden Jahren folgten dann Publikationen zur i.t. Anwendung im Bronchialtrakt (Grah, Matthes 2005; 2006; Grah 2014) und den parabronchialen Lymphknoten (Grah *et al.* 2009). Eine Analyse zur i.t. Mistelanwendung zeigte, dass dieser Gebrauch sicher und effektiv ist (Steele *et al.* 2015).

Aufgrund dieser guten Daten für eine i.t.-Applikation der Mistel in Tumorläsionen hat sich die Kombination von thermoablativer Tumortherapie (multipolare Radiofrequenzablation, RFITT) und gleichzeitiger i.t. Mistelapplikation ergeben. Bei nicht resektablen bzw. multiplen Metastasen stellt die RFITT eine gute Therapieoption dar. Limitierend für eine RFITT bei großen Metastasen ist die Gefahr, dass einschmelzende Tumornekrosen sich infizieren und abszedieren. Eine andere Limitation sind Rezidive an den Metastasenrändern durch Abnahme der Ablationstemperatur der bipolaren Elektroden an den Rändern. Wird nach der thermischen Ablation Mistel hochdosiert in die abladierte Läsion eingespritzt, so verweilt diese lange in der Läsion, da keine Durchblutung mehr gegeben ist und kann einen zytotoxischen Effekt ausüben. Gleichzeitig führt die Mistel durch ihren immunstimulierenden Effekt zu einem vermehrten Einströmen eines gemischtzelligen Infiltrates, was den Abbau der Tumornekrose deutlich beschleunigt und damit die Abszessrate reduziert. Ferner wird die Tumorablationsrate meist auf einen Durchmesser von 5 cm wegen der Abszessgefahr beschränkt, so konnten in der Kombination RFITT und i.t. Mistel Läsionen bis 12 cm Durchmesser ohne Abszedierung abladiert werden (Matthes 2006).

Zukunftspotentiale einer Misteltherapie

Alle derzeitigen am Markt befindlichen Mistelpräparate sind wässrige Auszüge des Mistelkrautes und der Mistelbeeren. Dabei werden die lipophilen Substanzen der Mistel in dem wässrigen Gesamtextrakt nicht verwendet.

Untersuchungen zu lipophilen Mistelextrakten zeigen, dass diese pentazyklische Triterpene enthalten (Oleanolsäure, Betulinsäure) (Jäger *et al.* 2007), welche einen immunstimulierenden Effekt, eine antitumoröse Aktivität, eine Wundheilungsaktivität, eine antioxidative Aktivität und einen Apoptose-induzierenden Effekt aufweisen (Urech *et al.* 2005; Vicas *et al.* 2009; Kuonen *et al.* 2013).

Erste *in vitro*-Experimente mit einem patentierten Gesamtextrakt von wässrigen und lipophilen *Viscum*-Extrakt (sog. *Viscum*-TT / Mistel-TT-Präparat) wurden 2012 publiziert und zeigten synergistische Effekte bzgl. einer Tumor-/Proliferationshemmung, Zytotoxizität und einer Apoptoseinduktion (*via* Caspasekaskade) (Delebinski *et al.* 2012; 2015).

Bei diesen *in vitro*-Zellkulturversuchen wurden auch Tumorzelllinien von Tumorentitäten gewählt, die bisher für den wässrigen Mistelgesamtextrakt als weniger wirksam galten. So zeigte der *Viscum*-TT-Extrakt beim Ewing Sarkom (Twardziok *et al.* 2016; 2017), beim Osteosarkom (Kleinsimon *et al.* 2017), bei der akuten myeloischen Leukämie (AML) sowie der akuten lymphoblastischen Leukämie (ALL) (Seifert *et al.* 2008; Delebinski *et al.* 2012) beachtliche Effektstärken und war teilweise den konventionell eingesetzten Zytostatika überlegen oder erbrachte darüber hinaus einen proliferationshemmenden Zusatzeffekt.

Trotz dieser vielversprechenden Grundlagendaten wird derzeit nicht an einer Zulassung eines *Viscum*-TT-Präparates für die Humanmedizin gearbeitet, so dass große Potenziale einer Misteltherapie in der Onkologie noch nicht gehoben sind.

Indikationen der Mistel außerhalb der Onkologie

Der Einsatz der Mistel in Studien bezieht sich fast ausschließlich auf onkologische Fragestellungen, inkl. der immunologischen Wirkungen der Lektine (Apoptose, T-Zellaktivierung etc.). Der antiinflammatorische Effekt (Lavastre *et al.* 2004; Hegde 2013; Nicoletti 2023) und der immunmodulatorische Effekt im Einsatz bei Autoimmunerkrankungen und rheumatischen Erkrankungen findet sich häufiger in der Praxis (2017), jedoch fehlen systematische Studien zu diesen Indikationen. Erste interessante

Erfahrungen für Mistelextrakte liegen in der Behandlung des Post-Covid- und Post-Vac-Syndroms vor (Soldner *et al.* 2021).

Das Potenzial der Misteltherapie, insbesondere, die Verabreichungswege und die Indikationen außerhalb der Onkologie müssen in Zukunft weiter erforscht werden.

Interessenkonflikt

Der Autor erklärt, dass keine konkurrierenden Interessen bestehen. Es erfolgten keine Zuwendungen von Mistelherstellern in den letzten Jahren. Es bestehen keine anderen Beziehungen/ Bedingungen/ Umstände, die einen potenziellen Interessenkonflikt darstellen. Der Autor hat eine Stiftungsprofessur an der Charité, die durch die Software AG Stiftung finanziert ist. Er ist im Verwaltungsrat der Weleda AG (Schweiz), die kein Mistelpräparat vertreibt, tätig.

Literatur

Axtner J, Steele M, Kroz M, Spahn G, Matthes H, Schad F: Health services research of integrative oncology in palliative care of patients with advanced pancreatic cancer. BMC Cancer. 2016; 16: 579.

Bar-Sela, G, Wollner M, Hammer L, Agbarya A, Dudnik E, Haim N: Mistletoe as complementary treatment in patients with advanced non-small-cell lung cancer treated with carboplatin-based combinations: a randomised phase II study. Eur J Cancer. 2013; 49 (5): 1058–1064.

Bonamin LV, de Carvalho AC, Waisse S: Viscum album (L.) in experimental animal tumors: A meta-analysis. Exp Ther Med. 2017; 13 (6): 2723–2740.

Büssing A: Immune modulation using mistletoe (Viscum album L.) extracts Iscador. Arzneimittelforschung. 2006; 56 (06): 508–515.

Büssing A, Raak C, Ostermann T: Quality of life and related dimensions in cancer patients treated with mistletoe extract (iscador): a meta-analysis. Evid Based Complement Alternat Med 2012: 219402.

Cleophas JT, Zwinderman HA: Modern meta-analysis: Review and update of methodologies. Springer; 2017.

Cogo E, Elsayed M, Bhardwaj S et al.: Mistletoe Extracts during the Oncological Perioperative Period: A Systematic Review and Meta-Analysis of Human Randomized Controlled Trials. Current Oncology. 2023; 30 (9): 8196–8219.

Delebinski CI, Jaeger S, Kemnitz-Hassanin K et al.: A new development of triterpene acid-containing extracts from Viscum album L. displays synergistic induction of apoptosis in acute lymphoblastic leukaemia. Cell Prolif. 2012; 45 (2): 176–187.

Delebinski CI, Twardziok M, Kleinsimon S et al.: A Natural Combination Extract of Viscum album L. Containing Both Triterpene Acids and Lectins Is Highly Effective against AML In Vivo. PLoS One. 2015; 10(8): e0133892.

Fachgesellschaften, A. d. W. M.: S3-Leitlinie Komplementärmedizin in der Behandlung von onkologischen PatientInnen (Stand: 02. August 2021).

Freuding M, Keinki C, Kutschan S et al.: Mistletoe in oncological treatment: a systematic review: Part 2: quality of life and toxicity of cancer treatment. J Cancer Res Clin Oncol. 2019a; 145 (4): 927–939.

Freuding M, Keinki C, Micke O, Buentzel J, Huebner J: Mistletoe in oncological treatment: a systematic review: Part 1: survival and safety. J Cancer Res Clin Oncol. 2019b; 145 (3): 695–707.

GAÄD (Hrsg.): Vademecum Anthroposophische Arzneimittel, 4. Auflage 2017.

Grah C: Immunmodulatorische Wirkung von Misteltherapie (Viscum album L. Extrakten) beim Lungenkarzinom. Atemwegs- und Lungenkrankheiten. 2014; 40 (1): 31–39.

Grah C, Matthes B: Fall-Kontrollanalyse zur intraläsionalen Viscum-Therapie bei endobronchial erreichbarem Bronchialkarzinom. In: Scheer R, Bauer R, Becker H et al. (Hrsg.): Fortschritte in der Misteltherapie. Essen: KVC; 2005: 499–506.

Grah C, Matthes B: Fall-Kontrollanalyse zur intraläsionalen Viscum-Therapie bei endobronchial erreichbarem Bronchialkarzinom. Pneumologie. 2006; 60 (S 1): P58.

Grah C, Matthes B, Griff S, Mairinger T: Sicherheit und Machbarkeit von endosonographisch gesteuerter transbronchialer Nadelinstillation von Viscum album zur Induktion von Apoptose in Lymphknotenmetastasen. Pneumologie. 2009; 63 (S 01): P155.

Hegde P: Therapeutic intervention in inflammatory pathologies and cancer: understanding the anti-inflammatory properties of Viscum album, Université de Technologie de Compiègne. 2013.

Huber R, Schlodder D, Effertz C, Rieger S, Tröger W: Safety of intravenously applied mistletoe extract–results from a phase I dose escalation study in patients with advanced cancer. BMC complementary and alternative medicine. 2017; 17: 1–8.

Jäger S, Winkler K, Pfüller U, Scheffler A: Solubility studies of oleanolic acid and betulinic acid in aqueous solutions and plant extracts of Viscum album L. Planta Med. 2007; 73 (2): 157–162.

Kienle GS, Kiene H: Die Mistel in der Onkologie. Stuttgart, New York: Schattauer; 2003.

Kienle GS, Mussler M, Fuchs D, Kiene H: Intravenous Mistletoe Treatment in Integrative Cancer Care: A Qualitative Study Exploring the Procedures, Concepts, and Observations of Expert Doctors. Evidence-Based Complementary and Alternative Medicine. 2016(ID 4628287): 16.

Kleinsimon S, Kauczor G, Jaeger S et al.: ViscumTT induces apoptosis and alters IAP expression in osteosarcoma in vitro and has synergistic action when combined with different chemotherapeutic drugs. BMC Complement Altern Med. 2017; 17 (1): 26.

Kuonen R, Weissenstein U, Urech K et al.: Effects of Lipophilic Extract of Viscum album L. and Oleanolic Acid on Migratory Activity of NIH/3T3 Fibroblasts and on HaCat Keratinocytes. Evid Based Complement Alternat Med. 2013: 718105.

Lavastre V, Cavalli H, Ratthe C, Girard D: Anti-inflammatory effect of Viscum album agglutinin-I (VAA-I): induction of apoptosis in activated neutrophils and inhibition of lipopolysaccharide-induced neutrophilic inflammation in vivo. Clinical & Experimental Immunology. 2004; 137(2): 272–278.

Loef M, Walach H: Quality of life in cancer patients treated with mistletoe: a systematic review and meta-analysis. BMC Complement Med Ther. 2020; 20(1): 227.

Mabed M, El-Helw L, Shamaa S: Phase II study of Viscum Fraxini-2 in patients with advanced hepatocellular carcinoma. Br J Cancer. 2004; 90 (1): 65–69.

Macaskill P, Gatsonis C, Deeks J, Harbord R and Y Takwoingi: Cochrane handbook for systematic reviews of diagnostic test accuracy, Version 1.0. 2010.

Matthes H: Viscum album in the therapy of primary inoperable hepatocellular carcinoma (HCC). Gastroenterology. 2004; 126: A665.

Matthes H: Die Misteltherapie in der Onkologie „Stellenwert und Ausblick" Symposium medical – Naturheilkunde. 2006; 7: 10–14.

Matthes H, Buchwald D, Schad F, Jeschke E: Intratumorale Applikation von Viscum album L. (Mistelgesamtextrakt; Helixor M®) in der Therapie des inoperablen Pankreaskarzinom. Z Gastroenterologie. 2007; 45: doi: 10.1055/s-2007-988162.

Matthes H, Hofheinz RD, Bar-Sela G et al.: Letter to the editors of the Journal of Cancer Research and Clinical Oncology. J Cancer Res Clin Oncol. 2019; 145(9): 2405–2407.

Matthes H, Schad F, Buchwald D, Schenk G: Endoscopic Ultrasound-Guided Fine-Needle Injection of Viscum album L. (mistletoe; Helixor M) in the Therapy of Primary Inoperable Pancreas Cancer: a Pilot Study. Gastoenterology. 2005; 128 (4 Suppl. 2): 433: T 988.

Matthes H, Thronicke A, Hofheinz R-D et al.: Statement to an Insufficient Systematic Review on Viscum album L. Therapy. Evidence-Based Complementary and Alternative Medicine 2020: 1–9.

Nicoletti M: The Anti-Inflammatory Activity of Viscum album. Plants. 2023; 12 (7): 1460.

Oei SL, Thronicke A, Kröz M et al.: The Internal Coherence of Breast Cancer Patients Is Associated with the Decision-Making for Chemotherapy and Viscum album L. Treatment. Evid Based Complement Alternat Med. 2018: 1065271.

Oei SL, Thronicke A, Kröz M et al.: Supportive Effect of Viscum album L. extracts on the inner feeling of Warmth in Non-metastasized Breast

Cancer Patients. European Journal of Integrative Medicine. 2017; 27: 97–104.

Oei SL, Thronicke A, Kröz M et al.: Impact of Oncological Therapy and Viscum album L. Treatment on Cancer-Related Fatigue and Internal Coherence in Nonmetastasized Breast Cancer Patients. Integr Cancer Ther. 2020; 19: 1534735420917211.

Ostermann T, Appelbaum S, Poier D et al.: A Systematic Review and Meta-Analysis on the Survival of Cancer Patients Treated with a Fermented Viscum album L. Extract (Iscador): An Update of Findings. Complement Med Res. 2020; 27 (4): 260–271.

Piao BK, Wang YX, Xie GR et al.: Impact of complementary mistletoe extract treatment on quality of life in breast, ovarian and non-small cell lung cancer patients. A prospective randomized controlled clinical trial. Anticancer Res. 2004; 24 (1): 303–309.

Schad F, Axtner J, Buchwald D et al.: Intratumoral mistletoe (Viscum album L.) therapy in patients with unresectable pancreas carcinoma – a retrospective analysis. Integrative Cancer Therapies. 2013. doi: 10.1177/1534735413513637.

Schad F, Buchwald D, Merkle A, Popp S, Kroez M and H Matthes: Retrospective analysis of patients with advanced pancreatic cancer under palliative treatment and additive intratumoral application of Viscum album L. J Clin Oncol. 2011; 29(suppl): abstr e14538.

Schad F, Kästner A, Matthes B et al.: Health service research study with cohort design measuring survival of colorectal cancer (CRC) patients treated with and without Viscum album L. 1st European Congress for Integrative medicine. The future of comprehensive patient care. European Journal of Integrative medicine. 2008; 1 (Suppl. 1): S27.

Schad F, Thronicke A, Merkle A et al.: Implementation of an Integrative Oncological Concept in the Daily Care of a German Certified Breast Cancer Center. Complement Med Res. 2018; 25 (2): 85–91.

Schad F, Thronicke A, Steele M et al.: Overall survival of stage IV non-small cell lung cancer (NSCLC) patients treated with Viscum album L. in additon to standard care, under revision July 2018. PLOS ONE. 2017.

Schad F, Thronicke A, Steele ML et al.: Overall survival of stage IV non-small cell lung cancer patients treated with Viscum album L. in addition to chemotherapy, a real-world observational multicenter analysis. PLOS ONE. 2018; 1: 1–19.

Seifert G, Jesse P, Laengler A et al.: Molecular mechanisms of mistletoe plant extract-induced apoptosis in acute lymphoblastic leukemia in vivo and in vitro. Cancer Lett. 2008; 264 (2): 218–228.

Soldner G, Heine R, Matthes H et al.: Long-COVID aus Sicht der Anthroposophischen Medizin – Symptome und Behandlungsmöglichkeiten. Anthromedics, Gesellschaft Anthroposopischer Ärzte in Deutschland, Medizinische Sektion am Goetheanum. 2021.

Steele ML, Axtner J, Happe A et al.: Adverse Drug Reactions and Expected Effects to Therapy with Subcutaneous Mistletoe Extracts (Viscum album L.) in Cancer Patients. Evid Based Complement Alternat Med. 2014; 724258.

Steele ML, Axtner J, Happe A et al.: Safety of Intravenous Application of Mistletoe (Viscum album L.) Preparations in Oncology: An Observational Study. Evid Based Complement Alternat Med. 2014; 236310.

Steele ML, Axtner J, Happe A et al.: Use and safety of intratumoral application of European mistletoe (Viscum album L) preparations in Oncology. Integr Cancer Ther. 2015; 14 (2): 140–148.

Stumpf C, Ramirez-Martinez S, Becher A etz al.: Intratumorale Mistelapplikation bei stenosierendem Rezidiv eines Cardia-Carzinoms. Erfahrungsheilkunde. 1997; 46: 509–513.

Stumpf C, Ramirez-Martinez S, Becher A, Stein GM, Büssing A und M Schietzel: Intratumorale Mistelapplikation bei stenosierendem Rezidiv eines Cardia-Carcinoms. Der Merkurstab. 1998; 2(51): 85-88.

Thronicke A, Matthes B, von Trott P et al.: Overall survival of nonmetastasized NSCLC patients treated with add-on Viscum album L: a multicenter real-world study. Integrative cancer therapies. 2020; 19: 1534735420940384.

Thronicke A, Schad F, Debus M et al.: Viscum album L. therapy in oncology: An update on current evidence. Complementary Medicine Research. 2022; 29(4): 362-368.

Tröger W, Galun D, Reif M et al.: Viscum album [L.] extract therapy in patients with locally advanced or metastatic pancreatic cancer: a randomised clinical trial on overall survival. Eur J Cancer. 2013; 49 (18): 3788–3797.

Tröger W, Jezdic S, Zdrale Z et al.: Quality of life and neutropenia in patients with early stage breast cancer: a randomized pilot study comparing additional treatment with mistletoe extract to chemotherapy alone. Breast Cancer. 2009; 16 (3): 35–45.

Tröger W, Zdrale Z, Tišma N, Matijasevic M: Additional Therapy with a Mistletoe Product during Adjuvant Chemotherapy of Breast Cancer Patients Improves Quality of Life: An Open Randomized Clinical Pilot Trial. Evid Based Complement Altern Med. 2014; 2014:430518. doi: 10.1155/2014/430518.

Twardziok M, Kleinsimon S, Rolff J et al.: Multiple Active Compounds from Viscum album L. Synergistically Converge to Promote Apoptosis in Ewing Sarcoma. PLoS One. 2016; 11(9): e0159749.

Twardziok M, Meierhofer D, Borno S et al.: Transcriptomic and proteomic insight into the effects of a defined European mistletoe extract in Ewing sarcoma cells reveals cellular stress responses. BMC Complement Altern Med. 2017; 17 (1): 237.

Urech K, Scher JM, Hostanska K, Becker H: Apoptosis inducing activity of viscin, a lipophilic extract from Viscum album L. J Pharm Pharmacol. 2005; 57 (1): 101–109.

Vicas S, Prokisch J, Rugina OD, Socaciu C: Hydrophilic and Lipophilic Antioxidant Activities of Mistletoe (Viscum album) as determined by FRAP method. Notulae Botanicae Horti Agrobotanici Cluj-Napoca. 2009; 37 (2): 112–116.

Ziegler R, Grossarth-Maticek R: Individual Patient Data Meta-analysis of Survival and Psychosomatic Self-regulation from Published Prospective Controlled Cohort Studies for Long-term Therapy of Breast Cancer Patients with a Mistletoe Preparation (Iscador). Evid Based Complement Alternat Med. 2010; 7 (2): 157–166.

Zuzak TJ, Wasmuth A, Bernitzki S et al.: Safety of high-dose intravenous mistletoe therapy in pediatric cancer patients: a case series. Complement Ther Med. 2018; 40: 198–202.

Prof. Dr. med. Harald Matthes
Gemeinschaftskrankenhaus Havelhöhe gGmbH, Kladower Damm 221, 14089 Berlin, Deutschland
Medizinische Klinik für Gastroenterologie, Infektiologie und Rheumatologie CBF und Institut für Sozialmedizin, Epidemiologie und Gesundheitsökonomie CCM, Charité-Universitätsmedizin Berlin, Deutschland

Korrespondenzadresse:
hmatthes@havelhoehe.de

Das Meridiansystem als neue Basis für die Misteltherapie

The Meridian System as the New Basis of Mistletoe Therapy

Johannes Wilkens

Zusammenfassung
Wissenschaftliche Studien zur Misteltherapie streben normalerweise den Nachweis der Wirksamkeit auf Tumorzellen an. Dieses Vorgehen entspricht aber nur teilweise Rudolf Steiners Intentionen. Er postulierte, dass der Effekt der Mistel je nach Wirtsbaum stark variiert und dass die Mistel vor allem die Seele und das funktionelle System stärke. In der Anthroposophischen Medizin werden diese Kräfte als Astralleib und Ätherleib bezeichnet. Vor allem die Bedeutung des Ätherleibs ist auch der Traditionellen Chinesischen Medizin bekannt.
Der Autor zeigte, dass die 13 Mistel-Wirtsbäume mit 12 Meridianen aus dem System der TCM korrespondieren. Seine Forschung bestätigte, dass sich das Meridiansystem der TCM für die Suche nach dem geeigneten Wirtsbaum für den jeweiligen Patienten eignet. Die Eichenmistel korrespondiert mit dem Lebermeridian, die Bergahornmistel entspricht den Beschwerden, die mit dem Milz-Pankreas-Meridian assoziiert sind. Die Weidenmistel ist mit dem Blasenmeridian verbunden und daher für zahlreiche schwere Erkrankungen der Wirbelsäule geeignet. Das Meridiansystem eignet sich also sehr gut für die Suche nach der für den Patienten adäquaten Mistel und erweitert die Therapiemöglichkeiten.
Schlüsselwörter: Misteltherapie, Wirtsbaum, Meridiansystem, TCM

Summary
Scientific studies on mistletoe therapy usually aim to prove its efficacy on tumor cells. However, this approach only partially corresponds to Rudolf Steiner's intentions. He postulated that the effect of mistletoe varies greatly depending on the host tree and that mistletoe strengthens the soul and the functional system.

In Anthroposophic medicine, these forces are referred to as the astral body and etheric body. Above all, the importance of the etheric body is also known in Traditional Chinese Medicine.
The author showed that the 13 mistletoe host trees correspond to 12 meridians from the TCM system. His research confirmed that the meridian system of TCM is suitable for the search for the appropriate host tree for the respective patient. The oak mistletoe corresponds to the liver meridian, the sycamore mistletoe corresponds to the complaints associated with the spleen-pancreatic meridian. Willow mistletoe is connected to the bladder meridian and is therefore suitable for numerous serious diseases of the spine. The meridian system is therefore very well suited for the search for the mistletoe that is adequate for the patient and expands the treatment options.
Keywords: Mistletoe therapy, host trees, meridian system, TCM

Einleitung

Bisherige wissenschaftliche Studien zur Misteltherapie zielten auf den Nachweis der Wirksamkeit auf Tumorzellen ab. Auch wenn dies eine wichtige Grundlage für künftige Forschung darstellt, entspricht dieses Vorgehen nur teilweise Rudolf Steiners Intentionen. Der Begründer der Misteltherapie postulierte, dass der Effekt der Mistel je nach Wirtsbaum stark variiert und dass die Mistel vor allem die seelischen Qualitäten und das funktionelle System stärke. In der Anthroposophischen Medizin werden diese Kräfte als Astralleib und Ätherleib bezeichnet. Dass Verständnis vom Ätherleib ist auch in der Traditionellen Chinesischen Medizin gut bekannt und wird dort Chi genannt.

Der Autor zeigte vor 21 Jahren, dass die 13 Mistel-Wirtsbäume, die in der Onkologie eingesetzt werden, weniger mit den Körper-Organen als vielmehr mit den Qualitäten der 12 Meridiane aus dem System der TCM korrespondieren. Nach 2002 demonstrierte er die Bedeutung des jeweiligen Wirtsbaumes in Fallstudien und Baum-Darstellungen. Demnach eignet sich das Meridiansystem der TCM für die Suche nach dem geeigneten Wirtsbaum in der individualisierten Krebstherapie. Die Eichenmistel hat natürlich einen Effekt auf die Leber, korrespondiert aber noch mehr mit allen Beschwerden im Verlauf des Lebermeridians. Die

Bergahornmistel kann gegen neuroendokrine Tumoren eingesetzt werden, entspricht aber fast exakt den Beschwerden, die mit dem Milz-Pankreas-Meridian assoziiert sind. Die Weidenmistel wirkt spezifisch bei Blasenkarzinomen. Da der Blasenmeridian aber paravertebral verläuft, ist die Weidenmistel ebenso für zahlreiche schwere Erkrankungen der Wirbelsäule, z. B. Fibromyalgie, geeignet.

Das Meridiansystem eignet sich also sehr gut für die Suche nach der richtigen Mistel und erweitert zudem die Therapiemöglichkeiten. Das System der 12 Meridiane wird im Folgenden in seiner besonderen Beziehung zur Mistel vorgestellt.

Die Mistel in der anthroposophischen Krebstherapie

Dass die Mistel eine spezifische Heilpflanze gegen die Krebserkrankung darstellt, daran kann es letztlich wissenschaftlich kaum mehr einen Zweifel geben. Sie ist damit neben der Eibe eines der wenigen Heilmittel aus der Natur, denen eine Wirksamkeit bei dieser Erkrankung zugesprochen werden muss. Pflanzen, die so auffallend anders sind wie die Mistel, verfügen über besondere Inhaltsstoffe. So enthalten Mistelextrakte neben Schleim (und Mistelleim) unterschiedliche Eiweißverbindungen (Mistellektine, Viscotoxine), Mineral- und Farbstoffe sowie Hunderte anderer Substanzen. All diese Inhaltsstoffe – und die Mistellektine und Viscotoxine sind nur ein kleiner Teil davon – wirken zusammen, also synergistisch und als Gesamtextrakt.

So unzweifelhaft deren Bedeutung auch sein mag, man vergisst hier das eigentliche Agens der Misteltherapie: die Kräfte des jeweiligen Wirtsbaums. Der Begründer der Misteltherapie, Rudolf Steiner, äußert sich diesbezüglich eigentlich sehr unmissverständlich:

> „(...) die Mistel in entsprechender Weise nun so verarbeitet, daß sie dieses dem Baum Ätherische wirklich auf den Menschen übertragen kann, was unter Umständen durch Injektionen geschieht –, dieses sagt uns: die Mistel übernimmt als äußere Substanz dasjenige, was wuchernde Äthersubstanz beim Karzinom ist, verstärkt dadurch,

> daß sie die physische Substanz zurückdrängt, die Wirkung des astralischen Leibes und bringt dadurch den Tumor des Karzinoms zum Aufbröckeln, zum In-sich-Zerfallen. So daß, wenn wir die Mistelsubstanz in den menschlichen Organismus hineinbringen, wir tatsächlich die Äthersubstanz des Baumes in den Menschen hineinbringen, und die Äthersubstanz des Baumes also, auf dem Wege durch den Mistelträger in den Menschen übergeführt, wirkt verstärkend auf den astralischen Leib des Menschen." (Steiner 1923/1924)

Damit ist die Misteltherapie eigentlich eine Visco-Dendrologie, eine Therapie mit den jeweiligen Kräften des Wirtsbaums der Mistel. Die Mistel entspricht botanisch funktionell dem Krebsgeschehen, wie es bei Scheffler (2001) bereits ausführlich dargestellt worden ist.

Weniger Gedanken hatte man sich lange zu den Wirtsbäumen gemacht. Doch in den letzten Jahren zeigte es sich immer mehr: Der Wirtsbaum mit seinen Kräften entspricht dem jeweiligen Träger des Krebsprozesses. Die Mistelwirksamkeit ist schon in physiologischen Dosierungen je nach Wirtsbaum am betroffenen Menschen recht unterschiedlich, obwohl alle Wirtsbäume starke Rötungen und Schwellungen mit Fieber hervorrufen können. Schwere allergische Erscheinungen finden sich gehäuft nach einer Birkenmistelinjektion oder mehr blasenbildende Erscheinungen bei der Pappelmistel, hingegen eher schwache Reaktionen auf die Nadelbaummisteln. Diese physischen Reaktionen sind dennoch allgemein gehalten.

Das wird schon anders, wenn die Misteln homöopathisch potenziert werden, wie es von zwei Firmen, der Abnoba und der WALA, mit den Iscucinen erfolgt (Wilkens 2007; 2008a; 2008b; 2010; Wilkens, Mandera 2012; Mandera, Wilkens 2017; Wilkens, Meyer 2022). Je höher hier die Potenzierung, desto klarer bildet sich dabei ein jeweiliger Typus des Wirtsbaums aus. Abnoba führt diese Potenzierungen im Dezimalbereich bis zur D30 durch, die Iscucine werden hingegen im Verhältnis 1:20 über acht Stufen von H bis A potenziert. Das ist so auch von Rudolf Steiner und seiner ärztlichen Mitarbeiterin Ita Wegman gefordert worden (Wegman 2000).

Es geht natürlich auch bei einer Misteltherapie um das physische Zerstören des Tumors, mehr aber um die Stärkung der übergeordneten Ebenen des Ätherleibs, des Astralleibs und der Ich-Ebene.

Die Wirkung einer Misteltherapie ist entsprechend vor allem an einer Steigerung der Lebensqualität erkenntlich, was so ja auch wissenschaftlich vielfältig bestätigt worden ist (Loef, Walach 2020; Brandenburger *et al.* 2013). Das „Zerbröseln" eines Tumors ist hingegen eher selten und setzt meistens – wo dieses erfolgreich ist – heftige Fieberzustände (von Schoen-Angerer *et al.* 2015) voraus.

Wesensmerkmale und Typologie der Bäume

Bei den aus der Mistel durch Potenzierung und andere Verfahren hergestellten Arzneimitteln lassen sich tatsächlich viele Wesensmerkmale der Bäume finden. Wir versuchen das Charakteristische ihrer Wirtsbäume anhand ihrer botanischen Phänomene zu begreifen, aber auch anhand der Phänomene, die uns unsere Patienten Tag für Tag liefern nach den Injektionen mit den entsprechenden Wirtsbäumen.

Vom Autor werden im Jahr ca. 500–700 Patienten auf eine Mistel eingestellt, und so lassen sich Phänomene am Patienten leicht beobachten und systematisieren.

Als Beispiel sehen wir unten Symptome, die Patienten nach Injektionen mit der Birkenmistel aufwiesen. Wer die Fähigkeit hat, etwas genauer auf die Erfahrungen der Patienten zu hören und diese Wirkungen zu dokumentieren, der sieht tatsächlich einen Strauß an Reaktionen, die sich nicht nur auf die Physis beziehen, sondern gerade funktionelle und seelische Veränderungen beinhaltet.

Kleine Auswahl von Reaktionen auf die Injektionen 20 mg – D30:

Fast regelmäßig allergische Erscheinungen
Allergische Reaktionen, Schwellung der Brust auf doppelte Größe, Fließschnupfen, tränende Augen, Hautjucken, Allergie mit Schüttelfrost, Nesselfieber, Gelenkschmerzen.

Todesaspekte
Früher Angst vor dem Sterben, schon als Kind Angst vorm Tod.
Träumt nur schrecklich, nie schön, Träume vom Tod.
Nach den Birkeninjektionen verschwinden diese seelischen Erlebnisse.

Hautveränderungen
Pityriasis nach Tod des 3. Kindes
Heißer roter Fleck am Sitzbein.
Gefühl, Haare werden wieder brauner.
Will keine dunklen Farben mehr tragen und auch kein Make-up (nach 30 Jahren).

Alte Liebe, falscher Ehemann
Träumt seit mehr als 30 Jahren jede Nacht von ihrem ersten Freund.
Im Traum wurde ihr klar, dass sie den falschen Mann geheiratet hat.
Ehemann ist wie eine dunkle Wolke, zu hart.

Aus diesen und vielen anderen Symptomen ergibt sich dann eine Art „idealer Typus“, der besonders auf diesen Mistelbaum reagiert. Am Beispiel Birkenmistel ergibt sich:

> Die Birkenmistel repräsentiert den ästhetisch feinsinnigen Typus mit zahlreichen Allergien und/oder Heuschnupfen. Bei Tumoren der Haut und der Mamma sowie dem Ovar. Bei weißem und schwarzem Hautkrebs. Konstitutionsbezogen bei eher nordischem, hellhäutigem Typus, v.a. bei feingliedrigen, dennoch tatkräftigen und empfindsamen Patienten. Neigung zu chronischen Blasenentzündungen oder Nierenbeckenentzündungen. Auf der Suche nach der richtigen Liebe selbst noch im Alter.

In dieser Weise ließ sich vom Autor in den letzten 21 Jahren eine Typologie von allen 13 aktuell auf dem Markt erhältlichen Mistelbäumen durchführen (Wilkens, Böhm 2015) und damit eine individualisierte Krebstherapie erarbeiten.

Diese Typussuche erscheint aber auch wieder etwas subjektiv einseitig und lässt sich nur schwer operationalisieren.

Es war dem Autor schon 2002 (Wilkens 2003) aufgefallen, dass die jeweiligen erarbeiteten Typusideen sich recht genau auch in der chinesischen Medizin in der Lehre von den Meridianen wiederfinden. Die 12 (13) Mistelbäume stellen sich exakt als einseitige Ausprägung eines Meridians dar. Diese Erkenntnisse haben sich in den letzten zwei Jahrzehnten sowohl bei mir als auch bei Mitarbeitern des Instituts für Naturheilkunde und Traditionelle Chinesische Medizin der Universität Essen bestätigt.

Erleichtert wird diese Suche nach dem richtigen Typus nun durch ein zugelassenes Medizinprodukt, das die Meridiane sehr genau und reliabel zu messen vermag. Das System PROGNOS® gehört zu den Methoden der Elektro-Akupunktur-Diagnostik, d. h., auf Grund der Erfassung der elektrophysiologischen Eigenschaften der Haut im Areal der Akupunkturpunkte werden die verschiedenen Aspekte des Gesundheitszustandes ausgewertet. Schon allein durch eine derartige Untersuchung können Schwachpunkte im Bereich des Chi oder des Ätherleibes erkannt werden.

Es ist nun aber gelungen, die jeweiligen Misteln als Frequenz zu speichern und über einen Kopfhörer dem jeweiligen Patienten einzuspielen. In den meisten Fällen wird zu Beginn einer Misteltherapie das Meridianfeld sehr stark und von vielen unterschiedlichen Misteln verändert, so als ob zu Beginn vor allem die Wirksamkeit der Mistel im Vordergrund stehen würde. Im weiteren Verlauf sind es hingegen in der Regel spezifische Bäume, die stärker reagieren.

Die Ergebnisse dieser Untersuchungen in Verbindung mit dem Ort des Tumors und auch dem Typus des Patienten lassen in der Regel dann eine adäquate Zuordnung des „richtigen Mistelbaumes“ zu.

Der Vorteil in der Integration der Bedeutung des jeweiligen Mistelbaumes liegt auf der Hand: Mistel ist nicht gleich Mistel, und so verschieden wie die Tumoren sind eben die jeweiligen Patienten. Gleichwohl wird hierdurch auch die Planung von neuen Studien zur Mistel erleichtert. Auf der einen Seite bestätigen unsere Erfahrungen Studien zur Mistel an bestimmten Organen. Es ist kein Zufall, dass die Eichenmistel vor allem auf Lebermetastasen wie bei einem Pankreaskarzinom eine zentrale Rolle spielt. Diese Wirkung wäre vermutlich mit einer Kiefernmistel nicht annährend so gut ausgefallen.

Erst mit einer (Eichen-)Mistel verdoppeln sich die Überlebenszeiten beim Pankreaskarzinom (Tröger *et al.* 2013). Erst der Einsatz einer Ulmenmistel beim Pleuramesotheliom (Wilkens 2020) führt zu erstaunlichen Überlebenszeiten, die vorher kaum je erreicht wurden. So lässt sich unter Berücksichtigung der Mistelbaumvielfalt a priori sagen, dass aufgrund der Entsprechung von Milz-Pankreasmeridian und der Bergahornmistel diese sich vor allem für die Behandlung von neuroendokrinen Tumoren (Wilkens, Meyer 2022) eignet. In gleicher Weise konnte bestätigt werden, dass beim Blasenkarzinom die Weidenmistel von größter Wichtigkeit ist (von Schoen-Angerer *et al.* 2015), diese aber auch darüber hinaus vielen Menschen mit einer Fibromyalgie (Soldner *et al.* 2005) zu helfen vermag, da zahlreiche Triggerpunkte sich auf dem Blasenmeridian befinden.

Kurzum, erst durch die Anregungen bezüglich der Baumvielfalt kommt es zu einem lebendigen Austausch mit den Patienten, der über eine abstrakte nüchterne Beschreibung von Labordaten hinaus geht.

Aufgrund dieser vielfältigen Erfahrungen bestätigt sich, dass die Misteln echte Alleskönner sind und in ihren Fähigkeiten nicht nur auf die Endstadien von Krebserkrankungen zu reduzieren sind, wo sie in Deutschland aktuell noch als Kassenleistung bezahlt werden (palliative Situation).

Bereits Rudolf Steiner als Begründer der Misteltherapie in der Onkologie hat von den Ärzten gefordert, dass sie den Blick auf die Krebs-Prophylaxe, die Vorbeugung richten und sie angeregt, die Misteltherapie frühzeitig einzusetzen. Wenn der Krebs erst einmal da ist, dann kommt auch die Mistel oft zu spät. Aus den modernen Forschungen zur Krebserkrankung ist deutlich geworden, dass der Weg bis zum endgültigen Krebsgeschehen lang ist und oft jahrzehntelanger „Vorbereitung" bedarf. Es wird dieses in der modernen Forschung mit komplexen genetischen Prozessen und falschen Zellteilungen (Mutationen) erklärt. Fast immer gehen dem Krebs chronische Entzündungen voraus. Vielfach lassen sich diese Vorgänge durch gängige Laboruntersuchungen nicht nachweisen.

Umso wichtiger ist es für uns geworden, einen Blick und ein Gespür dafür zu entwickeln, wenn ein Mensch besonders gefährdet ist, Krebs zu entwickeln.

Bedeutende Einsichten verdanken wir heute der Statistik und der Einführung des Begriffes der Präkanzerose. Unter einer Präkanzerose versteht man eine Gewebeveränderung, die mit einem statistisch erhöhten Risiko für eine spätere krebsartige Entartung einhergeht. Darunter fallen Erkrankungen wie die Kolitis ulcerosa, die Leberzirrhose, sowie Krebsvorstufen wie die aktinische Keratose der Haut und die Leukoplakie der Mundschleimhaut. Diese Erkrankungen können nach einem gewissen Zeitraum in einer Krebserkrankung münden. Häufiger ist dies der Fall bei Erkrankungen wie der Dysplasie (Entartung) der Schleimhaut am Gebärmutterhals. Auch bei zahlreichen anderen Erkrankungen wie der Divertikulose oder selbst bei einem M. Parkinson ist ein gehäuftes Auftreten von bestimmten Krebserkrankungen belegt. Nicht zu vergessen sind die Autoimmunerkrankungen, die immunsuppressiv über einen längeren Zeitraum behandelt worden sind wie die rheumatoide Polyarthritis (Gelenkrheuma) und die multiple Sklerose. Bei diesen Erkrankungen sollte der Einsatz einer (homöopathisierten) Mistel ernsthaft erwogen und geprüft werden.

Da wir insgesamt in einer krebsfördernden, „karzinogenen" Gesellschaft leben, ist leider die Präkanzerose fast schon allumfassend ein gesellschaftliches Problem geworden. Wenn wir in einem modernen Auto mit Nanopartikelausstoß fahren, erhöht dieses ähnlich wie das Zigarettenrauchen das Lungenkarzinomrisiko. Wenn wir häufig mit dem Flieger von Ost nach West und *vice versa* fliegen, dann erhöht sich das Hautkrebsrisiko. Wer gerne ins Solarium geht steigert dieses Risiko fast ins Unverantwortliche hinein. Kurzum, überall lauert das Krebsrisiko und es ist kaum zu vermeiden. Insofern ist eine grundlegende Prophylaxe heutzutage geradezu eine medizinische Notwendigkeit.

Zur Vereinfachung in der Suche nach der richtigen Mistel kann neben den Meridianen auch dieses Schema aus einem Artikel (Abb. 1, Wilkens 2020) dienen. Je nach Temperament, das mit einem bestimmen Körperbau einhergeht, und dem Schwerpunkt der Beschwerden werden unterschiedliche Bäume notwendig sein. So bei Rheumatikern mit hagerer

Gestalt und traurigem Habitus eher die Weidenmistel, bei trägen adipösen Patienten mit Unterleibsbeschwerden (Obelixtypus) die Apfelmistel, hingegen bei temperamentvollem energischem Typus die Eiche (Asterixtypus). Miraculix wird hingegen eher von einer Birkenmistel profitieren.

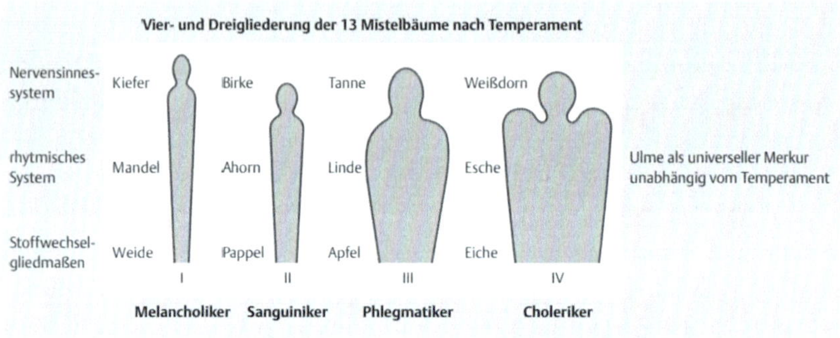

Abb. 1: Vier- und Dreigliederung der 13 Mistelbäume nach Temperament

Insgesamt ergibt sich, dass erst der vielfältige Einsatz unterschiedlicher Mistelbäume die Therapie wesentlich erleichtert, andererseits aber auch die Notwendigkeit eines Ausbruchs aus der Erstarrung bisheriger Denkgewohnheiten notwendig macht. Erste Schritte sind gemacht. Es ist zu hoffen, dass weitere folgen werden.

Die Meridiane in Abbildung 2 stehen für bestimmte Kräfte, aber auch seelische Sachverhalte. In Kombination mit den anderen dargestellten Schemata lässt sich ein Mistelbaum vergleichsweise einfach finden. Die Wirkung der Mistel wird durch den parallelen Einsatz von Metallzusätzen wie bei Iscador oder einer ergänzenden Metalltherapie wesentlich verbessert.

Meridian	Problem	Mistel	Ergänzendes Metall	System
Lunge	Innere unterdrückte Wut (Mandel), Misstrauen, Enttäuschung, Süchte (Ulme), Benebelung	Ulme bei extrovertiertem Typus Mandel bei Introversion	Ulme: Quecksilber und Zinn Mandel: Gold oder Silber	*Immunsystem*
Dickdarm	Schamgefühl, nicht zu sich stehen, Ideal versus Wirklichkeit	Apfel	Silber, Quecksilber, Antimon	*Lymphsystem*
Magen	Kühle Distanz, Starre, alles auf sich beziehen, Stolz, Hypochondrie	Tanne	Blei oder Silber	*Säure-Basen-Haushalt*
Milz-Pankreas	Pseudodemut, Grübeln, Entscheidungsschwäche, Hast und Hektik	Ahorn	Platin, Zink	*Blut, Nahrungsrhythmus, Kohlenhydratstoffwechsel*
Herz	Gestaute oder unterdrückte Gefühle, Workaholic, Reizbarkeit	Weißdorn	Gold	*Rhythmen, Gefühle*
Dünndarm	Überhöhte Ansprüche, sich nichts gönnen, Schuldgefühle, Zwänge	Kiefer	Arseneisen, Eisen Kupfer	*Resorption*
Blase	Melancholie, nicht vergeben können, wie außen vor, Groll, Neid	Weide	Silber	*Sexualität, Vitalität*
Niere	Extrovertiertheit, starke seelische Beeinflussbarkeit, auf der Suche nach Liebe	Birke	Kupfer	*Flüssigkeit, Elektrolyte*
Kreislauf	Erregbar, unstet, Oberflächlichkeit	Pappel	Silber	*Blutdruck, Durchblutung*
Dreifacher Erwärmer	Opferbereitschaft, Diakonissensyndrom, Erschöpfung	Esche	Gold	*Endokrinum (Hormonhaushalt)*
Galle	Verkrampfungen, familiäre Harmoniestörungen, Verdrängungen, Nachgiebigkeit	Linde	Kupfer, Quecksilber, Silber	*Fettstoffwechsel*
Leber	Verharren, nichts ändern wollen, innere Verarmung, Alkoholsucht	Eiche	Eisen und Kupfer	*Eiweißstoffwechsel*

Abb. 2: Meridiane und Mistelwirtsbäume

Interessenkonflikt

Johannes Wilkens erhielt Vortragshonorare von der Firma WALA.

Literatur

Brandenburger M, Simões-Wüst A P, Rostock M et al.: Lebensqualität von Krebspatienten währen der Misteltherapie – Eine explorative Studie mit dem zusätzlichen Einsatz von Fragebögen. In: Scheer R, Alban S, Becker H et al. (Eds): Die Mistel in der Tumortherapie 3. Essen: KVC; 2013: 379–388.

Loef M, Walach H. Quality of life in cancer patients treated with mistletoe: a systematic review and meta-analysis. BMC Complement Med Ther. 2020; 20 (1): 227. doi: 10.1186/s12906-020-03013-3.

Mandera R, Wilkens J: Die Bergahornmistel. Der Merkurstab. 2017; 70 (3): 200–220.

Scheffler A: Heilpflanzenerkenntnis aus Sicht der anthroposophischen Medizin am Bespiel der Mistel Viscum album L. In: Scheer R, Bauer R, Becker H et al. (Hrsg.): Die Mistel in der Tumortherapie. Essen: KVC; 2001: 519–558.

von Schoen-Angerer T, Wilkens J, Kienle GS et al.: High-Dose Viscum album Extract Treatment in the Prevention of Recurrent Bladder Cancer: A Retrospective Case Series. Perm J. 2015; 19 (4): 76–83.

Soldner G, Sommer M, Teut M, Wilkens J: Die Behandlung des Fibromyalgiesyndroms mit Weidenmistelextrakten. Der Merkurstab. 2005; 4: 264–271.

Steiner R: Gesamtausgabe 319: Anthroposophische Menschenerkenntnis und Medizin. Elf Vorträge gehalten in verschiedenen Städten 1923/1924.

Tröger W, Galun D, Reif M et al.: Viscum album [L.] extract therapy in patients with locally advanced or metastatic pancreatic cancer: a randomised clinical trial on overall survival. Eur J Cancer. 2013; 49 (18): 3788–3797.

Wegman I: Beiblätter der Zeitschrift Natura Nr. 1–2, September 1927. Dornach: Natura; 2000.

Wilkens J: Die Differenzierung der Wirtsbäume der Mistel nach homöopathischem Typus, Temperament und Meridian. Erfahrungsheilkunde. 2003; 52 (6): 404–412.

Wilkens J: Die Weidenmistel beim Blasenkarzinom. Der Merkurstab. 2007; 60 (5): 446–449.

Wilkens J: Die Eschenmistel. Der Merkurstab. 2008a; 61 (1): 68–76.

Wilkens J: Die Weißtannenmistel. Der Merkurstab. 2008b; 61 (6): 570–583.

Wilkens J: Die Mandelmistel. Der Merkurstab. 2010; 63 (1): 29–45.

Wilkens J, Mandera R: Die Ulmenmistel. Der Merkurstab. 2012; 65 (5): 432–447.

Wilkens J, Böhm G: Misteln – kraftvolle Krebsheiler aus der Natur. Aarau: AT; 2015.

Wilkens J, Meyer F: Die Birkenmistel. Der Merkurstab. 2022; 75 (1): 42–51.

Wilkens J: Homöopathisierte Misteltherapie beim CUP-Syndrom Können homöopathisierte Misteln eine Therapieoption beim CUP-Syndrom bilden? Erfahrungsheilkunde. 2020; 69 (05): 260–264.

Wilkens J, Steuer G, Meyer F: The Importance of Elm Mistletoe in the Therapy of Malignant Pleural Mesothelioma. Clinical Case Reports International. 2020; www.clinicalcasereportsint.com/open-access/the-importance-of-elm-mistletoe-in-the-therapy-of-malignant-5805.pdf (Stand: 1.3.2024).

Wilkens J: Die neun Mistelwirtsbäume von abnobaVISCUM. Öschelbronner Akzente; 2023/2024.

Dr. Johannes Wilkens
Ärztlicher Direktor der Alexander von Humboldtklinik, Bad Steben, Deutschland

Korrespondenzadresse:
Dr.wilkens@humboldtklinik.de

Die klinische Studienlage zur Misteltherapie in der Onkologie – in systematischen Reviews, Metaanalysen und Leitlinien

Current State of Clinical Studies on Mistletoe Therapy in Oncology – Including Systematic Reviews, Meta-Analyses and Guidelines

Matthias Rostock, Mirjam Wüsthof, Alena Krause, Alina Busch

Zusammenfassung

Die aktuell vorliegenden systematischen Reviews haben zu sehr unterschiedlichen Einschätzungen der Misteltherapie in der Behandlung von Menschen mit einer Krebserkrankung geführt. Freuding *et al.* (2019) haben in zwei systematischen Reviews zur Bewertung der antitumoralen Wirksamkeit und zur Bewertung der Wirksamkeit auf die Lebensqualität keinerlei Vorteil für die Misteltherapie gesehen. Ostermann *et al.* (2020) haben in ihrem systematischen Review der kontrollierten Studien mit fermentiertem Mistelextrakt eine antitumorale Wirksamkeit konstatiert. Loef und Walach (2020; 2022) sehen in ihren Reviews sowohl eine antitumorale Wirksamkeit der untersuchten nicht fermentierten Mistelextrakte als auch eine Wirksamkeit hinsichtlich einer Verbesserung der Lebensqualität bezogen auf sämtliche Mistelextrakte, die in ihrem zweiten systematischen Review untersucht worden sind.

Als Beispiel für die Anwendung der Mistel in der adjuvanten Therapiesituation sind wiederholt bei Patientinnen mit Mamma-Ca randomisierte kontrollierte Therapiestudien (RCTs) begleitend zur adjuvanten Chemotherapie durchgeführt worden. Es konnte eine Verbesserung der Lebensqualität mit verschiedenen QoL-Messinstrumenten gezeigt werden, auch in zwei großen placebokontrollierten Studien 2004 und 2006. Diese Ergebnisse wurden aber bisher nur in zwei kleineren RCTs mit aktuellen Chemotherapie-Konzepten repliziert.

Als Beispiel für die Anwendung in der palliativen Therapiesituation konnte in einem RCT mit Patientinnen und Patienten mit fortgeschrittenem Pankreas-Karzinom mit Mistelextrakt plus Best Supportive Care gegenüber alleinigem Best Supportive Care sowohl eine Verbesserung der Lebensqualität als auch eine Verbesserung des Overall Survival gezeigt werden. Es ist abzuwarten, ob der kürzlich abgeschlossene Replikationsversuch mit einer randomisierten Doppelblindstudie in Schweden gelingt. Eine Publikation der Ergebnisse steht aktuell noch aus.
Die 2021 erstmals veröffentlichte S3-Leitlinie zur Komplementärmedizin in der Behandlung onkologischer Patienten hat entsprechend der Bewertung der Datenlage keine Empfehlung für oder gegen eine Verordnung von Mistelgesamtextrakt mit dem Ziel der Verlängerung der Überlebenszeit ergeben. Aber gemäß Leitlinie besteht eine „kann“-Empfehlung für die subkutane Gabe von Mistelgesamtextrakt mit dem Ziel einer Verbesserung der Lebensqualität bei Patienten mit einer Krebserkrankung.
Eine fortlaufende Evaluation der Misteltherapie über methodisch hochqualitative Studien ist wesentlich. Hierbei müssen die sich seit einigen Jahren rasch verändernden Therapiekonzepte in der Onkologie berücksichtigt werden. U.a. interessiert hier auch die Sicherheit und Wirksamkeit bei kombinierter Anwendung mit Immun-Checkpoint-Inhibitoren.
Schlüsselwörter: *Viscum album* L., klinische Studien, systematischer Review, Lebensqualität, Überlebenszeit

Summary

Extant systematic reviews have led to very different assessments of treating cancer patients with mistletoe extract. In two systematic reviews evaluating efficacy of mistletoe extracts on survival and tumor response or quality of life in cancer patients, Freuding *et al.* did not find a benefit (2019). Ostermann *et al.* (2020), on the other hand, confirmed antitumor efficacy in their systematic review of controlled studies with fermented mistletoe extract. In two other systematic reviews, Loef and Walach (2020; 2022) saw, firstly, antitumor efficacy of the investigated non-fermented mistletoe extracts and, secondly, efficacy in improving quality of life under treatment with fermented as well as non-fermented mistletoe extracts.
As an example of the use of mistletoe extract in the adjuvant therapy situation, randomized controlled trials (RCTs) have been repeatedly carried out in breast cancer patients in addition to adjuvant chemotherapy. An improvement in quality of life has been shown with various QoL measurement instruments, including in two large placebo-controlled studies 2004 and 2006.

However, these results have so far only been replicated in two smaller RCTs with current chemotherapy concepts.
As an example of the application in the palliative therapy situation, an RCT with advanced pancreatic cancer patients with mistletoe extract plus best supportive care compared to best supportive care alone showed both, an improvement in quality of life and an improvement in overall survival. A recently completed replication attempt with a randomized double-blind study in Sweden is currently pending.
The S3 guideline on complementary medicine in the treatment of oncology patients, published for the first time in 2021, did not – according to the evaluation of the existing data – give any recommendation for or against prescribing mistletoe extract with the aim of improving survival time. However, the guidelines recommend the subcutaneous administration of mistletoe extract with the aim of improving quality of life in cancer patients.
Ongoing evaluation of mistletoe extract using methodologically high-quality studies is essential. The rapidly changing therapy concepts in oncology in recent years must be taken into account here. Of particular interest is the safety and effectiveness of mistletoe therapy when used in combination with immune checkpoint inhibitors, to give one example.
Keywords: *Viscum album* L., clinical trials, systematic review, quality of life, survival

Hintergrund

Seit mittlerweile über 100 Jahren wird Mistelextrakt als Injektionspräparat in erster Linie für subkutane Injektionen bei Patienten mit Tumorerkrankungen eingesetzt. In einer ersten Publikation berichtete Ita Wegman 1921 über ihre ersten Erfahrungen mit dieser Therapie: „Absolute einwandfreie Heilungen (...) sind bis jetzt noch nicht erreicht (...). Eine Besserung des subjektiven Befindens tritt immer ein. Die Schlaflosigkeit und Müdigkeit gehen allmählich zurück, so dass man sogar sprechen kann von einer Euphorie nach der Injektion. Die Patienten bekommen wieder Mut zu leben und mir persönlich kommt es sogar vor – ich will mich hier nur vorsichtig ausdrücken – als ob die Schmerzen im letzten Stadium bedeutend vermindert werden“ (Wegman 1921).

Leitlinie zur Komplementärmedizin in der Onkologie

Die erstmals im September 2021 online publizierte S3-Leitlinie zur Komplementärmedizin in der Behandlung von onkologischen Patienten urteilt nicht weit davon entfernt: „Es liegen unterschiedliche Ergebnisse aus 3 Übersichtsarbeiten / Metaanalysen und einzelnen RCTs zur Wirksamkeit von Mistelgesamtextrakt (*Viscum album* L.) zur Verlängerung der Gesamtüberlebenszeit von Krebspatienten verschiedener Entitäten vor, die z.T. positive Ergebnisse, z.T. keine statistisch signifikante Wirksamkeit zeigen. Die Daten reichen für eine klare abschließende Bewertung nicht aus. Es kann keine Empfehlung für oder gegen eine Verordnung von Mistelgesamtextrakt (*Viscum album* L.) enthaltenden Präparaten mit dem Ziel der Verlängerung der Überlebenszeit gegeben werden". Die Bewertung der Wirksamkeit bzgl. einer Verbesserung der Lebensqualität kam in dieser Leitlinie zu einem anderen Ergebnis: „Es liegen heterogene Daten aus systematischen Übersichtsarbeiten/Metaanalysen und RCTs mit der subkutanen Gabe von Mistelgesamtextrakt (*Viscum album* L.) enthaltenden Arzneimitteln bei Patienten mit soliden Tumoren zur Verbesserung der Lebensqualität vor. Die subkutane Gabe von Mistelgesamtextrakt (*Viscum album* L.) kann für den therapeutischen Einsatz zur Verbesserung der Lebensqualität bei Patienten mit soliden Tumoren erwogen werden" (https://www.leitlinienprogramm-onkologie.de/home 2024) Mit dieser Beurteilung ist die Mistel eine von nur vier Heilpflanzen (bzw. sechs Heilpflanzen in der überarbeiteten Version, deren Publikation für Mitte 2024 erwartet wird), die von der Expertenkommission dieser S3-Leitlinie mit einer positiven Bewertung eingeschätzt worden ist.

Zwischen diesen beiden Beurteilungen der Misteltherapie in der therapeutischen Anwendung bei Patienten mit Tumorerkrankungen, deren zentrale Aussagen doch relativ nahe beieinander liegen, sind einhundert Jahre klinischer Anwendung und klinischer Forschung vergangen. Zunächst wurden Einzelfall- und Kollektivberichte und retrospektive Studien in den 40er, 50er und 60er Jahren des 20. Jahrhunderts veröffentlicht (Kienle, Kiene 2003). Erste prospektive randomisierte Studien folgten in den 80er Jahren und werden mit zunehmender methodologischer Qualität auch heute weiterhin durchgeführt.

Systematische Reviews und Metaanalysen

Erste systematische Übersichtsarbeiten wurden 1989 (Kiene 1989) und 1994 (Kleijnen, Knipschild 1994) veröffentlicht. Nachfolgende systematische Reviews, z. T. mit Metaanalyse führten zu sehr unterschiedlichen Bewertungen der klinischen Wirksamkeit der Misteltherapie und sollen im Folgenden näher dargestellt werden.

Ein erster systematischer Review für die Cochrane Collaboration, der 2008 veröffentlicht worden war (Horneber *et al.* 2008), hatte die bis zu diesem Zeitpunkt vorliegenden 21 prospektiv randomisierten Studien mit insgesamt n = 3484 Patienten eingeschlossen. Die Autoren kritisierten bei einem Großteil der Studien eine mangelhafte methodologische Qualität, die mittels Jadad Score, Delphi List und Approach der Cochrane Collaboration eingeschätzt worden war. Die Arzneimittelsicherheit der s.c. applizierten Mistelextrakte war in 12 RCTs untersucht worden, und es war in allen 12 Studien eine gute Verträglichkeit der Therapie beschrieben worden. 13 Studien hatten den Einfluss der verabreichten Mistelextrakte auf das Überleben der Patienten untersucht. Davon fanden 6 Studien einen Hinweis auf einen Benefit durch die verabreichte Therapie, 7 Studien fanden diesbezüglich keinen signifikanten Unterschied zur Kontrollgruppe. Die methodologische Qualität in diesen 7 Studien wurde höher eingeschätzt, und die gewonnenen Daten wurden als nicht ausreichend für eine insgesamt positive Bewertung angesehen. Eine bessere Bewertung erfolgte für die in 16 Studien untersuchte Lebensqualität und Beeinflussung von Nebenwirkungen der begleiteten antitumoralen Therapien. Hier fanden die Autoren in 14 dieser 16 Studien zumindest einen Hinweis auf das Vorliegen eines Benefits. Lediglich 2 dieser 14 Studien waren von höherer methodologischer Qualität – ein Prädikat, das quasi ohne Doppelverblindung der Studie nicht erreicht werden konnte, nur diese beiden Studien waren placebokontrolliert und doppelblind durchgeführt worden – und beide waren mit Patientinnen mit einem Mamma-Karzinom erfolgt. Placebokontrolle und Verblindung ist bei Verwendung höher dosierter Mistelextrakte nicht einhaltbar, da Patienten bei Überschreiten individueller Dosisgrenzen eine Lokalreaktion an der Injektionsstelle entwickeln, die den Patienten auf einfachem Weg eine Einschätzung erlaubt, ob sie sich in der Verum- oder in der Placebogruppe befinden. Nur die beiden Studien von Semiglasov *et al.* (2004; 2006) mit Patientinnen mit einem Mamma-Karzinom waren mit einem Extrakt mit einem relativ niedrigen Mistellektin I Gehalt durchgeführt worden, der eine nachvollziehbar funktionierende Verblindung bei einem größeren Teil der teilnehmenden Patientinnen erlaubt hatte.

In zwei weiteren systematischen Reviews, die in diesem Zeitraum publiziert worden waren (Melzer *et al.* 2009; Kienle, Kiene 2010), waren nicht ausschließlich nur RCTs eingeschlossen worden. Hier waren u.a. auch Retrolektivstudien ausgewertet worden, deren Aussagekraft durchaus kontrovers diskutiert wird. Beide Arbeiten kommen zu dem Schluss, dass die vorliegenden Daten für eine Verbesserung der Lebensqualität unter dieser Therapie sprechen könnten.

Ein aktueller systematischer Review mit Metaanalyse wertete die Daten von 32 kontrollierten Studien mit insgesamt n = 13745 Patienten aus, in denen die Behandlung mit einem fermentierten Mistelextrakt und ihre Auswirkung auf das Gesamt- bzw. ereignisfreie Überleben der Patienten untersucht worden war (Ostermann *et al.* 2020). In der Metaanalyse dieser Untersuchung wurde eine Hazard Ratio von 0,59 (95 %CI:[0.53;0.65], $p < 0{,}0001$) zugunsten der Misteltherapie errechnet bei moderater Heterogenität der Studienergebnisse ($I^2 = 50{,}9$ %; $p < 0{,}0001$, $T^2 = 0{,}053$). Die Autoren betonen, dass zwischen einzelnen Tumorentitäten erheblich unterschiedliche Therapieeffekte gesehen wurden mit einer HR von 0,43 beim Zervix-Karzinom und von 0,84 beim Bronchialkarzinom. Es muss darauf hingewiesen werden, dass in dieser Metaanalyse lediglich 14 Studien prospektiv randomisierte Studien waren. 8 Studien hatten ein Matched-Pair-Design, 2 ein retrolektives und 12 ein retrospektives Design. Die Autoren beschreiben in einer Subgruppen-Analyse der randomisierten Studien einen geringeren Therapieeffekt (HR = 0,68; CI: [0,55; 0,83], aber ohne Signifikanz gegenüber den nicht randomisierten Studien.

Ein nachfolgender systematischer Review mit Metaanalyse untersuchte die Daten aus klinischen Studien, die mit nichtfermentierten Mistelextrakten durchgeführt worden waren (Loef, Walach 2022). Auch hier wurden randomisierte (n = 11) und nichtrandomisierte Studien (n = 8) eingeschlossen. Die Autoren geben für die randomisierten Studien eine Hazard Ratio von 0,81 (95 % CI 0,69-0,95, p = 0,01) für die mit nichtfermentiertem Mistelextrakt behandelten Patienten gegenüber der Kontrolle an. In zwei Studien (jeweils eine randomisierte und eine nicht randomisierte Studie) wurde gegen eine aktive Kontrolle (einmal BCG und einmal ein chemoimmuntherapeutisches Gesamtkonzept) geprüft, weshalb diese nicht in die Gesamtauswertung für den HR aufgenommen wurden. Die Autoren geben außerdem einen moderaten bis hohen Risk of Bias an und die Gewichtung der in die Metaanalyse eingeschlossenen randomisierten Studien ist nicht gut nachvollziehbar.

Die Autoren haben außerdem einen systematischen Review mit eingeschlossener Metaanalyse durchgeführt, der in einer gemeinsamen Auswertung Effekte fermentierter und nichtfermentierter Mistelextrakte auf die Lebensqualität von Krebspatienten untersucht (Loef, Walach 2020). Es wurden insgesamt 26 Publikationen mit 30 Datensätzen zu prospektiv kontrollierten Studien gefunden und ausgewertet. Der Großteil dieser Studien war prospektiv randomisiert, lediglich 5 Studien waren nicht randomisiert durchgeführt worden. In der Gesamtauswertung lag die pooled standardized mean difference (SMD) für die globale Lebensqualität gegenüber der Kontrolle bei d = 0,61 (95 % CI 0,41-0,81, p < 0,00001).

Eine weitere Arbeitsgruppe führte zwei systematische Reviews zur Anwendung von Mistelextrakten bei Patienten mit Tumorerkrankungen durch (Freuding *et al.* 2019a; 2019b). Die Autoren beschränkten sich bei der Suche nach entsprechenden publizierten Studien auf den Zeitraum nach 1994, wodurch ein nicht unwesentlicher Teil der wissenschaftlichen klinischen Untersuchungen nicht mit in die Auswertungen aufgenommen worden ist. Die Arbeitsgruppe wertete insgesamt 28 Publikationen mit 2639 in diese Studien eingeschlossenen Patienten aus. Es handelte sich um Studien mit Mistelextrakt bei Patienten mit Krebserkrankungen der Harnblase, Mamma-Karzinom, weitere gynäkologische Karzinome (Zervix-Ca, Endometrium-Ca, Ovarial-Karzinom), Kolorektal-Ca, weitere gastroenterologische Tumoren (Magen-Karzinom, Pankreas-Karzinom), Gliom, Kopf-Hals-Karzinom, Bronchial-Karzinom, Melanom und Osteosarkom). Im systematischen Review zur Bewertung einer möglichen antitumoralen Wirksamkeit von Mistelextrakt wurde in 14 Studien mit n = 1054 Patienten das Gesamtüberleben und in 10 Studien mit n = 1091 Patienten das progressions- oder erkrankungsfreie Überleben oder die Tumor Response untersucht. Die Autoren beschreiben, dass in 5 von 14 Studien unter Anwendung von Mistelextrakt Effekte auf das Gesamtüberleben gesehen worden sind, und zwar beim Mamma-Karzinom (Grossarth-Maticek, Ziegler 2006a), beim kolorektalen Karzinom (Cazacu *et al.* 2003), beim fortgeschrittenen Gliom (Lenartz *et al.* 1996), beim nicht-metastasierten Endometrium-Karzinom (Grossarth-Maticek, Ziegler 2008) und beim Pankreas-Karzinom (Tröger *et al.* 2013). Bei den übrigen Untersuchungen wurde diesbezüglich kein Effekt gesehen. Bzgl. progressionsfreiem, krankheitsfreiem bzw. krankheitsspezifischem Überleben wurde in 3 von 9 Studien von den Autoren positive Effekte durch Mistelextrakt beschrieben, und zwar beim Osteosarkom (Longhi *et al.* 2014), Mamma-Karzinom (Grossarth-Maticek, Ziegler 2006b) sowie beim malignen Melanom (Grossarth-Maticek, Ziegler 2007). In der Conclusion wie im Abstract ihres Artikels fassen die Autoren ihre Ergebnisse jedoch dahingehend zusammen, dass in den meisten Studien keine Effekte durch Mistelextrakte auf das Überleben beobachtet werden, und dass insbesondere Studien höherer methodologischer Qualität keinen Benefit zeigen würden.

Auch im systematischen Review zu Mistelextrakt und therapeutischen Effekten auf Lebensqualität und Nebenwirkungen antitumoraler Therapien fassen die Autoren in ihrem Abstract zusammen, dass Studien besserer methodologischer Qualität weniger oder gar keine Effekte auf die Lebensqualität bei Patienten mit Tumorerkrankungen zeigen würden, und dass ihr Review keine Indikation zur Verschreibung von Mistelextrakt bei Krebspatienten ergeben hätte. Im Text selbst wird dann aber in diesem Kontext von signifikanten Therapieeffekten bei Patienten mit Mamma-Karzinom, Kolorektal-Karzinom und Pankreas-Karzinom sowie Gliom, Osteosarkom, Bronchialkarzinom und Magenkarzinom berichtet. Auch bezüglich Selbstregulation sehen die Autoren in der Mehrzahl der hier untersuchten Tumorentitäten günstige Effekte bei den Studienteilnehmer. Genannt werden hier Mamma-Karzinom, gynäkologische Tumoren und malignes Melanom. In der Begleitbehandlung zur Reduktion von Nebenwirkungen der Chemotherapie finden die Autoren in den meisten Studien positive Wirkungen der Misteltherapie. So berichten Bar Sela *et al.* (2013) über signifikant weniger nichthämatologische adverse events unter begleitender Misteltherapie, und bei signifikant weniger Patienten hatte die Dosis der Chemotherapie toxizitätsbedingt reduziert werden müssen (p = 0,005). In der Begleitbehandlung zur Chemotherapie beim Kolorektal-Karzinom wurde in zwei RCTs über eine geringere Häufigkeit von Nebenwirkungen berichtet, u.a. weniger Mukositiden Grad 3 (Cazacu *et al.* 2003; Heiny, Albrecht 1997). In einer chinesischen Studie wurden in der begleitend mit Mistelextrakt behandelten Therapiegruppe 28 adverse events gemeldet gegenüber 77 adverse events in der Kontrollgruppe (Piao *et al.* 2004).

Auch ihre Diskussion beginnen die Autoren mit dem Statement, dass sie in der Mehrzahl der untersuchten Studien positive Effekte der Misteltherapie auf die Lebensqualität der untersuchten Krebspatienten gefunden haben, so wie es auch in den vorhergehenden systematischen Reviews der Fall gewesen sei. Die folgende Diskussion, dass diese therapeutischen Effekte bedingt durch die Schwierigkeit, die Misteltherapie nicht adäquat verblinden zu können, nicht akzeptiert werden könnten, führt leider zu keinem konstruktiven Umgang mit der beschriebenen Situation.

Pelzer *et al.* (2022) haben in einem systematischen Review die klinische Forschungslage zur Anwendung von Mistelextrakt bei Patienten mit Cancer-related Fatigue aufgearbeitet. Dieser Symptomkomplex wird heute von einer Mehrheit der Krebspatienten als größte Beeinträchtigung des Allgemeinbefindens im Kontext ihrer Erkrankung und der dagegen erfolgenden Therapien betrachtet. In ihrem systematischen Review mit eingeschlossener Metaanalyse werten Pelzer *et al.* 12 RCTs mit 1494 Teilnehmern und 7 retrospektive Studien mit 2668 Teilnehmern aus. Sie zeigen in der Metaanalyse für die RCTs eine SMD von -0,48 (95 % CI -0,82 to -0,14; p = 0,006) und für die retrospektiven Studien eine Odds Ratio von 0.36 (95 % CI 0,20 to 0,66; p = 0,0008). Bis heute ist der Effekt von Mistelextrakt auf Cancer related Fatigue in den in diesem Review beschriebenen klinischen Studien ausschließlich als sekundärer Zielparameter untersucht worden. So liegt heute mit diesem systematischen Review ein starker Hinweis auf eine für Patienten möglicherweise sehr hilfreiche Wirksamkeit der Misteltherapie vor, aber noch kein Wirksamkeitsbeleg. Dies sollte möglichst in einer konfirmatorischen randomisierten Therapiestudie als primärer Zielparameter aufgegriffen werden.

Diskussion

In der gemeinsamen Betrachtung der heute vorliegenden systematischen Reviews zur Misteltherapie bei Patienten mit Tumorerkrankungen fallen z. T. sehr divergierende Beurteilungen der Autoren auf, die sich insbesondere erschließen, wenn sich die Auseinandersetzung auf die zusammenfassenden Abstracts der Publikationen reduziert. Es drängt sich dabei die Frage auf, inwiefern „objektive" Ergebnisse und Schlussfolgerungen ganz entscheidend von mehr „subjektiven" Auswahl- und Beurteilungskriterien der Autoren abhängen.

Einen zentralen Aspekt nimmt dabei die Beurteilung der methodologischen Qualität der einzelnen Studien ein. Die unterschiedliche Einschätzung der internen Validität der untersuchten Studien anhand des risk of bias als auch wesentlicher Ergebnisse ist bereits ausführlich öffentlich diskutiert worden (Matthes *et al.* 2019) und soll hier nicht erneut aufgegriffen werden. Eindrücklich ist, dass eine Arbeitsgruppe in ihrem systematischen Review zur Untersuchung der klinischen Effekte von Mistelextrakten auf die Lebensqualität von Krebspatienten in den meisten untersuchten Studien signifikante Therapieeffekte konstatiert, ihren Abstract aber mit folgender Conclusion abschließt: „With respect to quality of life or reduction of treatment-associated side effects, a thorough review of the literature does not provide any indication to prescribe mistletoe to patients with cancer" (Freuding *et al.* 2019b). Begründet wird dies im Review vor allem mit einem hohen Risiko für performance und detection bias durch die fehlende Verblindung.

Es ist richtig, dass für einen definitiven Wirksamkeitsnachweis bei subjektiven Beschwerden wie einer reduzierten Lebensqualität Placebo-kontrollierte Studien erwartet werden. Auch bei den im Cochrane Review durchgeführten Untersuchungen zur methodologischen Qualität der Studien anhand Jadad Score und Delphi List führte die fehlende Verblindung im Gros der untersuchten Studien dazu, dass die methodologische Qualität nicht als hoch bewertet werden konnte (Horneber *et al.* 2008). Abgesehen davon, dass eine Verblindung einer subkutan verabreichten Misteltherapie zumindest bei der üblichen Gabe ansteigender Dosierungen weitgehend unmöglich ist (Rostock, Huber 2004), reduziert sie auch den therapeutischen Wert allein auf den pharmakologischen Effekt. Inwiefern hierdurch eine wesentliche Reduktion der therapeutischen Wirksamkeit in Kauf genommen werden müsste, sollte kritisch diskutiert werden.

In aktuellen Diskussionen wird wiederholt in Frage gestellt, ob die therapeutische Anwendung von Mistelextrakten angesichts der sich erheblich wandelnden therapeutischen Vorgehensweisen in der modernen Onkologie weiterhin ein zeitgemäßes und hilfreiches Therapiekonzept darstellt. Auch vor diesem Hintergrund wurde sehr bewusst für die Einleitung dieser Arbeit der Bericht von Ita Wegman über die ersten Therapieerfahrungen mit der Misteltherapie von vor über 100 Jahren gewählt. Die Beschwerden, für die sie damals eine therapeutische Wirksamkeit der Misteltherapie beobachtet hatte – das eingeschränkte Allgemeinbefinden mit Schlafstörungen, ausgeprägter Fatigue, Inappetenz und Gewichtsverlust, Schmerzen und psychischen Beeinträchtigungen – sind nach wie vor die Beschwerden, für die Ärzte in der heutigen Zeit nach hilfreichen therapeutischen Möglichkeiten für ihre Patienten suchen.

Interessenkonflikt

Die Autoren geben keine Interessenkonflikte an; lediglich die vom Universitären Cancer Center Hamburg veranstaltete Fortbildung zur Komplementärmedizin in der Onkologie, verantwortet durch M. Rostock, ist in den letzten Jahren durch verschiedene Firmen geringfügig für Kosten der Durchführung gefördert worden, u.a. durch die Firma Helixor.

Literatur

Bar-Sela G, Wollner M, Hammer L et al.: Mistletoe as complementary treatment in patients with advanced non-small-cell lung cancer treated with carboplatin-based combinations: a randomised phase II study. Eur J Cancer. 2013; 49: 1058–1064.

Cazacu M, Oniu T, Lungoci C et al.: The influence of Isorel on the advanced colorectal cancer. Cancer Biotherapy and Radiopharmaceuticals. 2003;18: 27–34.

Freuding M, Keinki C, Micke O, Buentzel J, Huebner J: Mistletoe in oncological treatment: a systematic review : Part 1: survival and safety. J Cancer Res Clin Oncol. 2019a; 145: 695–707.

Freuding M, Keinki C, Kutschan S: Mistletoe in oncological treatment: a systematic review : Part 2: quality of life and toxicity of cancer treatment. J Cancer Res Clin Oncol. 2019b; 145: 927–939.

Grossarth-Maticek R, Ziegler R: Randomized and non-randomized prospective controlled cohort studies in matched-pair design for the long-term therapy of breast cancer patients with a mistletoe preparation (Iscador): a re-analysis. Eur J Med Res. 2006a;11: 485–495.

Grossarth-Maticek R, Ziegler R: Prospective controlled cohort studies on long-term therapy of breast cancer patients with a mistletoe preparation (Iscador). Forsch Komplementarmed. 2006b;13: 285–292.

Grossarth-Maticek R, Ziegler R: Efficacy and safety of the long-term treatment of melanoma with a mistletoe preparation (Iscador). Schweiz Z Ganzheitsmedizin. 2007;19: 325–332.

Grossarth-Maticek R, Ziegler R: Randomized and non-randomized prospective controlled cohort studies in matched-pair design for the long-term therapy of corpus uteri cancer patients with a mistletoe preparation (Iscador). Eur J Med Res. 2008;13: 107–120.

Horneber MA, Bueschel G, Huber R, Linde K, Rostock M: Mistletoe therapy in oncology. Cochrane Database Syst Rev. 2008; CD003297.

Heiny BM, Albrecht V: Complementary modes of therapy with mistletoe lectin-1. Medizinische Welt. 1997;48: 419–423.

Kiene H: Klinische Studien zur Misteltherapie karzinomatöser Erkrankungen. Eine Übersicht. Therapeutikon. 1989; 3: 347–353.

Kienle GS, Kiene H: Die Mistel in der Onkologie: Fakten und konzeptionelle Grundlagen. Stuttgart: Schattauer; 2003.

Kienle GS, Kiene H: Influence of Viscum album L. (European mistletoe) extracts on quality of life in cancer patients: a systematic review of controlled clinical studies. Integr Cancer Ther. 2010; 9: 142–157.

Kleijnen J, Knipschild P: Mistletoe treatment for cancer review of controlled trials in humans. Phytomedicine. 1994; 1: 255–260.

Lenartz D, Stoffel B, Menzel J, Beuth J: Immunoprotective activity of the galactoside-specific lectin from mistletoe aftertumor destructive therapy in glioma patients. Anticancer Res. 1996; 16: 3799–3802.

Loef M, Walach H: Quality of life in cancer patients treated with mistletoe: a systematic review and meta-analysis. BMC Complementary Medicine and Therapies. 2020; 20: 227.

Loef M, Walach H: Survival of cancer patients treated with non-fermented Mistletoe extract: A systematic review and meta-analysis. Integrative Cancer Therapies. 2022; 21: 1–10.

Longhi A, Reif M, Mariani E, Ferrari S: A Randomized Study on Postrelapse Disease-Free Survival with Adjuvant Mistletoe versus Oral Etoposide in Osteosarcoma Patients. Evid Based Complement Alternat Med. 2014:210198.

Matthes H, Hofheinz R-D, Bar-Sela G et al.: Letter to the editors of the Journal of Cancer Research and Clinical Oncology. J Cancer Research Clin Oncol. 2019; 145: 2405–2407.

Melzer J, Iten F, Hostanska K, Saller R: Efficacy and safety of mistletoe preparations (Viscum album L.) for patients with cancer diseases. A systematic review. Forsch Komplementmed. 2009; 16: 217–226

Ostermann T, Appelbaum S, Poier D, Boehm K, Raak C, Bussing A: A systematic review and meta-analysis on the survival of cancer patients treated with a fermented Viscum album L. extract (Iscador): An update of findings. Comp Med Research. 2020: 1–9.

Pelzer F, Loef M, Martin DD, Baumgartner S: Cancer-related fatigue in patients treated with mistletoe extracts: a systematic review and meta-analysis. Supportive Care in Cancer. 2022; 30: 6405–6418.

Piao BK, Wang YX, Xie GR et al.: Impact of complementary mistletoe extract treatment on quality of life in breast, ovarian and non-small cell lung cancer patients. A prospective randomized controlled clinical trial. Anticancer Res. 2004; 24: 303–309.

Rostock M, Huber R: Randomized and double-blind studies – demands and reality as demonstrated by two examples of mistletoe research. Forsch Komplementarmed. 2004; Supp l:18–22.

Semiglasov VF, Stepula VV, Dudov A, Lehmacher W, Mengs U: The standardised mistletoe extract PS76A2 improves QoL in patients with breast cancer receiving adjuvant CMF chemotherapy: a randomised, placebo-controlled, double-blind, multicentre clinical trial. Anticancer Res. 2004; 24: 1293–1302.

Semiglazov VF, Stepula VV, Dudov A et al.: Quality of life is improved in breast cancer patients by standardised Mistletoe extract PS76A2 during chemotherapy and follow-up: a randomised, placebo-controlled, double-blind, multicentre clinical trial. Anticancer Res. 2006; 26: 1519–1529.

Tröger W, Jezdić S, Zdrale Z et al.: Quality of life and neutropenia in patients with early-stage breast cancer: A randomized pilot study comparing additional treatment with Mistletoe extract to chemotherapy alone. Breast Cancer: Basic and Clinical Research. 2009; 3: 35–45.

Tröger W, Zdrale Z, Tišma N, Matijasevic M: Additional Therapy with a Mistletoe Product during Adjuvant Chemotherapy of Breast Cancer Patients Improves Quality of Life: An Open Randomized Clinical Pilot Trial. Evid Based Complement Altern Med. 2014; 2014:430518. doi: 10.1155/2014/430518.

Tröger W, Galun D, Reif M, Schumann N, Stanković N, Milićević M: Viscum album [L.] extract therapy in patients with locally advanced or metastatic pancreatic cancer: A randomised clinical trial on overall survival. Eur J Cancer. 2013; 49: 3788–3797.

Tröger W, Galun D, Reif M, Schumann A, Stankovic N, Milićević M: Quality of life of patients with advanced pancreatic cancer during treatment with mistletoe – a randomized controlled trial. Dtsch Aerztebl Int. 2014; 111: 493–502.

Wegman I: Die ersten Krebsbehandlungen mit Viscum album (1921). Beiträge zu einer Erweiterung der Heilkunst. 1987; 40: 233–238.

Office des Leitlinienprogramms Onkologie c/o Deutsche Krebsgesellschaft e.V.: S3-Leitlinie Komplementärmedizin in der Behandlung onkologischer PatientInnen: Komplementärmedizin bei onkologischen PatientInnen (leitlinienprogramm-onkologie.de, Stand: 28.04.2024).

Prof. Dr. med. Matthias Rostock, Dr. med. Mirjam Wüsthof,
Dr. rer. nat. Alena Krause, Dr. med. Alina Busch
Universitäres Cancer Center Hamburg, 2. Medizinische Klinik,
Universitätsklinikum Hamburg-Eppendorf, Martinistrasse 52,
20246 Hamburg, Deutschland

Korrespondenzadresse:
m.rostock@uke.de

Die Mistel in der klinischen Anwendung – Real-World Data und Leitlinien

Mistletoe in Clinical Practice – Real-World Data and Guidelines

Friedemann Schad

Zusammenfassung

Die Versorgungsforschung gewinnt in der Onkologie, zunehmend an Bedeutung. Häufig wird der Begriff heute mit Real-World Data (RWD) oder Real-World Evidence (RWE) ersetzt. Die Versorgungsforschung hat sich mit zunehmender internationaler Anerkennung weiterentwickelt. Anhand des Beispiels des Netzwerk Onkologie (NO) Registers wird gezeigt, dass Versorgungsforschung in onkologischen Zentren erfolgreich etabliert werden und die Erfassung versorgungsnaher Daten generieren kann. Das NO ist eine wachsende klinische Registerdatenbank im Bereich integrativer Onkologie. Bis Juli 2022 wurden klinische Daten von über 22.000 Patienten erfasst. Das NO ist in neun Bundesländern aktiv und hat sich auf Themen wie Arzneimittelsicherheit und Nebenwirkungsprofile fokussiert, mit zahlreichen Publikationen zu integrativen Therapieverfahren, darunter auch der Misteltherapie. Psychometrische Inventare wurden im NO schrittweise eingeführt, um selbstberichtete Lebensqualität (PROMs) systematisch zu erfassen sowie Analysen zum Gesamtüberleben und zur Kosteneffektivität von Therapieverfahren aus dem NO. Es wird dargelegt, dass die Versorgungsforschung die Behandlungsqualität, Therapiesteuerung und Qualitätssicherung verbessern kann, indem sie patientenorientierte Ansätze und selbstberichtete Lebensqualität integriert sowie externe Validität in RCT-Daten ergänzt. Dies zeigt sich in der Zunahme registerbasierter Forschungsprojekte und der akademischen Anerkennung in Deutschland und Europa. Zukünftig könnten versorgungsnahe Daten regulatorische Verfahren beschleunigen und Kosten in der onkologischen Medikamentenentwicklung senken. Kombinierte Studiendesigns wie RRCT-Studien sind vielversprechend. In Zukunft könnte die Versorgungsforschung eine zunehmende Rolle in regulatorischen Verfahren und der evidenzbasierten Leitlinienentwicklung spielen.

Schlüsselwörter: Versorgungsforschung, Real-World Data, Real-World Evidence, *Viscum album* L., Netzwerk Onkologie

Summary
Health services research is gaining increasing importance in oncology. The term is often replaced today with Real-World Data (RWD) or Real-World Evidence (RWE). Health services research has continued to evolve with increasing international recognition. The example of Network Oncology (NO) registry illustrates that health services research can be successfully establish in oncological centers to generate Real-World Data. The NO is a growing clinical registry database in integrative oncology. By July 2022, clinical data from over 22,000 patients had been collected across nine federal states. NO focuses on drug safety, side effect profiles, and has numerous publications on integrative therapies, including mistletoe therapy. Psychometric inventories have been gradually introduced in NO to systematically assess patient-reported outcomes (PROMS), survival analyses, and cost-effectiveness of therapies. The article reveals how health services research can enhance treatment quality, therapy management, and quality assurance by integrating patient-centered approaches, self-reported quality of life, and complementing external validity in RCT data. This is also reflected in the increase of registry-based research projects and academic recognition in Germany and Europe. Moving forward, health services research could expedite regulatory processes and reduce costs in oncological drug development. Combined study designs such as RRCT studies show promise. Health services research is positioned to play an increasing role in regulatory processes and evidence-based guideline development in the future.
Keywords: Health services research, real-world data, real-world evidence, *Viscum album* L, Network Oncology

Einleitung

Die Versorgungsforschung hat in der Medizin und auch im Bereich der Onkologie zunehmend an Bedeutung gewonnen. Der Begriff Versorgungsforschung wurde bisher im Englischen mit „Health Services Research" übersetzt. In jüngerer Zeit wird dieser durch den Begriff Real-World Data (RWD) oder Real-World Evidence (RWE) ersetzt. Gemäß dem Rahmenprogramm der FDA (Food and Drug Administration, Amerikanische Zulassungsbehörde für Lebens- und Arzneimittel) werden Real-World Data wie folgt definiert: „Daten zum Gesundheitszustand der Patienten und/oder zur Gesundheitsversorgung, die routinemäßig aus einer Vielzahl von Quellen erhoben werden" (US Food & Drug Administration 2018). Die englische Zulassungsbehörde Medicines and Healthcare Products Regulatory Agency (MHRA) definiert RWD wie folgt: „Informationen, die aus routinemäßig erfassten Patientendaten gewonnen werden, z. B. aus elektronischen Gesundheitsakten sowie aus Krankheits- und Patientenregistern" (MHRA *et al.* 2021). Damit war und ist die Versorgungsforschung auf internationaler Ebene definiert und findet Einzug in regulatorische Verfahren. Eine Übersicht zu dieser Entwicklung ist 2022 von Schad und Thronicke publiziert worden (Schad, Thronicke 2022). Mit der zunehmenden administrativen Anerkennung dieser Methodiken hat sich die Versorgungsforschung auch in der klinischen Forschung weiterentwickelt. Sie ergänzt das bisher verfügbare wissenschaftliche Instrumentarium um einen wesentlichen Anteil. Wenn wir im gründlich durchgeführten, klassischen randomisiert kontrollierten Versuch (RCT) durch z. B. Randomisation, Verblindung und einer auf den Effekt berechneten adäquaten Fallzahl ein hohes Maß an **interner Evidenz** erreichen, so weist diese Methodik jedoch im Allgemeinen einen Mangel an **externer Evidenz** auf. Häufig entspricht z. B. die untersuchte Kohorte nicht dem medizinischen Alltag. Faktoren wie Multimorbidität, Polypharmazie, gleichzeitige komplexe Therapieverfahren oder auch die Gruppe von betagten Patienten oder solchen mit seltenen Erkrankungen können in diesem Setting wenig gut abgebildet werden. Auch stößt die RCT-Methodik an ethische Fragestellungen wie z. B. in der Neonatologie, Intensivmedizin und Palliativmedizin und es gehen mit ihr im Allgemeinen ein hoher organisatorischer und finanzieller Aufwand einher. Es stellt sich daher die Frage: Kann die Versorgungsforschung durch ein höheres Maß an externer Evidenz einen Beitrag zur Entwicklung von Leitlinien leisten? Ist sie eine adäquate Methode zur Überprüfung von Implementierung, Wirksamkeit und Nutzen wissenschaftlicher Erkenntnisse und Therapieempfehlungen? Und wird sie nicht zuletzt einen zunehmenden Stellenwert auch bei Zulassungsverfahren einnehmen?

Methoden

Das Netzwerk Onkologie (NO) ist eine wachsende klinische Registerdatenbank im Bereich integrativer Onkologie (Schad *et al.* 2013). Bis Juli 2022 wurden über 22.000 Patienten mit Verlaufsdaten im Netzwerk Onkologie erfasst. In der ersten Projektphase ging es neben der Datenbankentwicklung um die Etablierung von anerkannten Dokumentationsstandards. Dabei wurde zunächst auf den Erfassungsstandard der Arbeitsgemeinschaften deutscher Tumorzentren (ADT) bzw. der Basisdokumentation für Tumorkranke (BDT der Deutschen Krebsgesellschaft) aufgesetzt. Später wurde die Datenbank durch Items im Rahmen von Organzentrumszertifizierungen durch OnkoZert und Registermeldungsvorgaben ergänzt (Tab. 1).

Tab. 1: Entwicklungsschritte des Netzwerks Onkologie

	Schritte	**Beschreibung**
1.	Vernetzung aufbauen	Infrastruktur, Datenbank, Dokumentation, Rekrutierung, IT-Updates, Kooperation
2.	Qualitätsstandards etablieren	ADT/DKG/OnkoZert, Registermeldung, Ausbildung
3.	Arzneimittelsicherheit/Safety	Nebenwirkungen/Interaktionen ermitteln
4.	Patient-reported outcome measures (PROMs)	Selbstberichtete Lebensqualität, EORTC - QLQ C30, EQ-5D, SF-36, HADS, NCCN-Distress, MIDOS, MARS,MyCAW etc., Krankheit als Wachstumschance, Biographiearbeit, kulturelle Bedürfnisse
5.	Compliance/Therapieabbruch	Adhärenz zum Therapiekonzept
6.	Efficacy/Effectiveness	Progressionsfreies Überleben, Gesamtüberleben
7.	Konzeptvergleiche	Kosteneffektivität

Nach einer Phase von Aufbau und Vernetzung ist das Netzwerk Onkologie in neun Bundesländern mit einem Ethikvotum versehen und aktiv. Die inhaltlichen Projektebenen waren zu Beginn insbesondere zum Thema Arzneimittelsicherheit und Nebenwirkungsprofile. Hier konnten zahlreiche Publikationen im Bereich der Misteltherapie und kombinierten Therapieverfahren publiziert werden (Schad *et al.* 2024; Schad *et al.* 2023a; Thronicke *et al.* 2018a). Darüber hinaus sind im NO eine Reihe von psychometrischen Inventaren (Patientenfragebögen) über die Jahre schrittweise eingeführt worden, siehe Tabelle 1. Auch hier konnten zahlreiche Ergebnisse veröffentlicht werden (Schad *et al.* 2023b; Thronicke *et al.* 2023; Oei *et al.* 2023; Oei *et al.* 2018). Das NO ist damit eines der ersten Register, das systematisch selbstberichtete Lebensqualität von Patienten im Langzeit-Follow-up erfasst und damit die aktuell laufende Debatte um den wissenschaftlichen Wert von PROMs (Patient Reported Outcome Measures) nicht nur inhaltlich vorweggenommen, sondern diese frühzeitig eingeführt hat. Über die Jahre konnten darüber hinaus Auswertungen zum Gesamtüberleben und zur Kosteneffektivität von Therapieverfahren analysiert und publiziert werden (Thronicke *et al.* 2020a; Thronicke *et al.* 2020b). Tabelle 1 fasst die Reihenfolge der Entwicklungsschritte des Netzwerks Onkologie zusammen. Die Abbildung 1 fasst den Follow-up der psychometrischen Inventare/PROMs im Netzwerk Onkologie zusammen.

	Baseline	6m Follow-up	12m Follow-up	24m Follow-up	36m Follow-up	48m Follow-up
EORTC-QLQ C30	x	x	x	x	x	x
ICS	x	x	x	x	x	x
CFS-D	x	x	x	x	x	x
EQ5-D	x	x	x	x	x	x
HADS	x			x		x
Projektbezogene Fragebögen:						
NCCN Thermometer	X	und projektgebunden darüber hinaus				
MIDOS	X	und projektgebunden darüber hinaus				
MYCaW	X	und projektgebunden darüber hinaus				
MARS	X	und projektgebunden darüber hinaus				
SF-36	X	und projektgebunden darüber hinaus				

Abb. 1: Psychometrische Inventare zur Evaluierung patientenberichteter Ergebnismessungen (Patient-reported Outcome Measures – PROMs) im Netzwerk Onkologie

Ergebnisse

Die Bandbreite der aus dem Netzwerk Onkologie veröffentlichten Ergebnisse und Publikationen ist groß. In einer kleinen Pilotstudie an 35 Patienten konnte der Effekt von frühpalliativen/supportiven Therapieverfahren (EPC) auf den Distress von onkologischen Patienten mit hohen symptomatischen Beschwerden auf einer palliativen/früh-supportiven onkologischen Station erfasst werden. In 12 +/- 2 Tagen stationärer EPC-Behandlung zeigte sich sowohl im NCCN-Distress als auch in dem Symptomlast messenden Instrument MIDOS jeweils signifikante Verbesserungen der selbstberichteten Lebensqualität von Patienten mit fortgeschrittenen Tumorerkrankungen, siehe Abbildung 2 (Thronicke *et al.* 2022).

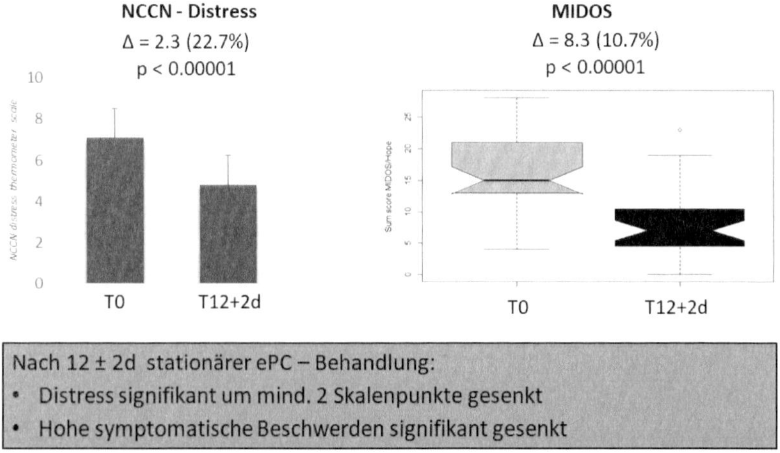

Abb. 2: Effekt von früh palliativer/supportiver Therapie (EPC, early palliative/supportive care) auf den Distress von onkologischen Patienten mit hohen symptomatischen Beschwerden

Ein Faktor, der in den letzten Jahren vielfach übersehen wurde, ist die Belastung von Krebspatienten durch ihr finanzielles Auskommen im Rahmen der Erkrankung und ihrer Behandlung. In einer Kohorte von 87 Lungenkrebspatienten konnten wir anhand des EORTC-QLQ-C30 Fragebogens und der Hospital Anxiety and Depression Scale (HADS), zeigen, dass über 30 % aller Lungenkrebspatienten von finanzieller Belastung (financial burden) berichteten. Insbesondere zeigte sich bei Patienten mit fortgeschrittenen Tumorstadien, dass die finanziellen Sorgen umso höher waren, je jünger sie waren. In frühen Tumorstadien I–II zeigte sich darüber hinaus ein signifikanter Zusammenhang von Schmerzen mit finanziellen Sorgen (Thronicke *et al.* 2020c).

Im Rahmen einer Befragung von chemotherapierten Patientinnen mit Brustkrebs im Stadium I–III bei Erstdiagnose zeigte sich (Thronicke *et al.* 2018b), dass ein intensives, offenes Gespräche (ECLR, Elaborate Life Review Consultation), welches den Patienten im Rahmen ihres ersten stationären Aufenthaltes angeboten wurde, nach 6 Monaten mit einer signifikant besseren globalen Gesundheit, besseren Rollenfunktion, besseren physischen Funktion und auch signifikant geringeren Angaben zur Fatigue assoziiert war (Abb. 3).

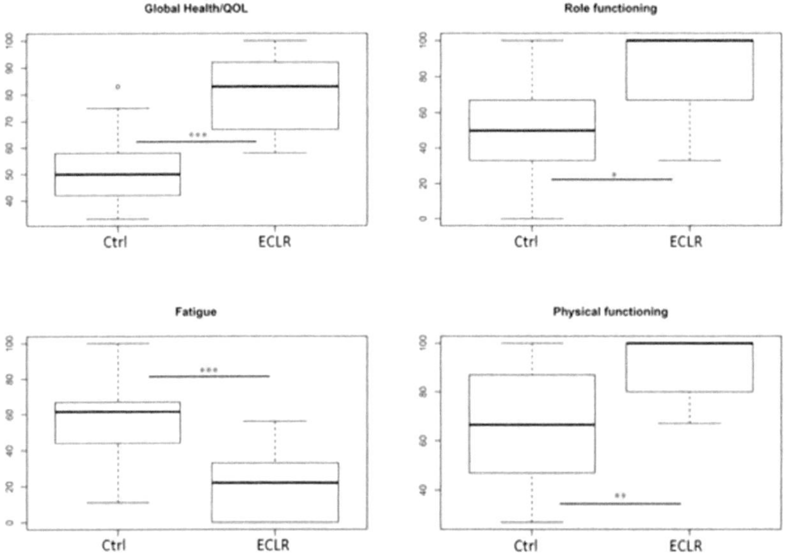

Abb. 3: Gesundheitsbezogene Lebensqualität in Chemotherapie-behandelten Patienten mit Stadium I-III Brustkrebs. ECLR, *elaborate life review consultation*, intensives, offenes Arztgespräch während des stationären Aufenthalts der Patienten

In einer Arbeit von Axtner *et al.* im British Medical Cancer 2016 (Axtner *et al.* 2016) zeigte sich an über 240 Patienten mit Pankreaskarzinom eine Verbesserung des Überlebens, wenn diese gegenüber best supportive care (bsc) Mistel erhielten bzw. wenn diese gegenüber der reinen Behandlung mit Chemotherapie letztere mit einer Misteltherapie ergänzten, siehe Abbildung 4. Interessanterweise führt die systematisch aufgebaute Nachsorgeambulanz am Onkologischen Zentrum Havelhöhe in Berlin mit der Einführung von Lebensqualitäts-Fragebögen (PROMS) zu einer hohen Compliance (Therapietreue). So besteht beispielsweise zu 93 % der Patienten im Brustkrebszentrum ein vollständiger Follow-up nach zwei Jahren (Schad *et al.* 2018).

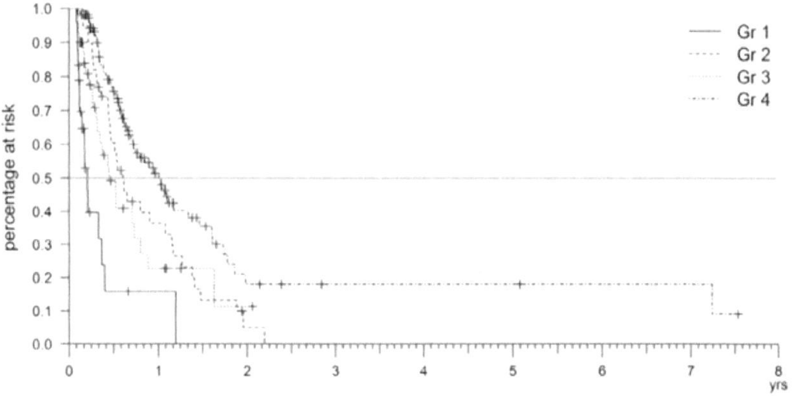

		N	Events	Median [months]	CI [months]
Gr 1:	No or < 1 week VA & no chemotherapy	24	16	2.5	1.7 – NA
Gr 2:	No or < 1 week VA & chemotherapy	40	33	7.3	5.6 – 14.0
Gr 3:	> 4 weeks VA & no chemotherapy	43	23	5.4	3.8 – 10.6
Gr 4:	> 4 weeks VA & chemotherapy	107	57	12.1	8.7 – 17.5

Abb. 4: Kaplan-Maier Überlebenskurve von UICC Stadium IV Patienten, stratifiziert nach Patienten, die Misteltherapie (keine oder weniger als 1 Woche; VA Therapie erhielten und die VA Therapie mehr als 4 Wochen) erhalten haben oder jene, die sowie Chemotherapie erhielten (keine Chemotherapie; Chemotherapie).

In Kooperation mit Autoren der Deutschen Krebsgesellschaft konnten Daten aus dem Netzwerk Onkologie zusammen mit 17 anderen zertifizierten Brustkrebszentren gepoolt werden (N = 3052) und erste Analysen zu Qualitätskriterien im Rahmen von der Deutschen Krebsgesellschaft zertifizierten Brustkrebszentren publiziert werden (Sibert *et al.* 2022). Dabei variierte die Übernahme von Leitlinienempfehlungen in den Zentren signifikant, war darüber hinaus stark altersabhängig und zeigte am Beispiel von Trastuzumab eine signifikante Steigerung der Umsetzungsempfehlung in den Jahren 2006-2019.

Diskussion und Schlussfolgerung

Am Beispiel der Netzwerk Onkologie Registerdatenbank und den hier gezeigten Auswertungen kann gezeigt werden, dass Versorgungsforschung in einem onkologischen Zentrum mit seinen zertifizierten Organzentren etabliert und versorgungsnahe Daten erfolgreich generiert werden können. Darüber hinaus kann im Rahmen des stationären Aufenthaltes sowohl bei Erstdiagnose, z. B. im Brustkrebszentrum, als auch bei fortgeschritten erkrankten Tumorpatienten, die selbstberichtete Lebensqualität (PROMS) systematisch erfasst, analysiert und publiziert werden. Auch sog. *unmet patient needs*, also Bedürfnisse oder Beschwerden von Patienten, die im klinischen Alltag, aber auch wissenschaftlich bisher nicht im Fokus standen, können über Versorgungsforschung detektiert werden. Das hier vorgestellte Netzwerk Onkologie kann nicht nur die jährliche Registermeldung generieren, sondern kann sich darüber hinaus mit anderen Registern vernetzten und Datenanalysen durchführen. Angeregt durch den ehemaligen Vorsitzenden der Deutschen Krebsgesellschaft Prof. Ortmann konnten Auswertungen aus 17 zertifizierten Brustzentren zusammen mit NO analysiert und publiziert werden. Weiterhin zeigen darüber hinaus Plattformen für molekulare Datenbanken, dass hier bundesweit in Tumorkonferenzen und zertifizierten Lungenkrebszentren Real-World Data/ Versorgungsforschungsdaten beispielsweise des nichtkleinzelligen Lungenkarzinoms im Stadium II und III bundesweit erfasst werden können. Die sog. CRISP-Studie (Klinische Forschungsplattform für molekulare Testung, Behandlung und Ergebnisse bei Patienten mit nichtkleinzelligem Lungenkarzinom – AIO-TRK-0315) hat in diesem Zusammenhang bereits über 800 Patienten erfasst. Das Lungenkrebszentrum Havelhöhe ist von 100 beitragenden Zentren das vierthäufigst rekrutierende Zentrum in diesem Projekt.

Darüber hinaus hat die Deutsche Krebsgesellschaft mittlerweile eine Fülle an Projekten in der Versorgungsforschung etabliert. Als Beispiel seien genannt eine Beobachtungsstudie zum Vergleich von Ergebnisqualität in Darmkrebszentren anhand von PROMs, die sog. EDEUM-Studie. Aber auch die Erfassung von Lebensqualität im Rahmen der PROB-Studie bei Patienten mit Brustkrebs in über 40 Zentren deutschlandweit. Auch die Industrie hat in den letzten Jahren Projekte in der Versorgungsforschung aufgebaut. Ein Beispiel ist das von dem Freiburger Forschungsinstitut IOMEDICO entwickelte Netzwerk, welches derzeit klinische Daten von über 50.000 onkologischen Patienten von 21 Tumorregister und -plattformen an über 738 Zentren sammelt und analysiert (www.iomedico.com).

Die vorgetragenen Beispiele zeigen, dass in der klinischen Praxis der Aufbau von prospektiven Registern möglich ist und diese mit vorhandenen Netzwerken und Registern gekoppelt werden können (OnkoZert Krebsregister, molekulare Datenbanken). Auch die systematische Erfassung von PROMS in zertifizierten und klinischen High-Volume-Centern ist möglich; dabei ist neben der patientenzentrierten Erfassung auch die wissenschaftliche Seite von Hypothesengenerierung und die Detektion von bisher nicht bekannten Faktoren gezeigt worden. Zu dem wichtigen Bereich von Unbedenklichkeit, der Medikamenteninteraktion bzw. dem Management von Nebenwirkungen kann das NO Register beitragen, es kann sich mit molekularen Datenbanken vernetzen und diese langfristig zu Outcome-Daten korrelieren. Darüber hinaus kann es den Versorgungsalltag abbilden, Behandlungsstandards evaluieren und im Rahmen der Langzeit-Nachverfolgung Daten zum Gesamtüberleben und Kosteneffektivität generieren.

Ausblick

Das Institut für Qualität und Wirtschaftlichkeit im Gesundheitswesen (IQWIG) äußerte sich bereits 2020 zu dem Stellenwert von Registerdaten für erweiterte Nutzenbewertungen von Arzneimitteln: „Oft fehlen Vergleiche mit dem deutschen Versorgungsstandard, um solche Evidenzlücken zu schließen, sollen künftig auch versorgungsnahe Daten in die frühe Nutzenbewertung von Arzneimitteln einfließen können" (IQWIG 2020). Registerdaten mit entsprechender Qualität können demnach wie im Rapid-Report des IQWIG im Auftrag des Gemeinsamen Bundesausschusses (GBA) als Zusatznutzen von versorgungsnahen Daten angesehen werden. Durch die Gründung einer Arbeitsgruppe zur Versorgungsforschung der Europäischen Krebsgesellschaft (ESMO) ist das Thema im Rahmen der onkologischen Fachgesellschaft auch auf europäischer Ebene angekommen. Die ESMO hat dazu im Herbst 2023 eine Richtlinie verfasst für die systematische Erfassung, Analyse und Publikation aus Versorgungsforschungsdaten in der Onkologie (Costelo-Branco *et al.* 2023).

Damit kann man zusammenfassen, dass die Versorgungsforschung einen Beitrag zur Verbesserung von Behandlungsqualitäten, Therapiesteuerung und Qualitätssicherung leisten, die Patientenorientierung unter Einbeziehung von selbstberichteter Lebensqualität in den Behandlungsablauf implementieren und das Defizit von externer Validität in RCT-Daten komplementieren kann. Das hat sich nicht nur an der Zunahme registerbasierter Forschungsprojekte gezeigt, sondern auch an ihrer fortschreitenden Akademisierung. Eine Auswertung zu Zulassungsverfahren der amerikanischen Zulassungsbehörde FDA zeigte für den Zeitraum 2015 bis 2020, dass bei 11 von 133 (8,3 %) Zulassungen onkologischer Medikamente Daten zur Wirksamkeit aus der Versorgungsforschung hinzugezogen wurden (Arondekar *et al.* 2022). Es bleibt abzuwarten, welche Anerkennung versorgungsnahe Daten im Rahmen regulatorischer Verfahren in Zukunft einnehmen werden. Sie scheinen jedenfalls ein praktikables und valides Instrument bei der Beschleunigung von Zulassungsverfahren und auch zur finanziellen Entlastung in der Produktentwicklung onkologischer Medikamente zu sein. Auch wären kombinierte Studiendesigns wie registerbasierte, kontrollierte Studien mit integrierten RCT-Armen, sog. RRCT-Studien von Interesse, in der sich beide Methodiken ergänzen können. Nicht zuletzt muss noch gezeigt werden, in welcher Weise Real-World-Daten bei der Evidenzbasierung in künftigen Leitlinien eine Rolle spielen und damit im Sinne von *Living Guidelines* zu mehr Wirklichkeitsnähe wissenschaftlicher Ergebnisse beitragen können.

Interessenkonflikt

Der Autor hat die folgenden Interessenkonflikte in Bezug auf die Forschung, die Autorenschaft und/oder Veröffentlichung dieses Artikels: FS berichtet über Zuschüsse von Astrazeneca (Reisekosten und Honorare für Vorträge), Helixor Heilmittel GmbH (Reisekosten und Honorare für Vorträge), Zuschüsse von der Abnoba GmbH und Zuschüsse von der Iscador AG, außerhalb der eingereichten Arbeit. Es wurden keine Zahlungen für andere Aspekte der eingereichten Arbeit erhalten. Es gibt keine Patente, Produkte in der Entwicklung oder vermarktete Produkte, die zu deklarieren sind. Es bestehen keine anderen Beziehungen/Bedingungen/Umstände, die einen potenziellen Interessenkonflikt darstellen.

Literatur

Arondekar B, Duh MS, Bhak RH et al.: Real-World Evidence in Support of Oncology Product Registration: A Systematic Review of New Drug Application and Biologics License Application Approvals from 2015-2020. Clin Cancer Res. 2022; 28 (1): 27–35. doi: 10.1158/1078-0432.CCR-21-2639.

Axtner J, Steele M, Kröz M et al.: Health services research of integrative oncology in palliative care of patients with advanced pancreatic cancer. BMC Cancer. 2016; 16: 579. doi: 10.1186/s12885-016-2594-5.

Bar-Sela G, Wollner M, Hammer L et al.: Mistletoe as complementary treatment in patients with advanced non-small-cell lung cancer treated with carboplatin-based combinations: A randomised phase II study. Eur. J. Cancer. 2013; 49: 1058–1064.

Castelo-Branco L, Pellat A, Martins-Branco D et al.: ESMO Guidance for Reporting Oncology Real-World Evidence (GROW). Ann Oncol. 2023; 34 (12): 1097-1112. doi: 10.1016/j.annonc.2023.10.001.

FDA's Real-World Evidence Program. December 2018. www.fda.gov (Stand: 20.6.2024).

IOMEDICO, International Organisation of Medical Oncology. https://www.iomedico.com/forschung/versorgungsforschung (Stand: 20.6.2024).

IQWIG: Registerdaten eignen sich – bei entsprechender Qualität – für die erweiterte Nutzenbewertung von Arzneimitteln. Pressemitteilung zum Rapid Report. Januar 2020. https://www.iqwig.de/presse/pressemitteilungen/pressemitteilungen-detailseite_9982.html (Stand: 20.6.2024).

Medicines and Healthcare products Regulatory Agency (MHRA) draft guidance on randomised controlled trials generating real-world evidence to support regulatory decisions, updated 2021.

Oei SL, Thronicke A, Groß J et al.: Does the Argentine Tango Sustainably Improve Cancer-Associated Fatigue and Quality of Life in Breast Cancer Survivors? Cancers (Basel). 2023; 15 (23): 5678. doi: 10.3390/cancers15235678.

Oei SL, Thronicke A, Kröz M et al.: Impact of Oncological Therapy and Viscum album L. Treatment on Cancer-Related Fatigue and Internal Coherence in Nonmetastasized Breast Cancer Patients. Integr Cancer Ther. 2020; 19: 1534735420917211. doi: 10.1177/1534735420917211.

Schad F, Thronicke A: Safety of Combined Targeted and Helixor® Viscum album L. Therapy in Breast and Gynecological Cancer Patients, a Real-World Data Study. Int J Environ Res Public Health. 2023a; 20 (3): 2565. doi: 10.3390/ijerph20032565.

Schad F, Thronicke A: Real-World Evidence-Current Developments and Perspectives. Int J Environ Res Public Health. 2022; 19 (16): 10159. doi: 10.3390/ijerph191610159.

Schad F, Thronicke A, Hofheinz RD, Matthes H, Grah C: Patients with Advanced or Metastasised Non-Small-Cell Lung Cancer with Viscum album L. Therapy in Addition to PD-1/PD-L1 Blockade: A Real-World Data Study. Cancers (Basel). 2024; 16 (8): 1609. doi: 10.3390/cancers16081609.

Schad F, Steinmann D, Oei SL, Thronicke A, Grah C: Evaluation of quality of life in lung cancer patients receiving radiation and Viscum album L.: a real-world data study. Radiat Oncol. 2023b; 18 (1): 47. doi: 10.1186/s13014-023-02234-3.

Schad F, Thronicke A, Merkle A et al.: Implementation of an Integrative Oncological Concept in the Daily Care of a German Certified Breast Cancer Center. Complement Med Res. 2018; 25 (2): 85–91. doi: 10.1159/000478655.

Schad F, Axtner J, Happe A et al.: Network Oncology (NO)--a clinical cancer register for health services research and the evaluation of integrative therapeutic interventions in anthroposophic medicine. Forsch Komplementmed. 2013; 20 (5): 353–360. doi: 10.1159/000356204.

Sibert NT, Wesselmann S, Breidenbach C et al.: Trastuzumab treatment of patients with early, HER2-positive breast cancer in 17 certified German breast cancer centers. J Cancer Res Clin Oncol. 2022; 148 (3): 719–726. doi: 10.1007/s00432-021-03651-1.

Thronicke A, Oei SL, Grieb G et al.: Self-Reported Baseline Quality of Life Mirrors Treatment-Specific Characteristics of Cancer Patients. Cancers (Basel). 2023; 15 (24): 5763. doi: 10.3390/cancers15245763.

Thronicke A, von Trott P, Grabowski P et al.: PACE: Effect of early palliative care on the distress of oncological patients with high symptomatic burden, a prospective pilot study. DKK, Berlin, September 2022.

Thronicke A, Reinhold T, von Trott P et al.: Cost-effectiveness of real-world administration of chemotherapy and add-on Viscum album L. therapy compared to chemotherapy in the treatment of stage IV NSCLC patients. PLoS One. 2020a; 15 (7):e0236426. doi: 10.1371/journal.pone.0236426.

Thronicke A, Reinhold T, von Trott P et al.: Cost-Effectiveness of Real-World Administration of Concomitant Viscum album L. Therapy for

the Treatment of Stage IV Pancreatic Cancer. Evid Based Complement Alternat Med. 2020b; 2020: 3543568. doi: 10.1155/2020/3543568. PMID: 32256640.
Thronicke A, von Trott P, Kröz M et al: Health-Related Quality of Life in Patients with Lung Cancer Applying Integrative Oncology Concepts in a Certified Cancer Centre. Evid Based Complement Alternat Med. 2020c; 2020: 5917382. doi: 10.1155/2020/5917382.
Thronicke A, Oei SL, Merkle A, Matthes H, Schad F: Clinical Safety of Combined Targeted and Viscum album L. Therapy in Oncological Patients. Medicines (Basel). 2018a; 5 (3): 100. doi: 10.3390/medicines5030100.
Thronicke A, Kröz M, Merkle A et al.: Psychosocial, Cognitive, and Physical Impact of Elaborate Consultations and Life Review in Female Patients with Non-Metastasized Breast Cancer. Complement Med Res. 2018b; 25 (2): 92–101. doi: 10.1159/000486672.
US Food & Drug Administration. Framework for FDA‘s Real-World Evidence Program. www.fda.gov.

PD Dr. Friedemann Schad
Interdisziplinäre Onkologie und Palliativmedizin, Gemeinschaftskrankenhaus Havelhöhe Berlin und Forschungsinstitut Havelhöhe Berlin, Deutschland

Korrespondenzadresse:
fschad@havelhoehe.de

Lebensqualität von Brustkrebspatientinnen unter Mistelextrakt-Behandlung: Eine systematische Übersichtsarbeit und Metaanalyse

Quality of Life in Breast-Cancer Patients Treated With Mistletoe Extracts: A Systematic Review and Meta-Analysis

Harald Walach, Daniela Paepke, Martin Loef

Dieser Buchbeitrag ist eine Zusammenfassung unseres Tagungsbeitrags, für Originalstudie siehe: Loef M, Paepke D, Walach H. Quality of Life in Breast Cancer Patients Treated with Mistletoe Extracts: A Systematic Review and Meta-Analysis. Integrative Cancer Therapies. 2023; 22. doi:10.1177/15347354231198074

Zusammenfassung

Brustkrebs ist die häufigste Krebsart bei Frauen und die Lebensqualität ein wesentlicher Bestandteil des Wohlbefindens der Patientinnen. Es ist umstritten, ob die pharmakologische Behandlung mit Mistelextrakten (ME) die Lebensqualität von Brustkrebspatientinnen verbessern kann.

Diese systematische Übersichtsarbeit umfasst randomisierte klinische Studien (RCTs) und nichtrandomisierte Interventionsstudien (NRSIs), in denen Brustkrebspatientinnen, die mit ME behandelt wurden, mit Kontrollgruppen verglichen wurden. Die Literatursuche umfasst frühere systematische Übersichten und mehrere Datenbanken bis Januar 2023. Analysiert wurden die Daten mittels Metaanalyse. Das Verzerrungsrisiko wurde mit RoB 2 und ROBINS-I und die Sicherheit der Evidenz mittels GRADE bestimmt.

Neun RCTs und sieben NRSIs mit 833 bzw. 2831 Teilnehmern wurden eingeschlossen. Die gepoolte standardisierte mittlere Differenz betrug SMD = 0,61 (95 % CI 0,47 bis 0,75; p < 0,0001) für RCTs und SMD = 0,46 (95 % CI 0,10 bis 0,82; p = 0,01) für retrospektive NRSIs.

Die Evidenz ist hauptsächlich aufgrund des Verzerrungsrisikos begrenzt. Unsere Ergebnisse deuten auf einen moderaten Effekt von ME auf die Lebensqualität von Brustkrebspatientinnen hin. Weitere RCTs und Real-World-Evidenz müssen dieses Ergebnis bestätigen und sollten klare Unterscheidungen zwischen verschiedenen Untergruppen und Stadien von Brustkrebs treffen.
Schlüsselwörter: Brustkrebs, Mistelextrakte, Metaanalyse, systematischer Review, Lebensqualität

Summary
Breast cancer is the most common cancer type in women and quality of life an essential part of the patients' well-being. It is a matter of debate whether the pharmacological treatment with mistletoe extracts (ME) can improve the quality of life of breast cancer patients
This systematic review includes randomized clinical trials (RCTs) and non-randomized studies of intervention (NRSIs) comparing breast cancer patients treated with ME to control groups. We searched previous systematic reviews and multiple databases until January 2023. We conducted a meta-analysis and assessed the risk of bias via RoB 2 and ROBINS-I and the certainty of evidence via GRADE, respectively.
Nine RCTs and seven NRSIs with 833 and 2831 participants, respectively, were included. The pooled standardized mean difference for RCTs was SMD = 0.61 (95 % CI 0.47 to 0.75; $p < 0.0001$) and for retrospective NRSIs was SMD = 0.46 (95 % CI 0.10 to 0.82; $p = 0.01$).
The risk of bias was medium to high for the RCTs and serious for all NRSIs. The GRADE was moderate for RCTs and very low for NRSIs.
Our results indicate a clinically relevant, medium effect of ME on the quality of life in breast cancer patients. The evidence is mainly limited due to the risk of bias. Further RCTs and real-world evidence need to confirm this result, especially in the setting of neoadjuvant chemotherapy and in breast cancer survivors.
Keywords: Mistletoe, breast cancer, quality of life, meta-analysis, systematic review

Einleitung

Brustkrebs ist die häufigste invasive Krebsart bei Frauen (Łukasiewicz *et al.* 2021). Im Jahr 2020 gab es weltweit 2,3 Millionen neue Fälle. Sie führten zum Verlust von 19,6 Millionen Lebensjahren, die um die Zeit der

Behinderung bereinigt sind und verursachten mehr als 680.000 Todesfälle (Łukasiewicz *et al.* 2021). Dabei ist die Lebensqualität (QoL) ein zentraler Parameter für das Wohlbefinden der Patientinnen, deren Verbesserung in pharmakologische und nichtpharmakologische Interventionen untersucht wird (Mokhatri-Hesari, Montazeri 2020).

Mistelextrakte (ME) werden häufig in der Krebsbehandlung eingesetzt (Kienle 1999). Übersichtsarbeiten haben gezeigt, dass ME eine breite Palette biologischer Aktivitäten wie krebshemmende, entzündungshemmende, antivirale, antibakterielle, angiogene, Apoptose-induzierende und immunmodulatorische Wirkungen entfalten. (Oei *et al.* 2019; Szurpnicka *et al.* 2020; Kleszken *et al.* 2022).

ME sind in mehreren Leitlinien enthalten, aber bestimmte Aspekte ihrer Wirksamkeit werden weiterhin diskutiert (Liedtke *et al.* 2014; Lyman *et al.* 2018; Deutsche Krebsgesellschaft 2023). Die Hauptdiskussionspunkte sind das Fehlen von doppelt verblindeten RCTs und die Heterogenität der Ergebnisse (Schnell-Inderst *et al.* 2021; Staupe *et al.* 2022), die sich u.a. durch die indikative Breite der bisherigen Überprüfungen erklären lässt: Keine der bisherigen Überprüfungen konzentrierte sich auf eine einzige Krebsentität (Loef, Walach 2020; Pelzer *et al.* 2022).

Ziel dieser Studie ist es daher, die Literatur zur ME-Behandlung bei Brustkrebspatientinnen systematisch zu sichten, speziell um den Einfluss auf die Lebensqualität zu dokumentieren, und sowohl RCT als auch NRSI metaanalytisch zu untersuchen.

Methodik

Das Review wurde gemäß PRISMA berichtet (Page *et al.* 2021), das Protokoll vorab in der PROSPERO-Datenbank registriert (CRD42023388900). Die Details der Methodik können der Originalarbeit entnommen werden (Loef *et al.* 2023)

Ergebnisse

Sechzehn Studien aus 15 Veröffentlichungen wurden einbezogen, von denen neun RCTs (Heiny 1991; Borrelli 2001; Semiglasov *et al.* 2004; 2006;

Grossarth-Maticek, Ziegler 2006a; 2006b, Büssing *et al.* 2008; Tröger *et al.* 2009; 2014) und sieben NRSIs (Schumacher *et al.* 2003; Grossarth-Maticek, Ziegler 2006a; Schmidt 2007; Beuth *et al.* 2008; Loewe-Mesch *et al.* 2008; Fritz *et al.* 2018; Oei *et al.* 2020) waren. Zwei RCTs waren doppelt verblindet (Semiglasov *et al.* 2004; 2006), sieben nicht verblindet. Zwei NRSI wurden prospektiv erstellt (Grossarth-Maticek, Ziegler 2006a; Loewe-Mesch *et al.* 2008) die übrigen fünf waren retrospektiv.

Für die RCTs wurde eine Metaanalyse mit einem Modell fester Effekte durchgeführt (siehe Abb. 1). Die geschätzte Effektgröße betrug SMD = 0,61 (95 % CI 0,47 bis 0,75), die hochsignifikant ist (p < 0,0001). Die Heterogenität zwischen den Studien wurde mit I2 = 12,3 % (95 % KI 0,0 % bis 54,1 %) geschätzt und das Vorhersageintervall reichte von 0,31 bis 0,86, was weder auf Heterogenität noch auf negative Interventionseffekte für zukünftige Studien hindeutet. Die Sensitivitätsanalysen und die Subgruppenanalysen zeigten, dass die Analyse gegenüber alternativen Bedingungsgruppen und in Teilbereichen der Gesamtpopulation robust ist.

Study	SMD	SE	Weight	Std. Mean Difference IV, Fixed, 95% CI
Borrelli 2001	0.4000	0.3740	3.6%	0.40 [-0.33; 1.13]
Büssing 2008	0.1900	0.2501	8.0%	0.19 [-0.30; 0.68]
Grossarth-Maticek, 2006a1	0.5200	0.2309	9.4%	0.52 [0.07; 0.97]
Grossarth-Maticek, 2006b	0.6600	0.3416	4.3%	0.66 [-0.01; 1.33]
Heiny 1991	0.8300	0.3214	4.9%	0.83 [0.20; 1.46]
Semiglasov 2004	0.5000	0.1760	16.2%	0.50 [0.16; 0.84]
Semiglazov 2006	0.8200	0.1148	38.1%	0.82 [0.60; 1.04]
Tröger 2009	0.2900	0.2525	7.9%	0.29 [-0.20; 0.78]
Tröger 2014	0.5900	0.2575	7.6%	0.59 [0.09; 1.09]
Total (95% CI)			**100.0%**	**0.61 [0.47; 0.75]**

Heterogeneity: $Tau^2 = 0.0071$; $Chi^2 = 9.13$, df = 8 (P = 0.33); $I^2 = 12\%$

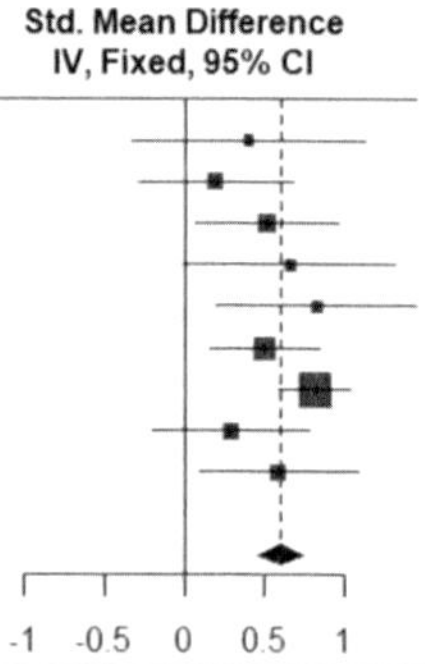

Abb. 1: „Fixed-Effect"-Metaanalyse über standardisierte Mittelwertunterschiede (RCT) zum Effekt von Mistelextrakten im Vergleich zur Kontrolle auf die Lebensqualität von Brustkrebspatientinnen

Für die retrospektiven NRSI wurde die gepoolte Effektgröße anhand eines Modells zufälliger Effekte berechnet, weil die Heterogenität groß war. Diese Analyse ergab eine signifikante SMD von 0,46 (95 % KI 0,1 bis 0,82; p = 0,01). Die Heterogenität zwischen den Studien wurde mit

$I2 = 96{,}5\,\%$ (95 % KI 94,1 % bis 97,9 %) geschätzt und das Vorhersageintervall reichte von -0,92 bis 1,84.

Das Risiko einer Verzerrung war bei den RCTs mittel bis hoch und bei allen NRSIs „serious“. Der GRADE-Wert war für die RCTs mittel und für die NRSIs sehr niedrig. Die Verlässlichkeit der Evidenz wurde mit dem GRADE-Ansatz bewertet und als „moderat“ für RCT und als „sehr niedrig“ für NRSI geschätzt.

Diskussion

Unsere Analyse zeigt einen mittleren Effekt von ME auf die Lebensqualität von Brustkrebspatientinnen, wobei die statistische Heterogenität zwischen den Studien gering ausgeprägt war. Das Verzerrungsrisiko ist bei Mistelstudien inhärent hoch, da die Anwendungen kaum ethisch verblindet werden können. Denn Mistelinjektionen lösen i.d.R. lokale Effekte, manchmal auch systemische Effekte aus, die nicht verblindet werden können, ohne dass man ein aktives Placebo verwenden würde. Das ist wiederum ethisch bedenklich. Dies muss bei der Interpretation des Verzerrungsrisikos berücksichtigt werden. Daher ist auch die Abschätzung des Risikos für eine Verzerrung bei der Messung interventionsbedingt relativ hoch. Denn Lebensqualität ist definitionsgemäß ein subjektives Maß, das durch Patienten bewertet wird, die in aller Regel wissen, in welcher Gruppe sie waren. Bei nichtrandomisierten Studien kommt designbedingt hinzu, dass durch die mangelnde Randomisierung ein Abschlag bei der Vergleichbarkeit der Gruppen gemacht werden muss. Diese inhärenten Probleme sind auch durch eine größere Zahl an Studien kaum zu lösen. Sie wären allenfalls durch andere Formen der Outcome-Messung behebbar, wenn beispielsweise externe, verblindete Personen Outcomes wie Funktionstüchtigkeit im Alltag bewerten würden, oder objektive Maße für Schlafqualität z. B. durch ambulantes Monitoring erhoben würden. Eine andere Möglichkeit wären pragmatische Vergleiche mit anderen Therapien.

Wir waren nicht in der Lage, Aussagen für einzelne Mistelpräparate zu extrahieren, weil dazu zu wenig Studien vorlagen.

In diesem Sinne müssen unsere Ergebnisse im Lichte zukünftiger Studien überprüft werden. Wenn diese große Beobachtungsstudien einschließen, kann gefolgert werden, welche Patientinnen, z. B. welches Krebsstadium und welcher Brustkrebs-Subtyp, von einer ME-Behandlung besonders profitieren.

Inzwischen folgern wir: Mistelextrakte leisten einen klinisch bedeutsamen Beitrag zur Verbesserung der Lebensqualität bei Brustkrebspatienten. Die Effekte sind statistisch sehr deutlich und damit nicht durch Zufall erklärbar. Die oben genannten methodischen Probleme schränken die Sicherheit dieser Aussage ein.

Interessenkonflikt

Die Studie wurde gefördert von der Stiftung „Integrative Medizin und Pharmazie (Stuttgart)". Es bestehen keine Interessenkonflikte.

Literatur

Beuth J, Schneider B, Schierholz J: Impact of complementary treatment of breast cancer patients with standardized mistletoe extract during aftercare: a controlled multicenter comparative epidemiological cohort study. Anticancer Res. 2008; 28 (1B): 523–527.

Borrelli E: Evaluation of the quality of life in breast cancer patients undergoing lectin standardized mistletoe therapy. Minerva Medica. 2001; 92 (Suppl 1 Nr 3): 105–107.

Büssing A, Bückner U, Enser-Weis U et al.: Modulation of chemotherapy-associated immunosuppression by intravenous application of Viscum album L. extract (Iscador): a randomised phase II study. Eur J Integr Med. 2008; 1: 2–3.

Deutsche Krebsgesellschaft: Leitlinienprogramm Onkologie (Deutsche Krebsgesellschaft, Deutsche Krebshilfe, AWMF): Komplementärmedizin in der Behandlung von onkologischen PatientInnen, Langversion 1.1, 2021, AWMF Registernummer: 032/055OL. https://www.leitlinienprogramm-onkologie.de/leitlinien/komplementaermedizin (accessed March 31, 2023).

Fritz P, Dippon J, Mueller S et al.: Is Mistletoe Treatment Beneficial in Invasive Breast Cancer? A New Approach to an Unresolved Problem. Anticancer Res. 2018; 38 (3): 1585–1593.

Grossarth-Maticek R, Ziegler R: Prospective controlled cohort studies on long-term therapy of breast cancer patients with a mistletoe preparation (Iscador®). Complement Med Res. 2006a; 13 (5): 285–292.

Grossarth-Maticek R, Ziegler R: Randomised and non-randomised prospective controlled cohort studies in matched-pair design for the long-term therapy of breast cancer patients with a mistletoe preparation (Iscador): a re-analysis. Eur J Med Res. 2006b; 11 (11): 485.

Heiny B: Additive Therapie mit standardisiertem Mistelextrakt reduziert die Leukopenie und verbessert die Lebensqualität von Patientinnen mit fortgeschrittenem Mammakarzinom unter palliativer Chemotherapie (VEC-Schema). Krebsmedizin. 1991; 12: 1–14.

Kienle GS: The story behind mistletoe: a European remedy from anthroposophical medicine. Altern Ther Health Med. 1999; 5 (6): 34.

Kleszken E, Timar AV, Memete AR et al.: On Overview Of Bioactive Compounds, Biological And Pharmacological Effects Of Mistletoe (Viscum album L). Pharmacophore. 2022; 13 (1): 10–26.

Liedtke C, Thill M, Hanf V et al.: AGO recommendations for the diagnosis and treatment of patients with early breast cancer: update 2014. Breast Care. 2014; 9 (3): 189–200.

Loef M, Paepke D, Walach H: Quality of Life in Breast Cancer Patients Treated With Mistletoe Extracts: A Systematic Review and Meta-Analysis. Integr Cancer Ther. 2023; 22: 15347354231198074.

Loef M, Walach H: Quality of life in cancer patients treated with mistletoe: a systematic review and meta-analysis. BMC Complement Med Ther. 2020; 20 (1): 1–14.

Loewe-Mesch A, Kuehn J, Borho K et al.: Adjuvante simultane Mistel-/Chemotherapie bei Mammakarzinom–Einfluss auf Immunparameter, Lebensqualität und Verträglichkeit. Complement Med Res. 2008; 15 (1): 22–30.

Łukasiewicz S, Czeczelewski M, Forma A et al.: Breast Cancer—Epidemiology, Risk Factors, Classification, Prognostic Markers, and Current

Treatment Strategies – An Updated Review. Cancers. 2021; 13 (17): 4287.

Lyman GH, Greenlee H, Bohlke K et al.: Integrative therapies during and after breast cancer treatment: ASCO endorsement of the SIO clinical practice guideline. J Clin Oncol. 2018; 36 (25): 2647–2655.

Mokhatri-Hesari P, Montazeri A: Health-related quality of life in breast cancer patients: review of reviews from 2008 to 2018. Health Qual Life Outcomes. 2020; 18 (1): 1–25.

Oei SL, Thronicke, Kröz M et al.: Impact of oncological therapy and Viscum album L. treatment on cancer-related fatigue and internal coherence in nonmetastasized breast cancer patients. Integr Cancer Ther. 2020; 19: 1534735420917211.

Oei SL, Thronicke A, Schad F: Mistletoe and Immunomodulation: Insights and Implications for Anticancer Therapies. Evid Based Complement Alternat Med. 2019; 2019: 5893017.

Page MJ, McKenzie JE, Bossuyt PM et al.: The PRISMA 2020 statement: an updated guideline for reporting systematic reviews. Systematic Reviews. 2021; 10 (1): 1–11.

Pelzer F, Loef M, Martin DD et al.: Cancer-related fatigue in patients treated with mistletoe extracts: a systematic review and meta-analysis. Support Care Cancer. 2022: 1–14.

Schmidt NE: Die postoperative komplementäre Therapie des primären Mammakarzinom mit lektinnormiertem Mistelextrakt – eine epidemiologische, kontrollierte retrolektive Kohortenstudie. Diss. Charité – Universitätsmedizin. 2007.

Schnell-Inderst P, Steigenberger C, Mertz M et al.: Additional treatment with mistletoe extracts for patients with breast cancer compared to conventional cancer therapy alone–efficacy and safety, costs and cost-effectiveness, patients and social aspects, and ethical assessment. Cologne: DIMDI. 2021: 0–80.

Schumacher K., Schneider B, Reich G et al.: Influence of postoperative complementary treatment with lectin-standardized mistletoe extract on breast cancer patients. A controlled epidemiological multicentric retrolective cohort study. Anticancer Res. 2003; 23 (6D): 5081–5087.

Semiglasov VF, Stepula VV, Dudov A et al.: The standardised mistletoe extract PS76A2 improves QoL in patients with breast cancer receiving adjuvant CMF chemotherapy: A randomised, placebo-controlled, double-blind, multicentre clinical trial. Anticancer Res. 2004; 24 (2C): 1293–1302.

Semiglazov VF, Stepula VV, Dudov A et al.: Quality of life is improved in breast cancer patients by Standardised Mistletoe Extract PS76A2 during chemotherapy and follow-up: a randomised, placebo-controlled, double-blind, multicentre clinical trial. Anticancer Res 2006; 26 (2B): 1519–1529.

Staupe H, Buentzel J, Keinki C et al.: Systematic analysis of mistletoe prescriptions in clinical studies. J Cancer Res Clin Oncol. 2022: 1–13.

Szurpnicka A, Kowalczuk A, Szterk A.: Biological activity of mistletoe: in vitro and in vivo studies and mechanisms of action. Arch Pharm Res. 2020; 43 (6): 593–629.

Tröger W, Jezdic S, Zdrale Z et al.: Quality of life and neutropenia in patients with early-stage breast cancer: a randomized pilot study comparing additional treatment with mistletoe extract to chemotherapy alone. Breast Cancer (Auckl.). 2009; 3 (1): 35–45.

Tröger W, Zdrale Z, Tišma N, Matijasevic M: Additional Therapy with a Mistletoe Product during Adjuvant Chemotherapy of Breast Cancer Patients Improves Quality of Life: An Open Randomized Clinical Pilot Trial. Evid Based Complement Altern Med. 2014; 2014:430518. doi: 10.1155/2014/430518.

Prof. Dr. Dr. Harald Walach[1, 3] , PD Dr. Daniela Paepke[2],
Dr. Martin Loef[1]

[1] Change Health Science Institute, Basel, Switzerland

[2] Spital Zollikerberg, Zürich, Switzerland

[3] Next Society Institute, Kazimieras Simonavicius University, Vilnius, Lithuania

Korrespondenzadresse:
hwalac@gmail.com

IV. Anwendung bei nichtonkologischen Erkrankungen

IV. Use in Non-oncological Diseases

Neue Therapie der Sarkoidose mit verdünnten Vielstoffgemischen, insbesondere Iscucin Salicis und *Ferrum chloratum* comp.

New Therapy of Sarcoidosis With Diluted Multi-Substance Mixtures, Especially Iscucin Salicis and *Ferrum chloratum* comp.

Christian Grah, Irina Gatov, Shiao Li Oei, Marcus Reif, Hannah Wüstefeld, Annika Marzok

Zusammenfassung

Hintergrund: Die Sarkoidose ist eine seltene entzündliche Systemerkrankung, die bevorzugt die Lunge, grundsätzlich aber alle Organe des Körpers befallen kann und durch eine überschießende Entzündungsreaktion gekennzeichnet ist. Etabliert ist eine Therapie mit oralen Glukokortikoiden (OCS), zum Teil in Kombination mit anderen Immunsuppressiva. In der Pneumologischen Abteilung am Gemeinschaftskrankenhaus Havelhöhe wurde seit 2003 die ergänzende Behandlung der Sarkoidose durch eine Vielstoffgemisch aus *Viscum album* L., und *Ferrum chloratum comp.* nach dem Havelhöher Sarkoidoseprotokoll (HSP) etabliert. Ziel dieser Studie war es, die Krankheitsverläufe von mit HSP behandelten Sarkoidosepatienten zu evaluieren.

Methoden: Gemäß Studienprotokoll und Ethikvotum wurde in einer systematischen Analyse eine Real-World-Datenanalyse durchgeführt, bei der der klinische Verlauf, die Lungenfunktion, Fatigue-Symptome und unerwünschte Wirkungen in einer Sarkoidose-Kohorte retrospektiv mittels deskriptiver Statistik evaluiert wurden.

Ergebnisse: 956 Sarkoidosepatienten wurden zwischen 2003 und 2022 mit HSP behandelt und die klinischen Verläufe von insgesamt 124 einwilligenden Patienten über insgesamt mehr als 500 HSP-Äquivalenzjahren wurden dokumentiert und konnten in einer umfassenden Analyse detailliert ausgewertet werden. Es konnten konsistente Daten zu Pharmakovigilanz, Compliance und Wirkungen der Therapie und Krankheitskontrolle erhoben werden.

Schlussfolgerungen: Die HSP ist eine sichere Therapie mit hoher Compliance. Hohe Ansprechraten, Krankheitskontrolle und Symptomverbesserung wurden beobachtet. Es wird daher empfohlen, die HSP-Therapie in den Behandlungsalgorithmus der chronischen Sarkoidose aufzunehmen und in prospektiven Studien weiter zu evaluieren.
Schlüsselwörter: Vielstoffgemisch, Sarkoidose, Fatigue, Mistel, *Ferrum chloratum*

Summary
Background: Sarcoidosis is a rare inflammatory systemic disease that primarily affects the lungs, but can affect any organ of the body, and is characterized by an excessive inflammatory response. Treatment with oral glucocorticosteroids (OCS), sometimes in combination with other immunosuppressive drugs, is well established. Since 2003, the Department of Pneumology at the Gemeinschaftskrankenhaus Havelhöhe has been treating sarcoidosis with a multi-component mixture of *Viscum album* L. and *Ferrum chloratum comp.* according to the Havelhöhe Sarcoidosis Protocol (HSP). The aim of this study was to evaluate the course of disease in sarcoidosis patients treated with the HSP.
Methods: In accordance with the study protocol and ethics approval, a real-world data analysis was performed in a systematic analysis retrospectively evaluating the clinical course, lung function, fatigue symptoms, and adverse effects in a sarcoidosis cohort using descriptive statistics.
Results: 956 sarcoidosis patients were treated with HSP between 2003 and 2022, and the clinical course of a total of 124 consenting patients over a total of more than 500 HSP-equivalent years was documented and could be evaluated in detail in a comprehensive analysis. Consistent data were collected on pharmacovigilance, compliance and effects of therapy and disease control.
Conclusions: HSP is a safe therapy with high compliance. High response rates, disease control and symptom improvement have been observed. Therefore, it is recommended that HSP therapy be included in the treatment algorithm for chronic sarcoidosis and further evaluated in prospective studies.
Keywords: Multi-component mixture, sarcoidosis, fatigue, mistletoe, *Ferrum chloratum*

Einführung

Die Sarkoidose ist eine granulomatöse Systemerkrankung unbekannter Ursache und zählt zu den sog. Orphan Diseases, mit einer Prävalenz von 46 pro 100.000 Einwohner (Polverino *et al.* 2020; Schulze 2019). Sie betrifft insbesondere junge und mittelalte Erwachsene. Typisch für die Lungensarkoidose sind eine beidseitige hiläre Lymphadenopathie und Lungeninfiltrate, die eine sehr unterschiedliche Röntgenmorphologie aufweisen können. Zudem können andere Organe betroffen sein, insbesondere Augen- und Hautveränderungen, Herz, Leber, Milz, Speicheldrüsen, Muskeln, Knochen, Nieren und das zentrale Nervensystem (Sève *et al.* 2021).

Zur Sicherung der Sarkoidose müssen zunächst andere granulomatöse Erkrankungen, Infektionserkrankungen und Autoimmunerkrankungen ausgeschlossen werden (Tab. 1). Die Diagnose der Sarkoidose ist eine Ausschlussdiagnose und wird neben typischen klinisch-radiologischen Befunden und ergänzend durch einen histologischen Nachweis von nichteitrigen (einschmelzenden) epitheloiden Granulomen und Riesenzellen, sowie ggf. mit dem Nachweis einer lymphozytären Alveolitis mit einem verschobenen Verhältnis von CD4/CD8 Lymphozyten zugunsten der CD4 Lymphozyten gestellt.

Die Prognose der Sarkoidose korreliert mit der Lokalisation der granulomatösen Entzündung, deren Ausmaß und dem initialen Krankheitsverlauf und der Krankheitsdynamik. Eine gesicherte Behandlung der Sarkoidose ist bis heute nicht definiert (Llabres *et al.* 2019).

Für orale Glukokortikoide (OCS) liegen nur wenige verblindete, randomisierte Studien vor, die darauf hindeuten, dass die Verabreichung von OCS mit einem Rückgang der Infiltrate in der Lunge korreliert (Polverino *et al.* 2020). Obwohl der Langzeiteffekt von OCS Krankheitsverlauf nicht geklärt ist, stellt die Gabe von OCS in der Regel die Standardtherapie bei symptomatischer Sarkoidose mit Organfunktionseinschränkung dar, auch wenn die klinische Evidenz nicht sehr hoch ist (Baughman *et al.* 2021). Die Therapie mit OCS wird in der Regel dann empfohlen, wenn entweder eine progrediente Organdysfunktion nachgewiesen ist, eine fibrosierende Verlaufsform mit Narbenbildung vorliegt, und/oder bei Beteiligung des Lungengewebes eine restriktive Ventilationsstörung besteht. Für die Beteiligung von Herz, Nieren, Haut und des Cerebrums liegen leicht abgewandelte – aber vergleichbare Empfehlungen vor (Baughman *et al.* 2021)

Tab. 1: Differenzialdiagnose der Granulomatosen der Lunge

Tuberkulose/atypische Mykobakteriose, Lepra
Aktinomykose, Aspergillose, Cryptococcose, Blastomykose, Borrelien, Histoplasmose, Mykoplasmen, Leishmaniose, Listeriose, Lues Nocardiose, Pneumocystis jirovecii, Schistosomiasis
Exogen-allergische Alveolitis/Whirlpool-Lunge
Pneumokoniose (Beryllium, Titan, Aluminium, Talkum)
Pulmonale Langerhanszellhistiozytose (PLCH)
Medikamente (MTX, Infliximab, Leflunomid, Sirolimus etc.)
Fremdkörperaspiration
Granulomatöse Polyangiitis (M. Wegner) Eosinophile Granulomatose mit Polyangiitis (Churg-Strauss – Syndrom)
Bronchozentrische Granulomatose
Nekrotisierende Granulomatose
Lymphomatoide Granulomatose
Kollagenose-assoziierte sarkoide granulomatöse Reaktion, Rheumaknoten bei RA
Immundefizienz-Syndrome (z. B. Common variable immundeficiency syndrome)
M. Crohn
Tumor-assoziierte sarkoide granulomatöse Reaktion
Granulomatous lesions of unknown significance (GLUS) (B-Zell-positiv)
Sarkoidose

Topische Steroide werden für die *Uveitis anterior* und ebenso für Hautläsionen empfohlen (Marchell, Judson 2010). Eine intensivierte Immunsuppression wird bei fortschreitenden Verläufen, insbesondere zum Einsparen von hohen OCS Dosen oder bei Versagen der Therapie mit OCS empfohlen. Mittel der ersten Wahl sind in diesen Fällen Methotrexat oder

Azathioprin (Baughman *et al.* 2021). Die Ansätze der zielgerichteten Blockaden in der pathobiologischen Kaskade des Inflammationsgeschehens der Erkrankung sind vielfältig (Polverino *et al.* 2020). Für diese Therapien liegen jedoch meist nur kleine Fallzahlen bzw. nichtrandomisierte Untersuchungen vor, und es gibt keine spezifische Zulassungen für Monosubstanzen (z. B. Leflunomide, Mycophenolat mofetil, Hydrochloroquine, Infliximab oder Adalimumab, Retuximab, Januskinase-Inhibitoren) (Baughman *et al.* 2021). Schwere Funktionsverluste bei pulmonaler oder kardialer Sarkoidose mit vitaler Bedrohung der Organfunktion stellen eine Indikation für eine Organtransplantation dar (Polverino *et al.* 2020). Regelmäßige Überwachungsuntersuchungen (alle 3, 6, 12 Monate) sind indiziert und unerwünschten Medikamentenwirkungen (insbesondere von OCS) sollten ärztlich erfasst und ggf. behandelt werden (Osteoporose, Hypertonie, Glaukom) (Beegle *et al.* 2013). Eine zusätzliche Herausforderung stellt die funktionelle und psychische Beeinträchtigung der Patienten dar. Neben der psychischen Belastung, die mit der Diagnosestellung einhergeht und häufig zur Angst vor einem Krankheitsprogress führt, steht vor allem ein begleitendes Fatigue Syndrom im Vordergrund, welches bei > 50 % der Betroffenen beschrieben wird (Drent *et al.* 2012).

In der Pneumologischen Abteilung am Gemeinschaftskrankenhaus Havelhöhe wurde seit 2003 die ergänzende Behandlung der Sarkoidose durch ein Vielstoffgemisch aus *Viscum album L.*, Mistelextrakten und *Ferrum chloratum* nach dem Havelhöher Sarkoidoseprotokoll (HSP) etabliert (Grah *et al.* 2008; 2014). Ziel der vorliegenden Studie war es, Daten zur Pharmakovigilanz, Compliance und Wirksamkeit der HSP-Therapie sowie zur Krankheitskontrolle in einem großen Sarkoidose-Kollektiv über einen sehr langen Zeitraum zu erheben.

Methode

Wir führten eine retrospektive monozentrische Studie durch, indem wir demographische Daten, Informationen zur Diagnose, zur Histologie der Sarkoidose (Scadding 1961) sowie zu Fatigue Symptomen und unerwünschten Ereignissen aus den Krankenakten von Sarkoidosepatienten, die eine schriftliche Einverständniserklärung abgegeben hatten, extrahierten und analysierten.

<table>
<tr><td>Woche des Zyklus:
Medikament:</td><td>1</td><td>2</td><td>3</td><td>4</td><td>5</td><td>6</td><td>7</td><td>8</td><td>9</td><td>10</td><td>11</td><td>12</td></tr>
<tr><td>I.</td><td colspan="12">Ferrum sesquichloratum D2 / Graphites D14 / Tartarus Stibiatus D4.
(Herstellung+Bezug über: Apotheke an der Weleda)
10 – 0 – 10 Tropfen für 12 Wochen</td></tr>
<tr><td>II.</td><td colspan="4">Phosphorus met. präparatum D5 (Weleda)
10 - 0 - 0 Tropfen für vier Wochen</td><td></td><td></td><td></td><td></td><td></td><td></td><td></td><td></td></tr>
<tr><td>III.</td><td></td><td></td><td></td><td></td><td colspan="8">Iscucin Salicis (Wala), subkutan (s.c.), Montag und Freitag wöchentl., z. Nacht fünfmal Stärke C, dann fünfmal Stärke D, dann fünfmal Stärke E</td></tr>
</table>

Abb. 1: Havelhöher Sarkoidose Protokoll

Die Präparate Iscucin Salicis (Firma Wala, PZN 03083512) in den Stärken A–G, und Phosphorus metallicum präparatum (PZN / EAN 01573146/4001638067416) sind über den Großhandel zu beziehen. Die Präparate Ferrum sesquichloratum D2, Graphites D14, Tartarus Stibiatus D4 werden über die Apotheke an der Weleda (https://apotheke-weleda.de) bezogen, wo sie aus der Herstellung der Einzelsubstanzen über die Firma Weleda gemäß dem HSP hergestellt werden.

Die Behandlung der Sarkoidose erfolgte nach den aktuellen Leitlinien (Baughman, Grutters 2015) und wurde durch eine zyklische Therapie mit HSP (Grah *et al.* 2008) ergänzt. Das HSP (Abb. 1) in einer graphischen Form, wie es auch den Patienten ausgehändigt wurde umfasst einen Behandlungszyklus über drei Monate und enthält Arzneimittel von drei verschiedenen Herstellern.

Ergebnisse

Insgesamt wurden zwischen 2003 und 2022 in der Abteilung für Pneumologie des GKH 956 Sarkoidosepatienten behandelt. Von 301 Patienten wurden Einverständniserklärungen unterzeichnet, und für 124 dieser Patienten waren vollständige Datensätze für die Analyse verfügbar (Abb. 2).

124 Sarkoidosepatienten (alle Stadien, 35 % Multiorgan-Sarkoidose, Durchschnittsalter 43 Jahre, 69 % weiblich) wurden nach einer mittleren Nachbeobachtungszeit von 23 Monaten hinsichtlich ihrer klinischen Ergebnisse untersucht. Zu Beginn der Behandlung erhielten 61 (49 %) OCS in Kombination mit HSP und 63 (51 %) erhielten ausschließlich HSP (Abb. 2).

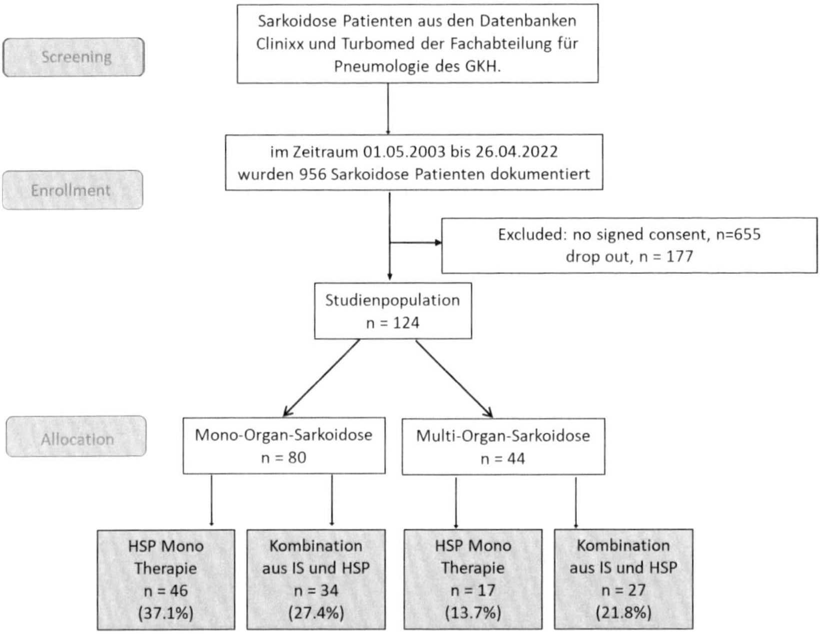

Abb. 2: Flussdiagramm der Studienpopulation.
HSP: Havelhöher Sarkoidose Protokoll; IS: Immunosuppressiva (Glukokortikosteroide, Methotrexat oder Azathioprin)

Bei der letzten Nachuntersuchung benötigten 103 (83 %) weder orale Glukokortikoide noch andere Immunsuppressiva (IS) und erhielten ausschließlich HSP. Ein HSP-Zyklus dauert drei Monate (Abb. 1), eine Standard-HSP-Therapie besteht aus zwei HSP-Zyklen pro Jahr und eine intensivierte HSP-Therapie aus vier HSP-Zyklen pro Jahr. Insgesamt beobachteten wir eine gute Compliance und Einhaltung des HSP-Protokolls (Tab. 2). Für die gesamte Studienkohorte von 124 Patienten wurden insgesamt 552 HSP-äquivalente Behandlungsjahre beobachtet und insgesamt 662 HSP-Zyklen verabreicht.

Tab. 2: HSP-Behandlungstherapie

n = 124	**n (%)**
Standard HSP (2 Zyklen/Jahr)	120 (97)
Intensivierte HSP (4 Zyklen/Jahr)	4 (3)
Gesamtzahl der HSP-Behandlungszyklen:	
1 HSP-Zyklus	8 (6)
2–5 HSP-Zyklen	69 (56)
6–10 HSP-Zyklen	29 (23)
> 10 HSP-Zyklen	14 (11)
HSP Unterbrechung	3 (2)
HSP Abbruch	6 (5)

Die Ansprechrate für die Krankheitskontrolle lag in dieser Studienkohorte bei 69 %. Bei der Erstuntersuchung zeigten 81 Patienten (65 %) klinisch relevante Fatigue Symptome, die sich bei 48 Patienten (59 %) im Verlauf der HSP-Therapie besserten. Die pharmakovigilante Überwachung zeigte ein sicheres therapeutisches Profil für das HSP, bei nur 10 (8 %) Patienten traten leichte unerwünschte Ereignisse (Grad 1) wie Lokalreaktionen wie Juckreiz oder Rötung auf.

Diskussion

Hier wurde eine große Sarkoidose-Kohorte mit vergleichbaren Ausgangscharakteristika, wie sie für andere Sarkoidose-Populationen beschrieben wurden (Schupp *et al.* 2018), über einen langen Behandlungszeitraum ausgewertet. Der hier abgedeckte Zeitraum umfasst mehr als 500 äquivalente HSP-Behandlungsjahre, was in kontrollierten randomisierten Studien kaum erreichbar wäre.

Das Havelhöhe Behandlungsprotokoll (HSP) ist ein Behandlungsansatz mit einem Multidrug-Protokoll, das dem Organismus eine zyklische Abfolge von Arzneimitteln in einem bestimmten Rhythmus anbietet. Diese zyklische Abfolge basiert auf der Hypothese, dass es sich ursächlich bei der Sarkoidose um eine funktionelle Störung von Prozessen im Atmungsrhythmus handelt. Damit ist eine Funktionsstörung adressiert, die in der konventionellen Medizin bislang keine pathophysiologische Bedeutung hat. In diesem Kontext stellt der Behandlungsansatz, wie er im HSP vorliegt, eine Brücke zu anderen Medizinsystemen und der modernen universitären Medizin dar (von Schoen-Angerer *et al.* 2023). Das HSP, erstmals 2003 definiert (Grah *et al.* 2008), im Laufe der Jahre leicht modifiziert, inzwischen seit mehr als 20 Jahren an über 1000 Patienten angewendet, ist bisher in medizinischen Fachkreisen noch unbekannt und wird auch in Übersichtsartikeln oder Empfehlungen von Fachgesellschaften, national wie international, noch nicht zitiert.

Die Sarkoidose-Fatigue ist ein schweres und häufiges Symptom der Sarkoidose, über das bis zu 80 % der Sarkoidosepatienten berichten (Drent *et al.* 2021; Drent *et al.* 2012). Die Sarkoidose Fatigue ähnelt in vielen Fällen dem Krankheitsbild des chronischen Fatigue-Syndrom (CFS) und schafft eine erhebliche Beeinträchtigung für betroffene Patienten (Drent *et al.* 2012) oft ohne relevante funktionelle Organbeeinträchtigung. Für Patienten mit Symptomlast Fatigue ohne progrediente Organdysfunktion sind OCS nicht indiziert. Die hierzu empfohlenen Therapievorschläge sind z. B. Armodafinil oder D-Methylphenidat (Psychostimunlanzien mit Stimulation von Neurotransmitterrezeptoren) oder Immuntherapeutika wie Infliximab, Adalimumab, ARA 290 oder auch physiotherapeutische Übungsprogramme (Atkins and Wilson 2017). Für die Behandlung des Sarkoidose-Symptoms Fatigue besteht daher derzeit ein sogenannter „unmet medical need", es liegen nur wenige Studien mit kleinen Fallzahlen vor (z. B. für Armodafinil (Lower *et al.* 2013)) und es besteht hier ein bislang zu wenig kommunizierter Forschungsbedarf (Atkins, Wilson 2017). Im Verlauf der HSP-Therapie wurden in dieser Studie eine hohe Ansprechrate, eine Verbesserung des Krankheitsverlaufs und auch eine deutliche Verbesserung der Fatigue-Symptomatik beobachtet. Es wird daher empfohlen, die HSP-Therapie in den Behandlungsalgorithmus der chronischen Sarkoidose aufzunehmen (Abb. 3). Zukünftig sollten weitere Evaluationen in prospektiven kontrollierten Studien im Vergleich zu einem Kontrollarm durchgeführt werden.

Zu den Limitationen vorliegender Analyse gehört das monozentrische, unkontrollierte, nicht randomisierte Studiendesign, das für verschiedene Verzerrungen anfällig ist, einschließlich der Selektion. Dennoch liefert diese Studie Hinweise auf die Sicherheit und klinische Wirksamkeit der HSP-Therapie bei Sarkoidosepatientinnen und -patienten. Die Stärke dieser Studie liegt in ihrem pragmatischen Design, einer großen Anzahl von untersuchten Patienten und einem sehr langen Beobachtungszeitraum.

Schlussfolgerungen

Es besteht ein ungedeckter Bedarf an wirksameren Therapien für die Sarkoidose selbst und das damit verbundene Fatigue Syndrom sowie zur Vermeidung der toxischen Wirkungen einer langfristigen Anwendung hochdosierter Glukokortikosteroide. Hier wurde eine große Sarkoidose-Kohorte mit ähnlichen Ausgangsmerkmalen wie bei anderen Sarkoidose-Populationen beschrieben. Die HSP ist eine sichere Therapie, die gut befolgt wird. Hohe Ansprechraten wurden beobachtet, die Krankheit konnte kontrolliert und die Symptome gebessert werden, so dass unsere Daten klinische Relevanz haben.

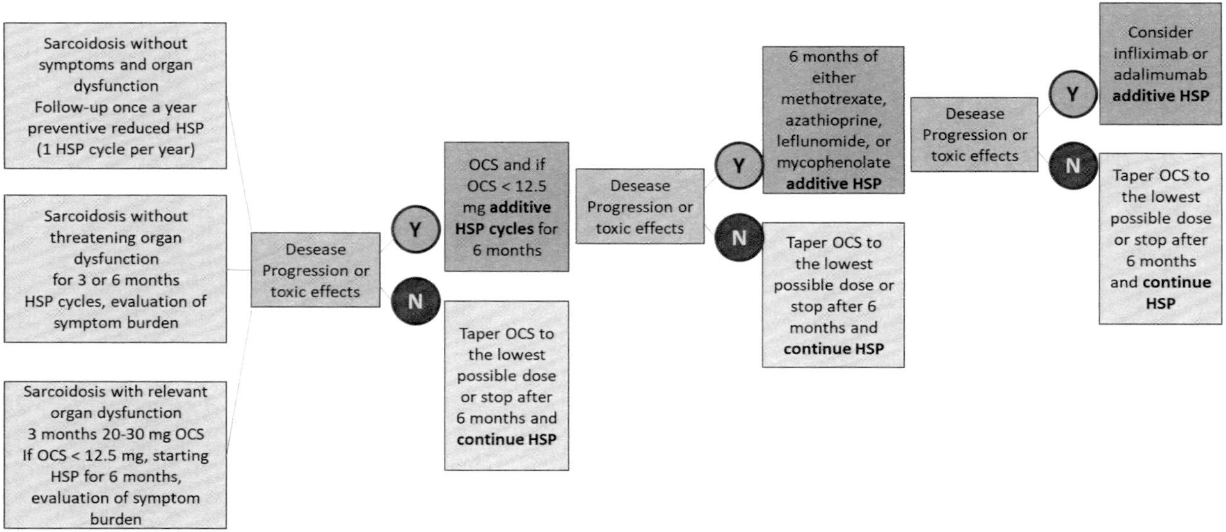

Abb. 3: Behandlungsalgorithmus zur Therapie der Sarkoidose
Modifiziert nach (Baughman, Grutters 2015) unter Hinzunahme der HSP-Therapie. HSP: Havelhöher Sarkoidose-Protokoll, OCS: orale Glukokortikosteroide wie Prednison oder Prednisolon; Y: ja; N: nein

Interessenkonflikte

CG berichtet über Zuschüsse von AstraZeneca, Takeda, Novartis, Chiesi, Iscador, außerhalb der eingereichten Arbeit. HW berichtet über Zuschüsse von AstraZeneca und Berlin-Chemie außerhalb der eingereichten Arbeit. Es bestehen keine weiteren relevanten Beschäftigungs- oder Beratungsbeziehungen.

Literatur

Atkins C, Wilson AM: Managing fatigue in sarcoidosis – a systematic review of the evidence. Chron Respir Dis. 2017; 14: 161–173.

Baughman RP, Grutters JC: New treatment strategies for pulmonary sarcoidosis: antimetabolites, biological drugs, and other treatment approaches. Lancet Respir Med. 2015; 3:813-822 doi:10.1016/s2213-2600(15)00199-x.

Baughman RP, Kotzin J, Lower EE: The Value of a Patient Global Assessment in Management of Sarcoidosis. Lung. 2021; 199: 357–362 doi:10.1007/s00408-021-00455-5.

Beegle SH, Barba K, Gobunsuy R, Judson MA: Current and emerging pharmacological treatments for sarcoidosis: a review Drug Design, Development and Therapy. 2013; 325–338.

Drent M, Crouser ED, Grunewald J: Challenges of Sarcoidosis and Its Management The New England journal of medicine. 2021; 385:1018-1032 doi:10.1056/NEJMra2101555

Drent M, Lower EE, De Vries J: Sarcoidosis-associated fatigue The European respiratory journal. 2012; 40:255–263. doi:10.1183/09031936.00002512.

Grah C, Happel H, Vogt J: Die Behandlung der pulmonalen Sarkoidose nach dem Havelhöher Sarkoidose-Therapieprotokoll Der Merkurstab Zeitschrift für Anthroposophische Medizin. 2008; 61:343–353 doi:10.14271/DMS-19286-DE.

Grah C, Thieme C, Seiberth R, Arne J, McCutcheon A, Schreiber S, Müller-Quernheim J: Benefit of steroid-free treatment compared to standard therapy (ST) in pulmonary sarcoidosis Eur Respir J. 2014; 44:P3765.

Llabres M, Brito-Zerón P, Ramos-Casals M, Sellares J: Synthetic pharmacotherapy for pulmonary sarcoidosis Expert Opinion on Pharmacotherapy. 2019; 20:1397–1404.

Lower EE, Malhotra A, Surdulescu V, Baughman RP: Armodafinil for sarcoidosis-associated fatigue: a double-blind, placebo-controlled, crossover trial. J Pain Symptom Manage. 2013; 45:159–169

Marchell RM, Judson MA: Cutaneous sarcoidosis. In: Seminars in respiratory and critical care medicine. Semin Respir Crit Care Med. 2010; 31 (04): 442–451.

Polverino F, Balestro E, Spagnolo P: Clinical presentations, pathogenesis, and therapy of sarcoidosis: state of the art. J Clin Med. 2020; 9: 2363.

Scadding JG: Prognosis of intrathoracic sarcoidosis in England. A review of 136 cases after five years' observation. BMJ. 1961; 2: 1165–1172.

Schulze F: Die Versorgungssituation von Patienten mit refraktärer Atemnot: eine qualitative Interviewstudie zu Status Quo und Perspektiven. Dissertation, LMU München: Medizinische Fakultät. 2019; doi: 10.5282/edoc.25328.

Schupp JC et al.: Phenotypes of organ involvement in sarcoidosis. Europ Respir J. 2018; 51 (1):1700991. doi:10.1183/13993003.00991-2017

Sève P et al.: Sarcoidosis: a clinical overview from symptoms to diagnosis. Cells. 2021; 10: 766.

von Schoen-Angerer T et al.: Traditional, complementary and integrative healthcare: global stakeholder perspective on WHO's current and future strategy. BMJ Glob Health. 2023; 8 (12): e013150. doi:10.1136/bmjgh-2023-013150.

Dr. Christian Grah[1, 2], Dr. Hannah Wüstefeld[1, 2], Dr. Shiao Li Oei[2], Dr. Marcus Reif[3], Irina Gatov[3], Annika Marzok[4]

[1] Pneumologie, Gemeinschaftskrankenhaus Havelhöhe, Berlin, Germany

[2] Forschungsinstitut Havelhöhe, Berlin, Germany

[3] Gesellschaft für Klinische Forschung e.V., Berlin, Germany
[4] Universität Witten-Herdecke und Forschungsinstitut Havelhöhe, Berlin, Germany

Korrespondenzadresse:
christian.grah@havelhoehe.de

V. Anwendung bei Tieren

V. Use of Mistletoe in Animals

Therapy Response of Equine Sarcoid-bearing Horses When Treated With Orally Administered Mistletoe Extract Compared to Administration by Subcutaneous Injection or Placebo, Respectively

Ansprechen von Pferden mit equinen Sarkoiden auf die Behandlung mit oral eingenommenem Mistelextrakt im Vergleich zur subkutanen Injektion oder einem Placebo

Anke Beermann, Ulrike Biegel, Marcus Reif, Lucia Unger, Ophélie Clottu, Christoph Koch

The authors wish to transparently declare that a full version of this article has previously been published in the *Journal of Veterinary Internal Medicine*. Article doi: 10.1111/jvim.17052.

Summary

Background: Equine sarcoids are the most common equine skin tumors. Their treatment can be challenging. Repeated subcutaneous injections of mistletoe extract (Iscador P®, manufacturer and marketing authorization holder Iscador AG, Arlesheim, Switzerland, fermented pine mistletoe available in ampoules with concentrations ranging from 0.1 mg/ml to 20 mg/ml) have already been successfully used in the therapy of sarcoids. However, repeated injections are inconvenient for the majority of horse owners, resulting in less frequent use of this therapy in practice.

Hypothesis: Oral administration of Iscador P® is as effective as subcutaneous injection and more effective than placebo. Furthermore, extending the duration of therapy from 15 to 28 weeks will shorten the time until remission and lead to a higher remission rate.

Animals: 45 privately owned horses with equine sarcoids (aged 5–12 years), in Switzerland.

Methods: A three-arm, randomized, prospective, parallel, placebo-controlled, double-blinded study in a double-dummy design was conducted. Horses were treated with Iscador P® (0.1–20 mg/ml) and/or placebo (1 ml sterile NaCl solution) for a duration of 28 weeks.
Results: The study did not observe any statistically significant differences in the overall outcomes among the three groups. A direct comparison between the oral VAE group and the placebo group yielded an odds ratio of 2.16 (95 % confidence interval: 0.45–10.42) with a p-value of 0.336.
Conclusion and Significance for Practice: The oral form of VAE was found to be safe for use. However, the study did not demonstrate a statistically significant benefit of systemic VAE treatment over placebo in treating equine sarkoids.
Keywords: Horse, mistletoe, equine sarcoid, *Viscum album* extract, randomized trial, immunotherapy

Zusammenfassung
Hintergrund: Equine Sarkoide sind die häufigsten Hauttumoren bei Pferden. Ihre Behandlung kann herausfordernd sein. Wiederholte subkutane Injektionen von Mistelextrakt (Iscador P®, Hersteller und Zulassungsinhaber Iscador AG, Arlesheim, Schweiz, fermentierter Kiefernmistel in Ampullen mit Konzentrationen von 0,1 mg/ml bis 20 mg/ml) wurden bereits erfolgreich in der Therapie von Sarkoiden eingesetzt. Jedoch sind wiederholte Injektionen für die Mehrheit der Pferdebesitzer unpraktisch, was dazu führt, dass diese Therapie in der Praxis seltener verwendet wird.
Hypothese: Die orale Verabreichung von Iscador P® ist genauso effektiv wie die subkutane Injektion und effektiver als ein Placebo. Darüber hinaus wird durch die Verlängerung der Therapiedauer von 15 auf 28 Wochen die Zeit bis zur Remission verkürzt und eine höhere Remissionsrate erzielt.
Tiere: 45 privat gehaltene Pferde mit equinen Sarkoiden (im Alter von 5–12 Jahren), in der Schweiz.
Methoden: Eine dreigliedrige, randomisierte, prospektive, parallele, placebokontrollierte, doppelt verblindete Studie im Double-Dummy-Design wurde durchgeführt. Die Pferde wurden mit Iscador P® (von 0,1 bis 20 mg/ml) und/oder Placebo (1 ml sterile NaCl-Lösung) über einen Zeitraum von 28 Wochen behandelt.

Ergebnisse: Die Studie beobachtete keine statistisch signifikanten Unterschiede in den Gesamtergebnissen zwischen den drei Gruppen. Ein direkter Vergleich zwischen der oralen VAE-Gruppe und der Placebogruppe ergab ein Odds Ratio von 2,16 (95 % Konfidenzintervall: 0,45–10,42) mit einem p-Wert von 0,336.
Schlussfolgerung und Bedeutung für die Praxis: Die orale Form von VAE wurde als sicher für die Verwendung befunden. Die Studie konnte jedoch keinen statistisch signifikanten Vorteil der systemischen VAE-Behandlung gegenüber Placebo bei der Behandlung von equinen Sarkoiden nachweisen.
Schlüsselwörter: Pferd, Mistel, equines Sarkoid, Viscum album Extrakt, randomisierte Studie, Immuntherapie

Conflict of interest

The authors declare no conflict of interest.

Dr. med. vet. Anke Beermann[1], Dr. med. vet. Ulrike Biegel[1], Dr. rer. nat. Marcus Reif[2], Dr. med. vet. Lucia Unger[3], Dr. med. vet. Ophélie Clottu[1], Dr. med. vet. Christoph Koch[3]
[1] Research Institute of Organic Agriculture (FiBL) Frick, Switzerland
[2] Society for Clinical Research (GKF e. V.), Berlin, Germany
[3] Swiss Institute of Equine Medicine, ISME, Vetsuisse Faculty, University of Bern, Bern, Switzerland

Korrespondenzadresse:
anke.beermann@fibl.org

Fallserie einer oralen Anwendung der Misteltherapie (Iscador® P) zur Behandlung von Equinen Sarkoiden

Case Series on the Oral Use of a Mistletoe Extract (Iscador® P) in Equine Sarcoid

Ophélie Clottu, Ulrike Biegel, Marcus Reif

Zusammenfassung

Hintergrund: Equines Sarkoid ist der häufigste Hauttumor bei Pferden und trotz einer großen Anzahl verfügbarer Therapien stellt die Behandlung dieser Krankheit weiterhin eine Herausforderung für den Praktiker dar. In einer RCT-Studie (Christen-Clottu *et al.* 2010) zeigten subkutane Injektionen von Mistelextrakten eine signifikant höhere Rate an kompletter und partieller Regression der Sarkoiden als eine Placebo-Behandlung.

Hypothese: Die orale Anwendung von Mistelextrakte könnte auch bei der Behandlung von Sarkoiden wirksam sein.

Ziel: Proof-of-Concept der oralen Anwendung von Mistelextrakt (ME_{oral}) (Iscador® P, Iscador AG, Arlesheim, Schweiz) in der Praxis und Vergleich mit der Placebo-Gruppe der RCT-Studie (PL_{RCT}).

Methoden: 9 Pferde und ein Esel, 3–10 Jahre alt, mit jeweils 1–10 Sarkoiden, wurden oral mit Mistelextrakt (Iscador® P, 0,1–20 mg wässriger Extrakt aus Kiefern-Mistel) nach dem gleichen RCT-Protokoll behandelt (3 Gaben/Woche für 15 Wochen + 1-jähriges Follow-up). Die Mistelextrakte wurden direkt ins Maul verabreicht oder mit dem Futter vermischt.

Ergebnisse: Fünf Pferde und ein Esel zeigten eine komplette Regression aller Sarkoide (60 %). Drei Pferde zeigten eine Abnahme der Anzahl der Sarkoide, ein Pferd eine Zunahme. Zum Vergleich: Von den 20 PL_{RCT} Pferden zeigten nur 3 Pferde eine komplette Regression (15 %).

Obwohl die beiden Pferdegruppen vor der Behandlung hinsichtlich der Anzahl der Sarkoide (Anzahl der ES, Mittelwert ± SD: PL_{RCT} 5,3 ± 3,2, ME_{oral} 5,0 ± 3,1) und der Tumorfläche (Fläche: PL_{RCT} 3,8 ± 2,1 cm^2, ME_{oral} 4,7 ± 2,6 cm^2) vergleichbar waren, wurden signifikante Unterschiede zwischen den beiden Gruppen in der Entwicklung der Sarkoide während der Behandlungszeit bis

zum Ende des Beobachtungszeitraums festgestellt (Veränderung der Anzahl der ES: PL_{RCT} +0,2 ± 2,5; ME_{oral} -2,3 ± 2,1; Veränderung der Fläche/Monat: PL_{RCT} +0,015 ± 0,248 cm^2; ME_{oral} -0,234 ± 0,220 cm^2).
Fazit: Diese Ergebnisse sind ein erster Hinweis auf die Verwendung von oralen Mistelextrakten als praktikable und effektive Methode zur Behandlung von Equinen Sarkoiden.
Schlüsselwörter: Mistel, Equines Sarkoid, Fallserie

Summary
Background: Equine sarcoid is the most common skin tumor in horses and despite a large number of available therapies, treatment of this disease continues to be a challenge for the practitioner. In an RCT study (Christen-Clottu *et al.* 2010) subcutaneous mistletoe injections showed a significantly higher rate of sarcoid regression than placebo treatment.
Hypothesis: Oral application of mistletoe treatment would also be effective in the treatment of sarcoid.
Purpose: Proof-of-Concept of the oral application of mistletoe extract (ME_{oral}) (Iscador® P Iscador AG, Arlesheim, Schweiz) in practice and comparison with the placebo group of the RCT study (PL_{RCT}).
Methods: 9 horses and one donkey, aged 3–10 years, with 1–10 sarcoids were treated orally with mistletoe extract (Iscador® P, 0.1–20 mg aqueous extract of pine mistletoe) in a manner similar to the RCT protocol (3 doses/week for 15 weeks + 1 year follow-up). The mistletoe extract was either administered directly into the mouth or mixed with food.
Results: Five horses and one donkey showed complete regression of all sarcoids (60 %). Three horses showed a decrease in the number of sarcoids, one horse an increase. In comparison, of the 20 PL_{RCT} horses, only 3 showed complete regression of sarcoids (15 %). Although the two groups of horses were comparable before treatment regarding the number of sarcoids (number of ES, mean ± SD: PL_{RCT} 5.3 ± 3.2, ME_{oral} 5.0 ± 3.1) and lesion area (area: PL_{RCT} 3.8 ± 2.1 cm^2, ME_{oral} 4.7 ± 2.6 cm^2), significant differences were found between the two groups in the evolution of sarcoids during the treatment period until the end of the observation period (change in number of ES: PL_{RCT} +0.2 ± 2.5; ME_{oral} -2.3 ± 2.1; decrease in area/month: PL_{RCT} +0.015 ± 0.248 cm^2; ME_{oral} -0.234 ± 0.220 cm^2).
Conclusion: These results are a first indication of the use of oral mistletoe extracts as a viable and effective method of treatment of sarcoid.
Keywords: Mistletoe, equine sarcoid, case series

Einleitung

Equine Sarkoide sind die häufigsten Hauttumoren bei Equiden. Diese weit verbreitete Krankheit betrifft mehr als 10 % der dreijährigen Pferde in der Schweiz (Mele *et al.* 2007; Studer *et al.* 2007). Das bovine Papillomavirus wird als Erreger des Sarkoids angesehen. Die DNA dieses Virus wird aber auch auf der gesunden Haut von fast 50 % der gesunden Pferde gefunden (Bogeart *et al.* 2008). Bei der Entstehung der Krankheit spielen also auch andere Faktoren eine Rolle: Genetische Veranlagung, ein schwaches Immunsystem, frühere Hautverletzungen, oder auch die Haltungs- und Fütterungsart vervollständigen die multifaktorielle Genese dieser Krankheit (Jandova *et al.* 2012; Chambers *et al.* 2003; Mele *et al.* 2007). Pferde zeigen häufig multiple Sarkoide unterschiedlicher Typen an verschiedenen Lokalisationen des Körpers auf, was eine chirurgische oder lokale Behandlung besonders schwierig machen kann. Obwohl die Rolle des Immunsystems bei der Entwicklung oder Rückbildung von Sarkoiden nicht vollständig geklärt ist, spielt es eine wichtige Rolle, weshalb Immuntherapien vor allem bei der Behandlung von Pferden mit multiplen Sarkoiden von Interesse sind (Martens *et al.* 2001; Haspeslagh *et al.* 2016). Immunmodulierende Präparate zur Behandlung von Sarkoiden stammen aus endogenen Quellen wie Interleukinen (Germann *et al.* 2006) oder autogenen Impfstoffen (Kinnunen *et al.* 1999; Mattil-Fritz *et al.* 2008) und aus exogenen Quellen wie dem BCG-Impfstoff (Martens *et al.* 2001) oder aus Pflanzen (Martens *et al.* 2000; Rush *et al.* 2000). Fermentierte Mistelextrakte (*Viscum album* L.) haben tumorhemmende (Kienle *et al.* 2003), antiangiogenetische (Duong Von Hungen *et al.* 2002), entzündungshemmende (Hedge *et al.* 2011) sowie immunmodulierende (Heinzerling *et al.* 2006) Eigenschaften gezeigt und werden als adjuvante Therapie in der humanen Onkologie (Kienle *et al.* 2007; Wode *et al.* 2020) sowie in der Veterinärmedizin (Biegel *et al.* 2022) bei Katzen (Biegel *et al.* 2013; Glardon *et al.* 2014) und Hunden (Biegel *et al.* 2017; Von Bodungen *et al.* 2017) eingesetzt. Mistelextrakte haben sich auch bei der Behandlung von Sarkoiden als wirksam erwiesen. In einer randomisierten Doppelblindstudie zeigten Mistelextrakte (Iscador P®), die dann in drei subkutanen Injektionen pro Woche über einen Zeitraum von 15 Wochen angewendet wurden, eine signifikant höhere Heilungs- und Verbesserungsrate bei Sarkoiden als die Placebogruppe (Christen-Clottu *et al.* 2010). Diese wiederholten Injektionen sind aber auch häufig der von den Besitzern angegebene Grund, diese Behandlung nicht durchzuführen. Aus diesem Grund wurde eine orale Anwendung der Mistelextrakte in Betracht gezogen. Die orale Anwendung von Mistelextrakten hat auch immunmodulatorische Eigenschaften gezeigt (Lavelle *et al.* 2000; Pryme *et al.* 2002) und wird zur Prophylaxe von Fibrosarkom-Rezidiven nach chirurgischer Entfernung bei Katzen eingesetzt (Biegel *et al.* 2013). Das Ziel dieser Fallserie im Vergleich zu einer historischen Placebogruppe war es, Hinweise auf eine Wirksamkeit von oral verabreichten Mistelextrakten (Iscador P®) bei der Behandlung von Equinen Sarkoiden in der Praxis zu finden.

Material und Methoden

Um zu testen, ob sich die orale Anwendung von Mistelextrakten auch bei der Behandlung von Equinen Sarkoiden als wirksam erweisen könnte, erhielten 10 an Sarkoiden erkrankten Equiden, die zwischen Januar 2017 und Februar 2020 in der Tierarztpraxis von Dr. Ophélie Clottu in Enges behandelt wurden, eine orale Behandlung mit Mistelextrakten der Kiefer (*Viscum album* ssp. *austriacus*, Iscador P®). Das Behandlungsprotokoll war das gleiche wie bei der Injektionstherapie (Iscador P® von 0,01 bis 20 mg/ml, 3 Einnahmen von 1 ml pro Woche während 15 Wochen gefolgt von einem Jahr Beobachtungzeit), um einen Vergleich mit der Placebogruppe der randomisierten Studie (PL_{RCT}) „Treatment of clinically diagnosed equine sarcoid with a mistletoe extract“, die 2010 veröffentlicht wurde (Christen-Clottu *et al.* 2010), zu ermöglichen. Die Anwendung der Mistelextrakte erfolgte entweder direkt ins Maul (N = 4) oder mit dem Futter vermischt (N = 6).

Die Sarkoide in der Gruppe, die die orale Therapie (ME_{oral}) erhielt, wurden klinisch, sowie nach dem von der Universität Bern vorgeschlagenen Diagnoseprotokoll (positiver Sarkoid-Befund bei einem Score grösser als 15) diagnostiziert (Haspeslagh *et al.* 2018). Die Diagnose der Sarkoide in der Kontrollgruppe war histologisch bestätigt worden. Bei jedem Equiden wurde die Anzahl der Sarkoide vor Beginn der Behandlung, sowie bei jedem folgenden Besuch alle 3 Monate während 14 Monaten bei der Kontrollgruppe und von 18 bis 21 Monaten bei den 10 oral behandelten Tieren erhoben. Außerdem wurden die 7 größten Sarkoide bei der Kontrollgruppe jeden Monat und bei der per oral behandelten Gruppe alle 3 Monate detailliert beobachtet (Lokalisation, Typ, Zustand), fotografiert und gemessen (Länge, Breite und Höhe). Für jedes Pferd wurde ein nach Mählmann *et al.* (2014) angepasster Score für den Schweregrad der Krankheit berechnet, der die Anzahl der Sarkoide, die Gesamtfläche der Sarkoide, den schwersten klinischen Typ (okkult, verrukös, nodulär, gemischt, fibroblastisch, maligne), die Anzahl der bereits erfolglos durchgeführten Behandlungen sowie die Wachstumsgeschwindigkeit in den letzten 6 Monaten umfasste (Score von 1 bis 23). Um die Entwicklung der Sarkoide zu vergleichen, wurde die Fläche der Sarkoide berechnet. Die Sarkoide werden als Halbellipsoide beschrieben und ihre jeweiligen Flächen werden nach Thomsen durch folgende Näherungsformel bestimmt:

$$A \approx \frac{1}{2} \cdot \left(4\pi \cdot (((a \cdot b)^{1.6075} + (a \cdot c)^{1.6075} + (b \cdot c)^{1.6075})/3)^{1/1.6075}\right)$$

wobei a, b und c die Radien der drei Achsen des Halbellipsoids darstellen und somit der halben Länge, der halben Breite und der gesamten Höhe in den Abmessungen eines Sarkoids entsprechen. Da die Flächenwerte durch die Multiplikation von Länge und Breite der Sarkoide stark rechtsverteilt sind, werden sie für die statistische Auswertung mit Hilfe der Quadratwurzel transformiert. Die so ermittelten Flächenwerte für die 7 größten einzelnen Sarkoide eines Pferdes werden für die Auswertung zu einem Gesamtwert addiert. Die primären Wirksamkeitsparameter in dieser Fallserie sind die Gesamtzahl der Sarkoide und die Fläche der 7 größten Sarkoide, die bei einem Pferd identifiziert wurden. Die primären Endpunkte der Behandlung sind die Unterschiede in der Anzahl und der Fläche der Sarkoide zwischen der ersten (Referenz-)Untersuchung zu Beginn der Behandlung und der Untersuchung 14 Monate nach Beginn der Behandlung.

Ergebnisse

Die Pferde, die oral mit Mistelextrakt behandelt wurden (ME_{oral}), 9 Pferde und ein Esel, waren zwischen 3 und 10 Jahren alt. Sie wiesen 1 bis 10 Sarkoide auf, die sowohl klinisch als auch nach dem von der Universität Bern vorgeschlagenen Diagnoseprotokoll (Score 15–21) diagnostiziert wurden. Der Score für den Schweregrad der Krankheit gemäß Mählmann *et al.* (2014) zeigte 4 leicht betroffene Pferde (Score 3–10), 2 mäßig betroffene Pferde (Score 11–14) und 4 schwer betroffene Pferde (Score 15–20).

Die Kontrollgruppe (PL_{RCT}) bestand aus 20 Pferden im Alter von 3 bis 17 Jahren, die an der Doppelblindstudie von 2010 teilgenommen hatten und damals subkutane Placebo-Injektionen (1 ml 0,9 %ige Kochsalzlösung) erhalten hatten. Sie hatten 1 bis 12 histologisch diagnostizierte Sarkoide. In dieser Gruppe waren 9, 7 und 4 Pferde leicht, mäßig bzw. schwer erkrankt.

Die beiden Pferdegruppen waren vor der Behandlung hinsichtlich Alter, Geschlecht, Schweregrad der Erkrankung, Art und Anzahl der Sarkoide (Mittelwert ± Standardabweichung: PL_{RCT} 5,3 ± 3,2, ME_{oral} 5,0 ± 3,1), sowie der Gesamtfläche der 7 größten Sarkoide (PL_{RCT} 3,8 ± 2,1 cm^2, ME_{oral} 4,7 ± 2,6 cm^2) vergleichbar.

In der Gruppe ME_{oral} zeigten fünf Pferde und ein Esel eine komplette Regression aller Sarkoide (60 %). Diese Pferde waren zwischen 3 und 7 Jahren alt und 3 waren leicht (Score 6–10), 2 mäßig (Score 12–13) und 1 schwer (Score 15) betroffen. Drei Pferde im Alter von 9 und 10 Jahren, die leicht (Score 8) und schwer (Score 16) betroffen waren, zeigten einen Rückgang der Sarkoidzahl. Ein schwer betroffenes 8-jähriges Pferd (Score 17) zeigte einen Anstieg der Sarkoidzahl.

Im Vergleich dazu zeigten von den 20 Kontrollpferden PL_{RCT}, nur drei eine komplette Regression der Sarkoiden (15 %). Diese drei Pferde waren 3, 5 und 7 Jahre alt und leicht erkrankt (Score 7–10).

Obwohl die beiden Gruppen vor der Behandlung keine signifikanten Unterschiede in der Anzahl der Sarkoide oder der Gesamtfläche der Sarkoide pro Pferd aufwiesen, zeigten sie signifikante Unterschiede in der Entwicklung der Sarkoide während des Behandlungszeitraums bis zum

Ende des Beobachtungszeitraums. Es wurde eine Abnahme der Anzahl der Sarkoide sowie der Sarkoidfläche in der oral behandelten Gruppe im Vergleich zur Placebogruppe signifikant nachgewiesen (Veränderung der Anzahl der ES, Mittelwert ± Standardabweichung: PL_{RCT} +0,2 ± 2,5; ME_{oral} -2,3 ± 2,1; Änderung der Fläche/Monat: PL_{RCT} +0,015 ± 0,248 cm^2; ME_{oral} -0,234 ± 0,220 cm^2) (siehe Abb. 1).

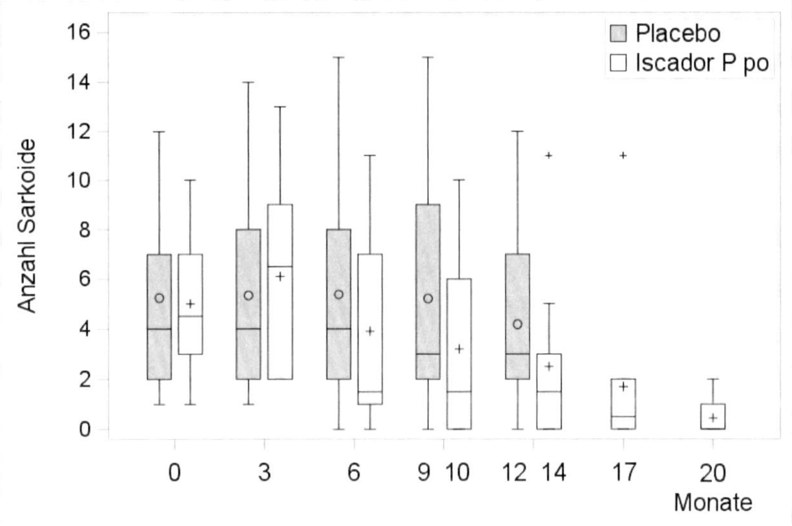

Abb. 1: Anzahl Sarkoide pro Pferd über die Untersuchungszeitpunkte (Querstrich: Median, Kreis: arithmetisches Mittel; Box: Interquartil-Range (IQR), Whisker: 1,5-facher IQR, Stern: Extremwert außerhalb des 1,5-fachen IQR)

Diskussion

Diese Fallserie aus der Praxis sollte eine mögliche Wirksamkeit der oralen Anwendung eines Extrakts aus der Kiefernmistel (Iscador P®) bei der Behandlung von Sarkoiden aufzeigen. Nach einer 14-monatigen Beobachtungszeit führten 15 Wochen Behandlung zu einem signifikant höheren Prozentsatz an komplette und partielle Regression von Sarkoiden im Vergleich zu einer Gruppe, die mit einem Placebo behandelt wurde.

Eine spontane komplette Regression (nach Verabreichung eines Placebos) wurde nur bei Pferden im Alter von 3 bis 7 Jahren und hauptsächlich bei Pferden mit 1 bis 2 Sarkoiden, also mit einem niedrigen Schweregrad der Erkrankung (Score 7–10), beobachtet. Eine vollständige Regression in der oral behandelten Gruppe wurde hingegen bei leicht, mäßig und schwer betroffenen Individuen (Score 6–17) mit 1 bis 9 Sarkoiden verzeichnet.

Die orale Misteltherapie wurde von allen Tieren gut vertragen. Um diese Ergebnisse genauer zu untersuchen, wurde eine breiter angelegte Studie als randomisierte, doppel-blinden, placebokontrollierte Studie mit 45 Pferden durchgeführt (Beermann *et al.* 2024). Diese Studie untermauert unsere Schlussfolgerung, wobei der Unterschied zwischen der oralen und der Placebogruppe dort nicht signifikant war.

Es gibt jedoch einige Einschränkungen bei dieser Fallserie. Der größte limitierende Faktor ist die geringe Anzahl der Pferde. Des Weiteren handelte es sich um Tiere aus der Praxis, bei denen die Sarkoide gerade erst aufgetreten waren und noch nicht für das Equine Sarkoid therapiert wurden, was die Chancen auf eine Heilung verbessert. Sarkoide, die nach einer Behandlung rezidivieren, sind oft schwieriger zu behandeln. In der Studie von Beermann *et al.* waren 50 % der Pferde schon erfolglos vorbehandelt. Da in der Fallserie keine Randomisierung vorgenommen wurde, kann es zu einer Verzerrung der Auswahl gekommen sein. Die Fälle in der Praxis wurden möglicherweise unbeabsichtigt als gute Kandidaten für eine Misteltherapie ausgewählt. In der Tat bei schwer erkrankten Tieren wurde dem Besitzer eine Alternative vorgeschlagen und die Pferde wurden zuerst chirurgisch in der Klinik behandelt und konnten nicht in diese Fallserie aufgenommen werden. Die Pferdegruppen waren jedoch hinsichtlich des Schweregrads der Krankheit, der Anzahl der Sarkoide und der Gesamtfläche der sieben größten Sarkoide vergleichbar mit den Placebo-Tieren.

Die Sarkoide wurden nur klinisch diagnostiziert. Es gab keine histologische Analyse in der Gruppe ME_{oral}. Allerdings wiesen alle Pferde einen Sarkoid-definierenden Score von über 15 in dem von der Universität Bern vorgeschlagenen Diagnoseprotokoll auf, das eine hohe Sensitivität aufzeigt (Haspeslagh *et al.* 2018).

Trotz dieser Einschränkungen zeigt diese Fallserie, dass Pferde, die oral mit Mistelextrakten behandelt wurden, mehr komplette und partielle Regressionen zeigten als die Placebogruppe. Dies ist in der täglichen Praxis bereits ein sehr interessantes Ergebnis, wenn man bedenkt, wie schwierig die Behandlung von Sarkoiden sein kann und dass immunmodulierende Behandlungen ohne Nebenwirkungen selten sind. Die orale Misteltherapie erleichtert die Motivation für die Behandlung und die Verabreichung der Therapie durch die Besitzer über einen längeren Zeitraum.

Interessenkonflikt

MR ist Mitarbeiter der Firma Iscador AG. Die übrigen Autoren erklären, dass kein Interessenkonflikt besteht.

Literatur

Beermann A, Clottu O, Biegel U et al.: A randomized placebo-controlled double-blinded study comparing oral and subcutaneous administration of mistletoe extract for the treatment of equine sarcoid disease. J Vet Intern Med. 2024. 38 (3): 1815–1824.

Biegel U, Mevissen M, Schuller S et al.: Viscum album L., a Therapeutic Option for Neoplastic Diseases in Companion Animals? A Systemic Review. Complement Med Res. 2022; 29(6): 465–482.

Biegel U, Stratmann N, Knauf Y et al.: Postoperative adjuvante Therapie mit einem Mistelextrakt (Viscum album ssp. album) bei Hündinnen mit Mammatumoren. Complement Med Res. 2017; 24 (6): 349–357.

Biegel U. et al.: Mistletoe extracts (Viscum album) as an adjuvant therapy concept in feline fibrosarcoma. In: Scheer R et al. (Eds): Die Mistel in der Tumortherapie 3. Essen: KVC; 2013: 475–485.

Bogaert L, Martens A, Van Poucke M et al.: High prevalence of bovine papillomaviral DANN in the normal skin of equine sarcoid-affected and healthy horses. Vet Microbiol. 2008; 126 (1–2): 58–68.

Chambers G, Ellsmore VA, O'Brien PM et al.: Association of bovine papillomavirus with the equine sarcoid. J Gen Virol. 2003; 84: 1055–1062.
Christen-Clottu O, Klocke P, Burger D et al.: Treatment of clinically diagnosed equine sarcoid with a mistletoe extract (Viscum album austriacus). J Vet Intern Med. 2010; 24: 1483–1489.
Christen-Clottu O. et al.: Eine randomisierte placebokontrollierte Studie zur Behandlung des Equinen Sarkoids bei Pferden mit Viscum album (Iscador® P). In: Scheer R et al. (Eds): Die Mistel in der Tumortherapie 3. Essen: KVC; 2013: 463–473.
Duong Van Huyen JP, Bayry J, Delignat S et al.: Induction of apoptosis of endothelial cells by Viscum album: a role for anti-tumoral properties of mistletoe lectins. Mol Med. 2002; 8: 600–606.
Germann, S.: Einsatz von Interleukin-12 und Interleukin-18 kodierender Plasmid-DNA zur Therapie Equiner Sarkoide, Dissertation Vetsuisse Fakultät Universität Zürich; 2006.
Glardon OJ, Pache V, Magnenat AL et al.: Viscum album L. (Iscador) in the cat: tolerance, adverse reactions and indications, Schweiz Arch Tierheilkd. 2014; 156 (8): 381–388.
Haspeslagh M, Gerber V, Knottenbelt DC et al.: The clinical diagnosis of equine sarcoids-Part 2: Assessment of case features typical of equine sarcoids and validation of a diagnostic protocol to guide equine clinicians in the diagnosis of equine sarcoids. Vet J. 2018; 240: 14–18.
Haspeslagh M, Vlaminck LE, Martens AM: Treatment of sarcoids in equids: 230 cases (2008-2013), J Am Vet Med Assoc. 2016; 249 (3): 311–318.
Hegde P, Maddur MS, Friboulet A et al.: Viscum album exerts anti-inflammatory effect by selectively inhibiting cytokine-induced expression of cyclooxygenase-2. PLoS One. 2011; 6: e26312.
Heinzerling L, von Baehr V, Liebenthal C et al.: Immunologic effector mechanisms of a standardized mistletoe extract on the function of human monocytes and lymphocytes in vitro, ex vivo, and in vivo. J Clin Immunol. 2006; 26: 347–359.

Jandova V, Klukowska-Rötzler J, Dolf G et al.: Whole genome scan identifies several chromosomal regions linked to equine sarcoids. Schweiz Arch Tierheilkd. 2012; 154: 19–25.

Kienle G. und Kiene H: Die Mistel in der Onkologie: Fakten und konzeptionelle Grundlagen. Stuttgart: Schattauer; 2003.

Kienle GS., Keine H: Complementary cancer therapy: a systematic review of prospective clinical trials on anthroposophic mistletoe extracts. Eur J Med Res. 2007; 12 (3): 103–119.

Kinnunen RE, Tallberg T, Stenback H et al.: Equine sarcoid tumour treated by autogenous tumour vaccine. Anticancer Res. 1999; 19: 3367–3374.

Lavelle EC, Grant G, Pusztai A et al.: Mucosal immunogenicity of plant lectins in mice. Immunology. 2000; 99 (1): 30–37.

Mählmann K, Hamza E, Marti E et al.: Increased FOXP3 expression in tumour-associated tissues of horses affected with equine sarcoid disease. Vet J. 2014; 202 (3): 516–521.

Martens A, De Moor A, Vlaminck L et al.: Evaluation of excision, cryosurgery and local BCG vaccination for the treatment of equine sarcoids. Vet Rec. 2001; 149: 665–669.

Martens A, De Moor A, Waelkens E et al.: In vitro and in vivo evaluation of hypericin for photodynamic therapy of equine sarcoids. Vet J. 2000; 159 (1): 77–84.

Mattil-Fritz S, Scharner D, Piuko K et al.: Immunotherapy of equine sarcoid: dose-escalation trial for the use of chimeric papillomavirus-like particles. J Gen Virol. 2008; 89(Pt1): 138–147.

Mele M, Gerber V, Straub R et al.: Erhebung der Prävalenz von Erbkrankheiten bei dreijährigen Pferden der Freiberger-Rasse. Schweiz Arch Tierheilkd. 2007; 149 (4): 151–159.

Pryme IF, Bardocz S, Pusztai A et al.: Dietary mistletoe lectin supplementation and reduced growth of a murine non-Hodgkin lymphoma. Histol Histopathol. 2002; 17 (1): 261–271.

Rush BR, Flaminio MJ: Immunomodulation in horses. Vet Clin North Am Equine Pract. 2000; 16 (1): 183–197.

Studer S, Gerber V, Straub R et al.: Erhebung der Prävalenz von Erbkrankheiten bei dreijährigen Schweizer Warmblutpferden. Schweiz Arch Tierhailkd. 2007; 149 (4): 161–171.
Von Bodungen U, Ruess K, Reif M et al.: Kombinierte Anwendung von Strahlentherapie und adjuvanter Therapie mit einem Mistelextrakt (Viscum album L.) zur Behandlung des oralen malignen Melanoms beim Hund: Eine retrospektive Studie. Complement Med Res. 2017; 24 (6): 358–363.
Wode K, Hök Nordberg J, Kienle GS et al.: Efficacy of mistletoe extract as a complement to standard treatment in advanced pancreatic cancer: study protocol for a multicentre, parallel group, double-blind, randomised, placebo-controlled clinical trial (MISTRAL). Trials. 2020; 21 (1): 783.

Dr. med. vet. Ophélie Clottu[1], Dr. med. vet. Ulrike Biegel[1], Dr. rer. nat. Marcus Reif[2]
[1] Forschungsinstitut für biologischen Landbau (FiBL), Frick, Schweiz
[2] Gesellschaft für klinische Forschung GKF, Berlin, Deutschland

Korrespondenzadresse:
ophelie.clottu@fibl.org

Could *Viscum album* L. Be a Therapeutic Option for Companion Animals Suffering From Neoplastic Diseases? A Systematic Review.

Könnte *Viscum album* L. eine therapeutische Option für Haustiere mit neoplastischen Erkrankungen sein? Eine systematische Literaturübersicht.

Ulrike Biegel, Meike Mevissen, Simone Schuller, Katja Ruess, Ophélie Clottu, Hannah Ayrle, Christoph Koch, Michael Walkenhorst

Summary

Background: Oncological diseases are common in companion animals. Their treatment confronts veterinarians with particular challenges. Pet owners are increasingly demanding complementary treatment options that reduce the treatment burden for their affected animals and improve the chances of successful treatment.

Objective: A systematic review (Biegel *et al.* 2022) was conducted to determine whether the use of preparations of European white-berried mistletoe is an effective therapy for neoplastic diseases in companion animals.

Methods: Only controlled studies (peer-reviewed) were considered according to the PRISMA criteria (Preferred Reporting Items for Systematic Reviews and Meta-Analyses) and the AMSTAR assessment tool (A Measurement Tool to Assess Systematic Reviews). All clinical studies, both *in vivo* and *in vitro*, were included to the extent that they allowed conclusions to be drawn regarding the efficacy of mistletoe extracts in the treatment of the most common neoplastic diseases of companion animals. The efficacy of each study was compared using a point system.

Results: A total of 6148 references were identified. After duplicate removal and additional screening steps, 114 of these were included in the full-text search and finally, 61 were included in the analysis. Of these, 25 references included in vitro experiments, 26 included *in vivo* or clinical experiments, and 10 included both *in vivo* and *in vitro* experiments.

Four controlled clinical veterinary studies were identified, including three studies in dogs (canine sarcoma (VAE adjuvant to chemotherapy), oral melanoma (VAE adjuvant to radiotherapy), mammary adenocarcinoma (VAE adjuvant to surgery)) and one study on mistletoe therapy for equine sarcoids (mistletoe therapy alone).
Based on the 61 references included (Biegel *et al.* 2022) the efficacy of mistletoe therapy was most pronounced in equine sarcoid (higher cure rate than placebo *in vivo*) and (based on results from *in vivo* and *in vitro* research) in melanoma, sarcoma, and mammary carcinoma.
Keywords: Systematic review, mistletoe therapy, companion animals, neoplastic diseases, immunotherapy

Zusammenfassung
Hintergrund: Onkologische Erkrankungen treten auch bei Haustieren häufig auf. Deren Behandlung stellt Tierärzte oft vor besondere Herausforderungen. Haustierbesitzer fordern zunehmend ergänzende Behandlungsoptionen, die die Behandlungsbelastung für ihre betroffenen Tiere reduzieren und gleichzeitig die Chancen auf eine erfolgreiche Behandlung verbessern.
Ziel: Anhand einer systematischen Literaturübersicht (Biegel *et al.* 2022) sollte analysiert werden, ob die Verwendung von Zubereitungen aus der europäischen weißbeerigen Mistel (*Viscum album* L.) eine wirksame Therapie für neoplastische Erkrankungen insbesondere von Hunden, Katzen und Pferden (sogenannte Companion Animals) sein könnte.
Methoden: Es wurden ausschließlich kontrollierte Studien (peer-reviewed) gemäß den PRISMA-Kriterien (Preferred Reporting Items for Systematic Reviews and Meta-Analyses) und dem AMSTAR-Bewertungstool (A Measurement Tool to Assess Systematic Reviews) berücksichtigt. Sowohl klinischen als auch *in vivo*- und *in vitro*-Studien wurden einbezogen, soweit sie eine Aussage zur Behandlung der häufigsten neoplastischen Erkrankungen von Haustieren zuließen. Die Wirksamkeit jeder Studie wurde mit einem Punktesystem bewertet.
Ergebnisse: Insgesamt wurden bei der systematischen Suche 6148 Referenzen identifiziert. Nach Entfernung von Duplikaten und zusätzlichen Screening-Schritten wurden 114 davon in die Volltextsuche einbezogen und schließlich 61 in die Analyse aufgenommen. Davon enthielten 25 Referenzen *in vitro*-Experimente, 26 enthielten *in vivo*- oder klinische Experimente und 10 enthielten sowohl *in vivo*- als auch *in vitro*-Experimente.

Insgesamt wurden vier kontrollierte klinische veterinärmedizinische Studien identifiziert, darunter drei bei Hunden (Stickersarkom (adjuvant zur Chemotherapie), orales Melanom (adjuvant zur Radiotherapie), Adenokarzinom der Mamma (adjuvant zur Chirurgie)) und eine Studie zur Misteltherapie bei Equinen Sarkoiden (alleinige Misteltherapie). Auf Basis der 61 einbezogenen Referenzen (Biegel *et al.* 2022) war die Wirksamkeit der Misteltherapie beim Equinen Sarkoid (höhere Heilungsrate als Placebo *in vivo*), sowie (basierend auf Ergebnissen aus der *in vivo* und *in vitro* Forschung) bei Melanomen, Sarkomen und Mammakarzinomen am deutlichsten ausgeprägt.
Schlüsselwörter: Onkologische Erkrankungen, Haustiere, Misteltherapie, Immuntherapie

Conflict of interest

The authors have no conflicts of interest to declare.

References

Biegel U, Mevissen M, Schuller S, Ruess K, Christen O, Ayrle H , Koch C, Walkenhorst M. Viscum album L., a Therapeutic Option for Neoplastic Diseases in Companion Animals? A Systematic Review. Complement Med Res. 2022; 29 (6): 465–482. doi: 10.1159/000525035.

Dr. Ulrike Biegel[1], Dr. Meike Mevissen[2], Dr. Simone Schuller[3], Dr. Katja Ruess[4], Dr. Ophélie Clottu[1], Dr. Hannah Ayrle[1], Dr. Christoph Koch[5], Dr. Michael Walkenhorst[1]

[1] Research Institute of Organic Agriculture (FiBL), Department of Livestock Sciences, Frick, Switzerland

[2] Department of Clinical Research and Veterinary Public Health, Division Veterinary Pharmacology and Toxicology, Vetsuisse Faculty, University of Bern, Switzerland

[3] Department of Clinical Veterinary Medicine, Division of Small Animal Internal Medicine, Vetsuisse Faculty, University of Bern, Switzerland

[4] Department Medical Oncology and Internal medicine, Center for Veterinary Medicine, Marigin AG, Feusisberg, Switzerland
[5] Department of Clinical Veterinary Medicine, Swiss Institut of Equine Medicine (ISME), Vetsuisse Faculty, University of Bern, Switzerland

Corresponding author:
ulrike.biegel@fibl.org

Autorenverzeichnis/ Contributing Authors

(Seitenzahlen in **Fettdruck**: Erstautorinnen und -autoren)

Arendt, Andreas	**325**
Ayrle, Hannah	467
Baumgartner, Stephan	13, 45, 103, 125, 251, 301
Beermann, Anke	**451**
Berg, Anton	57
Berger, Bettina	301
Biegel, Ulrike	451, 455, **467**
Bopp, Annette	**341**
Braun, Hans-Peter	35
Busch, Alina	391
Casteller, Alejandro	13
Chung, Sunjoo	227
Clottu, Ophélie	451, **455**, 467
Creutz v. Essen, Sibylle	215
da Costa Batista, João Vitor	45
Davis, Devra	**241**
de Almeida, Valter Pas	**45**
de Olalla, Eugenia Violeta Díez García	129
Debus, Marion	251, 315, 325
Delebinski, Catharina	19
Diehl, Andrea	251
Duncan, Lorna J.	301
Felenda, Jennifer E.	**185**
Franzén, Alexander Sebastian	129
Garnitschnig, Lydia	325
Garrett, Rafael	103
Gast, Martina	91
Gatov, Irina	435
Grabowski, Patricia	91, 163
Grah, Christian	135, 149, 173, **435**
Grazi, Mirio	45, 103

Gutenbrunner, Christoph	261
Gutsch, Johannes	325
Haeck, Timotheus	**215**
Heinze, Angelika	**57**
Hofheinz, Ralf	**357**
Holandino, Carla	45, 103
Huber, Roman	205
Hummel, Michael	91
Jones, Jeffrey A.	241
Kang, Chang Moo	**203**
Karutz, Markus	325
Kaufmann, Josanna	**67**, 79
Kergel, Maike	315
Kim, JongBae	227
Koch, Christoph	451, 467
Königsberger, Karolina	**251**
Kogan, Mikail	241
Krause, Alena	391
Kröz, Matthias	215, 261
Krüerke, Daniel	281
Kuck, Angela	325
Kunc, Klaudia	173
Lammert, Hedwig	91
Lederer, Ann-Kathrin	**205**
Leneweit, Gero	57, 67, **79**
Leonhard, Bettina	125
Loef, Martin	423
Lubitz, Larissa	79
Manfron, Jane	45
Martin, David D.	251, 301
Marzok, Annika	435
Mascher, Annika	**301**
Matthes, Harald	173, **361**
Meisermann, Thomas	251
Melo, Michelle Nonato de Oliveira	**103**

Melzig, Matthias F.	**19**
Mevissen, Meike	467
Meyer, Frank	**293**
Mörbt, Nora	117
Monchak, Irailson Thierry	45
Moody, Karen	333
Morash, Christopher	241
Ochioni, Alan Clavelland	103
Oei, Shiao Li	**135**, 149, 163, **173**, 435
Offer, Katharine	**333**
Oh, Inmyung	227
Oliveira, Adriana Passos	103
Paepke, Daniela	423
Park, Joon Beom (John)	**227**
Pecher, Gabriele	129
Pelzer, Florian	301
Raftery, Martin J.	129
Raman, Vijayasankar	45
Ramm, Hartmut	**3**
Reif, Marcus	173, 251, **261**, 333, 435, 451, 455
Rieger, Harden	67, 79
Rieger, Sabine	129, 205
Rostock, Matthias	**391**
Ruess, Katja	467
Sauer, Mathias	325
Schad, Friedemann	91, 135, **149**, 163, **315**, **407**
Schink, Michael	**129**, 205
Schläpfer, Dorothea	251
Schröder, Lucie	**35**
Schuller, Simone	467
Schwarz, Reinhard	325
Seely, Dugald	241
Seifert, Georg	19
Senkler, Jennifer	35

Simões-Wüst, Ana Paula 215, **281**
Soldner, Georg 315, 325
Sommer, Markus 325
Steinmann, Diana 149
Stintzing, Florian C. 117, 185
Stintzing, Sebastian 91
Strasser, Florian 215
Thronicke, Anja 135, 149, **163**, 315
Tröger, Wilfried 251
Turek, Claudia 117, 185
Unger, Lucia 451
Urech, Konrad 3, **13**, 251
Villegas, Yván 315
Vögele, Peter 117
Walach, Harald **423**
Walkenhorst, Michael 467
Weiß, Timo 173
Weissenstein, Ulrike **125**, 173
Wilkens, Johannes **377**
Winters, Nasha 241
Wolfshöfer, Sebastian **91**
Wüstefeld, Hanna 135, 173, 435
Wüsthof, Mirjam 391
Xie, Wenyan 19
Yoon, Taek Joon 227
Zancan, Patricia 103
Zerm, Roland 261
Zilkowski, Ilona **117**

Stichwortverzeichnis

Hinweis: Die Beiträge in diesem Buch sind entweder auf Deutsch oder auf Englisch, die Überschriften, Schlüsselwörter und Kurzfassungen sind zumeist in beiden Sprachen geschrieben. Daher gibt es ein englisches und ein deutsches Stichwortverzeichnis. Jedes Stichwort ist in beiden Verzeichnissen enthalten. Die Seitenzahlen geben jeweils die erste Seite des Beitrags an, zu dem das Stichwort gehört. In Einzelfällen wird direkt auf ein Stichwort verwiesen.

abnobaVISCUM	81, 203, 215, 227, 288, 297, 365
Aktinische Keratose	251
Antikörper, monoklonal (Therapie)	163
Anwendungsarten	
Hochdosis	227
intrapleural	135
intratumoral	125, 135, 227, 366
intravenös	135, 163, 173, 185, 205, 215, 227, 241, 365
intravesikal	241
oral (bei Pferden)	451, 455
paraurethral	185
subkutan	135, 173, 185, 203, 215, 241, 293, 301, 393, 435, 451
topische Anwendung	251
Anwendungsbeobachtung	siehe klinische Studien
Apoptose	26
Basalzellkarzinom	251
Beschichtung, immunprotektive	79
Bestrahlung, in Kombination mit einer Misteltherapie	149, 361
Blasenkarzinom	siehe Harnblasenkarzinom
Bronchialkarzinom	135, 149, 173, 293
Brustkrebs	siehe Mammakarzinom
Brustkrebs-Zelllinien	103, 125, 129

Cancer Fatigue Scale (CFS-D), deutsche Version	261
Cancer-related fatigue (CRF)	135, 215, 261, 399
Checkpoint-Inhibitoren	siehe Immun-Checkpoint-Inhibitoren (ICIs)
Chemotherapie, in Kombination mit einer Misteltherapie	361, 399, 414
CRF-Rehabilitationsinterventionen	215
CDK4/6 Inhibitoren	163
Chloroplasten	35
Chondrosarkom	227
Eiche, von Isigny le Buat	7
Einzelfallberichte	215, 227, 241, 293
Endoplasmatisches Retikulum (ER), Stressreaktion in Tumorzelllinien	125
Energiestoffwechsel	35
EORTC QLQ-C30 Fragebogen	135, 149, 185, 261
Equines Sarkoid	451, 455, 467
Fatigue (Sarkoidose)	435
Fatigue numerical scale (FNS)	261
Fehlanreize, finanzielle, in Kliniken und Praxen	341
Genom, *Viscum album*	35
Genotoxizität	117
Gliomzellen	67
Glykolytische Enzyme	103
Granulomatosen der Lunge	438
Gravitropismus	57
Gynäkologische Tumoren	163
Harnblasenkarzinom	185, 241
Hausärztliche onkologische Versorgung	293
Haustiere	467
Hautkrebs, nichtmelanomatöser	251
Havelhöher Sarkoidoseprotokoll (HSP)	435
Helixor	91, 129, 163, 205, 215, 241, 281, 293, 366
Hepatopathie, reversible	205

Hypokotyl 57
Immun-Checkpoint-Inhibitoren (ICIs) 129 135, 163, 173
Integrative Onkologie 241, 293, 357
Interviews, mit Patienten 301
Iscador 6, 125, 215, 281, 293, 301, 333, 451, 455
Iscucin 117, 185, 435
Keratinozyten, humane 105
Kinase Inhibitoren 135
Klinische Praxis, Umsetzung der integrativen Onkologie 357
Klinische Studien
- Anwendungsbeobachtung 173, 185
- doppelt-verblindete, randomisierte Studien 423, 451 (Pferde)
- Fallserie 455
- Metaanalysen 361, 391, 423
- nicht-interventionelle Studie (NIS) 185
- nicht-randomisierte interventionelle Studien (NRSI) 423
- Pharmakokinetikstudie 205
- Planung einer klinischen Studie für pädiatrische Osteosarkom-Patienten in den USA 333
- qualitative Studie 301
- randomisierte klinische Studien (RCTs) 363, 391, 423, 451 (Pferde)
- registerbasierte kontrollierte klinische Studien (RRCTs) 418
- Real-World Data (RWD)/ Real-World Evidence (RWE) 135, 149, 363, 407, 435
- retrospektive Studie 203, 251, 435
- systematische Reviews 361, 391, 423, 467
- Verblindung, Entblindung 391

Kolorektal-Zelllinien 91
Komplette Remission siehe Remissionen
Kosteneffektivität 407
Künstliche Intelligenz (KI) 341

Lebensqualität	135, 149, 185, 227, 293, 361, 391, 410, 423
Leitlinien	
medizinische	361, 391, 407
S3-Leitlinie Komplementärmedizin	364, 394
Liposomen	67, 79
Lokalreaktion	365, 395
Lunge, Granulomatosen	438
Lungenkrebs	siehe Bronchialkarzinom
Magenkarzinom	293
Mammakarzinom	163, 293, 361, 413, 423
Meridiansystem	siehe Misteltherapie
Metaanalysen	siehe klinische Studien
Metabolom	103
miRNA	19
Mistel	
geographische Verbreitung und Häufigkeit in Frankreich	13
geographische Verbreitung in Südwestdeutschland (1923)	8
Genom	35
Mikroskopische Charakterisierung	45
Mistelextrakt	
lipophiler	251, 368
Wirtsbaumeinfluss	108
Urtinkturen	103
Mistellektine	
frei und eingekapselt	67
Gehaltsbestimmung	235
Halbwertzeit (im Serum)	205
Pharmakokinetik	205
Stabilität	72
Mistelpräparate	
Anwendungsarten	siehe dort
individualisierte Behandlung	325

Produktnamen siehe abnobaVISCUM, Helixor, Iscador, Iscucin, *Viscum album Herba Extractum recinosum* 10% (Creme)

Misteltherapie
- Anwendung außerhalb der Onkologie 368, 435
- Anwendung bei Tieren 451, 455, 467
- aktueller medizinisch wissenschaftlicher Stand 315, 325, 391
- Evidenz- und Leitlinienbewertung 363
- Meridiansystem als Basis 377
- spirituelle Dimension 301, 355
- Zukunft 298, 361

Mitochondrien 35

Multimodale Behandlung 215

Mutagenität, *in vitro*, Bewertung 117

Myc Signalweg 91

Natürliche Killerzellen (NK)-Aktivitätstest 129

Nebenwirkungen 149, 163, 185, 251, 365, 391, 407, 435

Neoplastische Erkrankungen (bei Tieren) 467

Netzwerk Onkologie (NO) 135, 163, 363, 407

Nicht-kleinzelliges Lungenkarzinom (NSCLC) 173

Off-label 365

Osteosarkomzellen 19

Osteosarkom (Planung einer klinischen Studie für pädiatrische Osteosarkom-Patienten in den USA) 333

Ovarialkarzinom 293

Pankreaskarzinom 203

PARP-Inhibitoren 163

Partielle Remissionen siehe Remissionen

Patienten, pädiatrische 333

Patienten-berichtete Ergebnismessungen 407

Patientensicht, Patientenerleben zur Misteltherapie 301

Patientenzentrierter Ansatz 293
Pharmakokinetik von Mistellektinen 205
Pharmakovigilanz 281
PHOENIX-III-Studie 173
Photosynthese 35
Plattenepithelkarzinom, kutanes 251
Probanden, gesunde 205
Prostatakarzinom 185
Real-World Data (RWD)/
Real-World Evidence (RWE) siehe klinische Studien
Remission
komplette 241, 251, 365
partielle 227, 251, 365
Sarkoidose 435
Schlaftherapie 215
Schmerzlinderung 293
Schwangerschaft 281
Selbstbeobachtung, von Patienten 301
Sicherheit 185, 205, 227, 281, 395, 407
Spheroid-Modelle, 3D 129
Stärkekörner 48
Stärke, Statolithen- 57
Steiner, Rudolf 3, 377
S3 Leitlinie Komplementärmedizin in der Behandlung von onkologischen PatientInnen siehe Leitlinien
Systematischer Review siehe klinische Studien
Tubeuf, Karl von 3
Tumor-Stoffwechsel (*in vitro*) 111
Tyrosinkinaseinhibitoren 163, 329
Überleben
ereignisfreies Überleben 333, 396
Gesamtüberleben 203, 361, 391, 407
krankheitsfreies Überleben 203
Unerwünschte Ereignisse 163, 173, 211
Urogenitale Tumorerkrankungen 185
Urtinkturen, Mistel 103

Vademecum Anthroposophischer
Arzneimittel 281, 325
Versorgungsforschung 407
Verstopfung 135
Verträglichkeit 185, 385
Vesikel, extrazelluläre 19
Viscotoxine
Gehalt in Urtinkturen 103
Viscum album Herba Extractum recinosum
10% (Creme) 251
Viscum TT 368
Warburg Effekt 103
Webseite „www.mistel-therapie.de" 315
Wegman, Ita 6
Wirtsbäume
Einfluss auf Inhaltsstoffe von
Mistelextrakten und *in vitro*-Effekte 108
Wesensmerkmale, Typologie als
Basis für die Misteltherapie 377
Xenografts 24
Zellatmung 35
Zelltod, immonogener 125
Zelllinien
Brustkrebs 103, 125, 129
Glioma 67
Kolorektal 91
Melanom 125
Osteosarkom 19
Zielgerichtete Krebstherapie 79, 135, 163, 173
neuartige Formulierung 79
Risiko eines Therapieabbruchs 163
Zytotoxizität, *in vitro* 19, 67, 91, 105

Keyword Index

Please note: The articles in this book are written either in German or in English, the titles, keywords and abstracts mostly in both languages. Therefore, English and German keyword indices are available. You will find each keyword in both lists. The page numbers refer to the first page of the article to which the keyword belongs. In some instances, the page numbers refer directly to a keyword.

abnobaVISCUM 81, 203, 215, 227, 288, 297, 365
Actinic keratosis 251
Administration, method of
 high doses 227
 intrapleural 135
 intratumoral 125, 135, 227, 366
 intraveneous 135, 163, 173, 185, 205, 215, 227, 241, 365
 intravesical 241
 oral (horses) 451, 455
 paraurethral 185
 subcutaneous 135, 173, 185, 203, 215, 241, 293, 301, 393, 435, 451
 topical treatment 251
Adverse events (AEs) 163, 173, 211
Apoptosis 26
Antibodies, monoclonal 163
Artificial Intelligence (AI) 341
Basal cell carcinoma 251
Bladder carcinoma 185, 241
Breast cancer 163, 293, 361, 413, 423
Breast cancer cell lines 103, 125, 129
Cancer fatigue rehabilitative interventions 215
Cancer fatigue scale (CFS-D), German version 261
Cancer-related fatigue (CRF) 135, 215, 261, 399

Case reports 215, 227, 241, 293
CDK4/6 Inhibitors 163
Cell death, immunogenic 125
Cell lines
breast cancer 103, 125, 129
colorectal 91
glioma 67
melanoma 125
osteosarcoma 19
Cellular respiration 35
Checkpoint inhibitors see immune checkpoint inhibitors (ICIs)
Chemotherapy, combination with mistletoe therapy 361, 399, 414
Chloroplasts 35
Chondrosarcoma 227
Clinical practice, implementation of integrative oncology 357
Clinical studies
blinding, unblinding 391
case series 455
double-blinded, randomized trials 423, 451 (horses)
meta-analysis 361, 391, 423
non-interventional study (NIS) 185
non-randomized studies of intervention (NRSI) 423
observational study 173, 185
pharmacokinetic study 205
preparation of a clinical trial for pediatric osteosarcoma patients in the USA 333
qualitative study 301
randomized clinical trials (RCTs) 363, 391, 423, 451 (horses)
real-world-data (RWD)/ real-world-evidence (RWE) 135, 149, 363, 407, 435

register-based controlled clinical trials (RRCTs) 418
retrospective study 203, 251, 435
systematic reviews 361, 391, 423, 467
Coating, immune-protective 79
Colorectal cell lines 91
Companion animals 467
Complete remission (CR) see remissions
Constipation 135
Cost effectiveness 407
Cytotoxicity, *in vitro* 19, 67, 91, 105
Disincentives, financial in clinics and practices 341
Endoplasmatic reticulum (ER), stress response, cancer cell lines 125
Energy metabolism 35
EORTC QlQ-C30 questionnaire 135, 149, 185, 261
Equine sarcoid 451, 455, 467
Fatigue (Sarcoidosis) 435
Fatigue numerical scale (FNS) 261
Gastric cancer 293
Genome, *Viscum album* 35
Genotoxicity 117
Glioma cells 67
Glycolytic enzymes 103
Granulomatoses of the lung 438
Gravitropism 57
Guidelines
medical 361, 391, 407
S3 guideline complementary medicine 364, 394
Gynecological cancer 163
Havelhöhe Sarcoidosis Protocol (HSP) 435
Health service research 407
Helixor 91, 129, 163, 205, 215, 241, 281, 293, 366

Host trees
- characteristics, typology as basis for therapeutic treatment 377
- influence on the composition of mistletoe extracts and their *in vitro* effects 108

Hypocotyl 57
Immune checkpoint inhibitors (ICIs) 129, 135, 163, 173
Integrative oncology 241, 293, 357
Iscador 6, 125, 215, 281, 293, 301, 333, 451, 455
Iscucin 117, 185, 435
Keratinocytes, human 105
Kinase inhibitors 135
Liposomes 67, 79
Liver injury, reversible 205
Local reaction 365, 395
Lung cancer 135, 149, 173, 293
Lung, granulomatosis 438
Meridian system see mistletoe therapy
Meta-analysis see clinical studies
Metabolome 103
miRNA 19
Mistletoe
- geographic distribution, abundance in France 13
- geographic distribution in South-West-Germany (1923) 8
- genome 35
- microscopic characterization 45

Mistletoe extract
- host tree influence 108
- lipophilic 251, 368
- mother tinctures 103

Mistletoe lectins
- free and encapsulated 67

half-life (in serum) 205
measuring the content 235
pharmacokinetics 205
stability 72
Mistletoe preparations
individualized treatment 325
medicinal products see abnobaVISCUM, Helixor, Iscador, Iscucin, *Viscum album Herba Extractum recinosum* 10 % (Creme)
methods of administration see administration
Mistletoe therapy
current medical and scientific status 315, 325, 391
evidence and guideline evaluation 363
future 298, 361
meridian system as basis 377
spiritual dimension 301, 355
use in animals 451, 455, 467
use in non-oncological diseases 368, 435
Mitochondria 35
Mother tinctures, mistletoe 103
Multimodal therapy 215
Mutagenity, assessment *in vitro* 117
Myc signaling 91
Natural killer (NK) cytotoxicity test 129
Neoplastic diseases (animals) 467
Network oncology registry 135, 163, 363, 407
Non-small-cell-lung-cancer (NSCLC) 173
Oak, from Isigny le Buat 7
Off label use 365
Osteosarcoma cells 19
Osteosarcoma (preparation of a clinical trial for pediatric osteosarcoma patients in the US) 333
Ovarial cancer 293
Pain relief 293
Pancreatic cancer 203

PARP inhibitors	163
Partial remissions	see remissions
Patient-centered approach	293
Patient experience, levels of experience	301
Patients, pediatric	333
Patient-reported outcome measures (PROMs)	407
Pharmacokinetics of mistletoe lectins	205
Pharmacovigilance	281
PHOENIX-III study	173
Photosynthesis	35
Pregnancy	281
Primary care	293
Prostate carcinoma	185
Quality of life	135, 149, 185, 227, 293, 361, 391, 413, 423
Radiotherapy, combination with mistletoe therapy	149, 361
Real-world data (RWD)/ real-world evidence (RWE)	see clinical studies
Remissions	
complete	241, 251, 365
partial	227, 251, 365
Safety	185, 205, 227, 281, 395, 407
Sarcoidosis	435
Side effects	149, 163, 185, 251, 365, 391, 407, 435
Single cases	see case reports
Skin cancer, non-melanoma	251
Sleep therapy	215
Spheroid models, 3D	129
Squamous cell carcinoma, cutaneous	251
Starch grains	48
Starch, statolithic	57
Steiner, Rudolf	3, 377
Survival	
event-free survival	333, 396

disease-free survival (DFS) 203
overall survival (OS) 203, 361, 391, 407
Systematic reviews see clinical studies
S3 guideline complementary medicine in the treatment of oncological patients see guidelines
Targeted cancer therapies 79, 135, 163, 173
novel formulations 79
risk of termination 163
Tolerability 185, 395
Tubeuf, Karl von 3
Tumor metabolism 111
Tyrosinkinase inhibitors 163, 329
Urogenital tumor diseases 185
Use in animals 451, 455, 467
Vademecum Anthroposophical Medicines 281, 325
Vesicles, extracellular 19
Viscotoxins
content in mother tinctures 108
Viscum album Herba Extractum recinosum 10% (Creme) 251
Viscum TT 368
Volunteers, healthy 205
Warburg effect 103
Website "www.mistel-therapie.de" 315
Wegman, Ita 6
Xenografts 24